Springer Series on
Behavior Therapy and Behavioral Medicine

Series Editors: Cyril M. Franks, Ph.D., and Frederick J. Evans, Ph.D.

Advisory Board: John Paul Brady, M.D., Robert P. Liberman, M.D., Neal E. Miller, Ph.D., and Stanley Rachman, Ph.D.

Volume 1 **Multimodal Behavior Therapy**
Arnold A. Lazarus

Volume 2 **Behavior-Therapy Assessment**
Eric J. Mash and Leif G. Terdal, editors

Volume 3 **Behavioral Approaches to Weight Control**
Edward E. Abramson, editor

Volume 4 **A Practical Guide to Behavioral Assessment**
Francis J. Keefe, Steven A. Kopel, and Steven B. Gordon

Volume 5 **Asthma Therapy**
A Behavioral Health Care System
for Respiratory Disorders
Thomas L. Creer

Volume 6 **Behavioral Medicine**
Practical Applications in Health Care
Barbara G. Melamed and Lawrence J. Siegel

Volume 7 **Multimodal Handbook for a Mental Hospital**
Designing Specific Treatments for Specific Problems
Lillian F. Brunell and Wayne T. Young, editors

Volume 8 **Eating and Weight Disorders**
Advances in Treatment and Research
Richard K. Goodstein, editor

Volume 9 **Perspectives on Behavior Therapy in the Eighties**
Michael Rosenbaum, Cyril M. Franks, and Yoram Jaffe, editors

Volume 10 **Pediatric and Adolescent Behavioral Medicine**
Issues in Treatment
Patrick J. McGrath and Philip Firestone, editors

Volume 11 **Hypnosis and Behavior Therapy**
The Treatment of Anxiety and Phobias
J. Christopher Clarke, Ph.D., and
J. Arthur Jackson, M.B., Ch.B.

J. Christopher Clarke, Ph.D., received his clinical doctorate from the State University of New York at Stony Brook. He has taught at McMaster University in Canada and the Neuropsychiatric Institute at U.C.L.A. and is now at the University of New South Wales, Sydney, Australia, where he is involved in the clinical postgraduate program. His publications, research, and clinical interests are centered on the problems of anxiety, depression, and alcoholism and the development of ethological analyses and behavioral treatment for these disorders.

J. Arthur Jackson, M.B.,Ch.B., F.R.A.C.G.P., D. Obst., R.C.O.G., graduated from the University of Liverpool, U.K., following which he spent several years in general medical practice. For the past ten years, he has practiced medical hypnosis on a full-time basis and is clinical assistant in hypnosis to the Department of Pain Management at the Royal North Shore Hospital of Sydney, Australia, and visiting lecturer to the Cumberland College of Health Sciences, Sydney. He is a past president of the Australian Society for Clinical and Experimental Hypnosis and is a member of the editorial board of the *Australian Journal of Clinical and Experimental Hypnosis,* of which he was foundation editor. His research and publications cover a wide variety of areas associated with hypnosis, particularly endurance performance, pain, hypertension, family medicine, and hypnotic susceptibility.

HYPNOSIS AND BEHAVIOR THERAPY

The Treatment of Anxiety and Phobias

J. Christopher Clarke, Ph.D.
J. Arthur Jackson, M.B., Ch.B.

SPRINGER PUBLISHING COMPANY
New York

Springer Publishing Company, Inc.
200 Park Avenue South
New York, New York 10003

83 84 85 86 87 / 10 9 8 7 6 5 4 3 2 1

Library of Congress Cataloging in Publication Data

Clarke, J. Christopher.
  Hypnosis and behavior therapy.
  (Springer series on behavior therapy and behavioral
medicine ; 11)
  Bibliography: p.   Includes index.
  1. Hypnotism—Therapeutic use. 2. Behavior therapy. 3. Anxiety—Treatment. 4. Phobias—Treatment. I. Jackson, Arthur. II. Title. III. Series. [DNLM: 1. Anxiety—Therapy. 2. Phobic disorders—Therapy. 3. Hypnosis. 4. Behavior therapy. WI SP685NB v.11 / WM 415 C598h]
RC497.C55 1983   616.85′2206512   83-524
ISBN 0-8261-3450-5
ISSN 0278-6729

Printed in the United States of America

To Flossie and Fred,
without whose understanding, forbearance,
and support
this book could never have been written

Contents

Foreword by Fred H. Frankel   ix

Introduction by Leonard Krasner   xi

Preface   xiii

Acknowledgments   xvii

1.   Myths and Misconceptions   1

2.   The Nature of Hypnosis: A Perspective   15

3.   Hypnosis: Assessment and Modification   38

4.   Hypnosis: Preparation, Procedures, and Problems   61

5.   Hypnosis in Children   93

6.   Meditation: Its Relationship to Hypnosis   114

7.   The Nature and Practice of Self-hypnosis   144

8.   The Anxieties: Their Nature, Origin,
and Treatment Implications   167

9.   Phobic Anxiety: Management and Procedures   194

10.   Cognitive Anxiety: Management and Procedures   236

11.   Agoraphobia: Theory and Management   263

12.   Anxiety in Sports   289

Appendix A.   Techniques of Progressive Relaxation   305

Appendix B.   Sample Hierarchy Scenes   313

References and Bibliography   324

Index   351

Foreword

The authors demonstrate in these pages their serious concern with hypnosis and their deep commitment to understanding not only hypnosis per se but also how it articulates with the clinical needs of their patients and the techniques used in behavior therapy. Their priorities in the broad range of subjects covered are clear. It is not the advancement of one particular method or theory, but rather the clinical outcome that is held out to the reader as the goal. The authors, however, also carefully consider the relevant conceptual and theoretical issues and evaluate them. What emerges is a thoughtful treatise on hypnosis and behavior therapy with a wealth of useful information for the practitioner in addition to the necessary theoretical substrate.

While the past two decades have witnessed the growth of particularism in the field, with an emphasis on differences, territorial claims, and the invention of new labels, the authors from the perspective of their wide clinical experience demonstrate the close practical similarities between hypnosis and the meditative states and between several of the behavioral techniques. While explicitly in favor of conceptual clarity, they nonetheless demonstrate that what ultimately matters is how the various therapeutic procedures impinge on the cognitive, affective, and behavioral responses of patients.

Despite a clear-cut behavioral and non-Freudian bias, theirs is the flexibility that permits them to discuss the shades of gray in motivation, to live with clinical ambiguity, and to pay attention to feelings. Their work is the more admirable because they practice what they preach; the therapeutic outcome matters more than the consequences of an induction procedure or one's commitment to a theoretical position.

The authors have assembled a thoroughly informative overview of the field, which, combined with a sensitive clinical manual, provides a novel and comprehensive account of this area of therapy.

Fred H. Frankel, M.B.Ch.B., D.P.M.
Immediate Past President
International Society of Hypnosis;
Professor of Psychiatry
Harvard Medical School
Boston, Massachusetts

Introduction

Hypnosis is back! There are even some who will say it never really was very far away from a, perhaps *the*, central role in psychology. Hypnosis, whatever it is, articulates with virtually every aspect of the science and discipline of psychology.

It is always a pleasure to write an introduction to a book that enhances the creative process in the behavioral sciences. Behavioral science, indeed all of science, is a process of continual creation and integration of ideas, models, research, and theories. In this book, Clarke and Jackson take us through the whole gamut of both the process of hypnosis as a prototype of the broader behavior influence process and the intervention procedure, behavior therapy, which has become the prototype of the behavior change process. Because of its history, its public image, and the nature of the variables it involves, the study of hypnosis has all of the elements necessary to create interest, excitement, wonder, and bafflement: innocent people "forced" to do things that may be contrary to their moral code, spectacular "cures," systematic research, theoretical controversies, and evidence of the impact of social influence variables such as expectancy, social labeling, and demand characteristics.

The reemerging role of hypnosis as being virtually central to psychology is attested to by the statement of Donald Hebb in response to a question posed to a group of "distinguished psychologists" as to "What have we started to learn about human psychology that we didn't know 15 years ago?" (in *Psychology Today*, May 1982). Hebb's response is to cite Hilgard's recent work in bringing hypnosis "closer to everyday experiences." Hebb views the research as closely linking hypnosis with the rest of experimental psychology and casting "a new light on the functioning of the human mind." Indeed, this is strong support for the importance of the return of hypnosis, and Clarke and Jackson have put Hilgard (and the other current major hypnosis investigators) into historical and scientific perspective.

The approaches to human behavior fashionable in each era have been reflected in the procedures used and the explanations offered by the investigators of hypnosis. A good example of the historical integration of hypnosis research into the broader frame of psychology is offered in the recent paper of Triplet (1982) demonstrating the integral relationship between the hypnosis research of Clark Hull with the "behavioral orientation" of his enormously influential learning theory.

Thus, hypnosis as a procedure and as a social movement is a human behavior illustrative of the influencer influencing. As such, it is an appropriate historical and theoretical introduction to behavior therapy. This is very consistent with the historical development of behavior therapy. In the first *Annual Review of Psychology* article on "behavior therapy," (Krasner, 1971) I included research in "hypnosis" as among the streams of development that came together in the 1960s to form "behavior therapy."

> Investigations of the parameters of the social influence process have brought within its framework a series of human interactions previously seen as unique or discrete phenomena. This has included research on such clinical and social phenomena as hypnosis, placebo effect, demand characteristics, experimenter bias, subject and patient expectancy, and the effects of non-verbal cues in interviews. Investigators in these areas take the "skeptical" position that they are dealing with aspects of a broad social influence process and not with a unique phenomenon. (p. 490).

I call the reader's attention to some of the materials ahead which I found to be useful, exciting, and indispensable in a tome on hypnosis: the placing of hypnosis in a broader framework of developments in history, science, and psychology; the offering of a systematic theoretical framework for hypnosis; and a systematization of procedures, with reasonable rationales for each.

Enjoy your journey through the lands of "hypnosis" and of "behavior therapy." The two terms may well be alternative names for the same territory.

Leonard Krasner, Ph.D.
Professor
Department of Psychology
State University of
New York at Stony Brook

Krasner, L. Behavior therapy. In P. H. Mussen (Ed.), *Annual Review of Psychology* (Vol. 22). Palo Alto, CA: Annual Reviews, Inc., 1971, 483–532.

Triplet, R. G. The relationship of Clark L. Hull's hypnosis research to his later learning theory: the continuity of his life's work. *Journal of the History of the Behavioral Sciences*, 1982, *18*, 22–31.

Preface

Although the separate literatures on hypnosis and behavior therapy are vast, very little has been written about their integration. The simple reason for this is that there has been virtually no contact between research workers in the two areas. In view of their common commitment to the experimental method, and the fund of useful data on the modification of cognitive, emotional, and behavioral reactions gathered by investigators in both areas, this is indeed unfortunate.

When the circumstances of their respective histories and development are scrutinized, it is not difficult to see why hypnosis and behavior therapy have remained separate and distinct areas of endeavor. From the earliest days of Mesmer's magnetism and for a good part of its history since, hypnosis has attracted the attention of enthusiasts whose use of it was invariably idiosyncratic, unsystematic, and "clinical." Their legacy included little in the way of experimental data. In sharp contrast, behavior therapy had its origins in laboratory-based research of conditioning and learning, the goal of which was the careful study of environmental manipulations, their behavioral effects, and the laws relating the two. The experimental subjects in the classical theories of learning and, likewise, the clients in behavior therapy were believed to be the passive recipients of environmental stimuli; the data of interest were the overt responses made to them. Speculations about covert/cognitive events were proscribed as "subjective" and unscientific.

In its long-standing clinical orientation, hypnosis did not trouble to bring a systematic study of overt behavior into its range of concerns. And, as noted, behavior therapy was similarly uninterested in the study of cognition. Separated by this quite fundamental incompatability, they were destined to be kept apart by their partisan and parochial supporters. Disciplined skepticism was rare and outright credulity common in the annals of hypnosis, a state of affairs that gave weight to the charge that hypnosis has always been more in danger from its defenders than its detractors. Behavior therapy never lacked for scientific aspirations, but in its insistence on learning-theory answers for all questions of etiology and techniques, it, too, tended to become isolated from the mainstream of psychology.

In recent times, both areas have undergone important changes. The effects of these have been to open the door for fruitful interactions between behavior therapy and hypnosis. First, since the 1950s hypnosis has developed as an active area of research in university departments of psychology and psychiatry where a concern with methodological rigor replaced unbridled clinical speculation and hypnotic stagecraft. Second, while hypnosis was becoming established as a "respectable" field of study, forces were at work that opened up behavior therapy to other influences than those emanating from the conditioning laboratories. Indeed, conditioning itself was witnessing far-reaching changes under the impact of Kamin's (1969) work—which stimulated the interest of learning theorists in animal memory and cognition. In the late 1960s, the "cognitive revolution" finally began to make its impact upon behavior therapy. The work of Bandura, Cautela, Goldfried, and Meichenbaum, among others, alerted clinicians to the role of symbolic stimuli and mediating cognitive activities as key events in the modification of behavior. Researchers in hypnosis have, of course, long been occupied with these very matters. Thus, it is to be expected that in this new climate, cognitive-behavior therapists should turn to the literature on hypnosis for information and techniques.

One of the major aims in this book is to provide the reader with the information needed for the correct use of hypnotic techniques and a step-by-step account of the management of the hypnotic episode from induction to termination. As well as detailed presentation of a wide variety of standard and rapid induction techniques with adults (in the treatment of clinical problems and sports anxiety), we single out for special attention the use of hypnosis with children. We also give extensive coverage to the identification of the means of dealing with the prevalent myths and fears about hypnosis. Clinicians are inclined to overlook this aspect of technique, but we have always found it to be true that if anything useful is to be gained with hypnosis, the patient must first be put at ease.

In short, the focus throughout the book is on matters of technique and application. However, application cannot take place in a conceptual vacuum. For even the most pragmatic therapist, practice follows theory. Hence, any clinical handbook should contain a clear statement of the assumptions lying behind the recommended techniques. In constructing our perspective or model of hypnosis we have elected to side-step the long-standing state *versus* non-state controversies. Instead, we start with a close look at the commonalities in the operation and procedures of hypnosis which are visible behind the terminology differences that separate the different schools. The conclusion we reach is that hypnosis is one word for a configuration of cognitive changes, the most important of which is a focused attention.

In line with this we give considerable emphasis to the use of the methods of meditation as the techniques of choice for control of attention, which we consider to be *the* most important cognitive skill the patient can acquire. The connections between hypnosis and meditation are covered in some detail, and these provide a direct lead into the related topic of self-hypnosis. Self-hypnosis is an integral part of any hypnobehavioral program and can be fully exploited only by the person who has acquired the skills of attentional (self-) control.

An axiom which we favor is that people get treated *in* hypnosis but not *by* hypnosis. To say this another way, hypnosis is an adjunct to therapy and not a therapy itself. This brings us to the major aim and the second theme of the book: the application of hypnosis and the techniques that it can potentiate in the modification of maladaptive anxiety reactions. The central thesis of our argument in this section is that anxiety is not a unitary phenomenon. We present the evidence for a tripartite classification scheme composed of phobic, cognitive, and panic anxieties. The clinical implications of this analysis relate not only to the differences among these in terms of origin and nature but also, and most important, to the treatments to which they are responsive. To give an example, hypnobehavioral therapies for phobic anxiety should give center place to techniques of exposure, whereas for cognitive anxiety, exposure per se will accomplish little if negative self-statements and other kinds of self-defeating beliefs are left unchanged. In keeping with this perspective, we have given separate chapters to the combination of hypnosis with desensitization and other exposure techniques for phobic anxiety, and with rational-emotive therapy and a range of cognitive techniques for the management of non-phobic anxieties. To sum up, in this book we have tried to show in writing what we have discovered in our clinical practice and research—that an integrative hypnobehavioral approach is possible and valuable.

Before we close this preface we should make mention of some vexing questions of terminology. After experimenting with the counterbalanced use of she/he and he/she combinations, we gave up in frustration and chose the simpler path of referring to therapists and patients alike as "he," or "him." We hope that this will not be misunderstood as an open or tacit endorsement of sexist language. It is merely a tactic of convenience. Finally, we debated over the choice between "client" and "patient." With some misgivings we decided in favor of the latter. We are aware that some commentators believe that the word "patient" is weighted down with unfortunate associations (with medical models, and its suggestion, they say, of the passive role of a person seeking help). Nevertheless, we have chosen "patient" over "client" for it serves to remind us of the differences exhibited in severity of distress and degree of impairment between individuals studied in the great majority of (analogue) laboratory experiments and people who seek out help in the clinic. We agree wholeheartedly with Emmelkamp (1979) that the complexity of problems and the difficulty in generating clinically significant change justify the use of "patient" and the retention of the term "clinical phobias" and anxieties. We will have occasion throughout the book to remind the reader and ourselves of this.

Acknowledgments

We owe a special debt of gratitude to Sally Richardson, who has faced the formidable task of typing out the manuscript with unfailing good humor, patience, and expertise. In addition, we wish to express our thanks to Carolyn Bowyer for her library assistance, Greg Gass for his help with the artwork, and Don Davidson for his photography.

Finally, our thanks to the many colleagues who listened to our ideas and offered useful suggestions, criticisms, and support. We want to single out especially Fred Evans, Cyril Franks, Violet Franks, John Garcia, Bill Hardy, Syd Lovibond, Peter Suedfeld, and Fred Westbrook.

1
Myths and Misconceptions

Thus the unfacts, did we possess them, were too imprecisely few to warrant our certitude.

—James Joyce, *Finnegan's Wake*

Regardless of the disorders under consideration, or the modes of therapy employed, clinicians in general have to be alert to difficulties arising from a patient's misconceptions and misinformation about hypnosis. In this regard, it is probably true to say that hypnosis is clouded with more myths and misconceptions than any other form of psychological practice. Even though many of these misconceptions have their roots in long-distant history and have no foundation in fact, they exist in many minds as the conventional wisdom about hypnosis. It would appear that, for many, hypnosis is still surrounded by an aura of mystique and magic, and, interestingly, some individuals are often reluctant to relinquish these notions. For this reason, therapists should go to considerable lengths to seek the patient's views of hypnosis and, through discussion, to correct these impressions whenever necessary. In spite of such determined efforts to paint the correct picture, all too often the therapist will be told after terminating hypnosis that "I don't think I was hypnotized; I wasn't 'out of it,'" or alternatively, "I'm probably not such a good subject; I could hear everything you said." Frustrating though this may be for the therapist, this sort of thing is commonplace.

The expectancies that people have about treatments are known to exert an influence on how they respond (for example, Kazdin & Wilcoxin, 1976). It follows, therefore, that determining a patient's impressions of hypnosis and, where appropriate, spending sufficient time in correcting these are highly important if hypnosis is to be used effectively. If the conflict between the therapist's views and the patient's beliefs goes undetected or is unresolved, inevitably this will impede therapeutic progress. Ideally, this clarification of the true nature of hypnosis should be carried out before the first induction or assessment of hypnotizability. Even this preliminary discussion on the patient's misbeliefs may not be sufficient to allay his concerns and in that case will need to be dealt with again in later sessions.

In selecting the following myths and misconceptions, where possible we aim to present their historical derivation as well as the clinical and experimental evidence underpinning the correct position on these issues.

Myth: Hypnosis Is a Sleep State

One, if not *the* major misconception associated with hypnosis, is that it is a form of sleep or involves a loss of consciousness. Patients presenting for hypnotic treatment will frequently express the view that they expect not to be able to hear anything or, alternatively, expect to be unaware of what is going on. This particular misconception appears hard to ablate by prehypnosis discussion. Even after detailed discussion on the issue, we have observed that patients express the "but I could hear everything around me" view after termination of a successful hypnosis episode.

Why has this myth persisted? Well, for one thing, to the casual observer, hypnotized subjects, especially the highly susceptible ones, may show all of the outward appearances of being asleep. The other reason for the confusion between sleep and hypnosis is the result of beliefs long held by the practitioners of hypnosis themselves. Because the confusion between hypnosis and sleep can be traced to a much earlier period of hypnotic history, it is informative to study these earlier concepts in order to realize how this particular misconception has persisted in spite of an abundance of clinical and experimental evidence showing hypnosis to be a non-sleep state.

One of the earliest references to hypnosis being a form of sleep was made by de Puységur (1751–1825). Following his initial experiences with animal magnetism, de Puységur labeled the condition artificial somnambulism. He did this on two scores: first, because his subjects appeared to be asleep, and second, and most important, like sleepwalkers, they claimed that they had no memory of their experiences. Faria (1756–1819) also proposed a connection between hypnosis and sleep. He used the term *lucid sleep* to describe the hypnotic state. In 1819, Faria published a book entitled *De La Cause du Someil Lucide,* in which he described what we now understand as hypnosis as being ". . . this type of sleep, [that] is common to all human nature by dreams and to all individuals who get up, walk and talk in their sleep." Braid (1795–1860) was further responsible for the propagation of the sleep concept of hypnosis. He considered hypnosis as being similar to sleep, but being anxious to give a physiological explanation for the state, called it nervous sleep or *neurypnology.* Braid subsequently contracted this term to hypnosis, a word derived from the Greek word *hypnos,* meaning "to sleep." The use of this word cemented even more firmly the sleep–hypnosis association. In later years, Braid realized that hypnosis was a misnomer, and in an apparent effort to correct the error, propounded the theory of monoideism. This stated that hypnosis was a state of intense concentration in which the subject was more able to respond to dominant ideas because of the inhibitions of weaker, competing ones. Unfortunately, the association between hypnosis and sleep had by this time become so strong that Braid's efforts to correct his own error had no real impact on the perpetuation of this myth. More recently, yet another important historical figure worked to foster the hypnosis–sleep notion. This was August Liébault (1823–1904), who published his views in the book *Sleep, and the State Analogous to It, Specially Considered in the Action of the Morale of the Physique.*

Thus, it can be seen that many of the early influential workers assumed an identity between hypnosis and sleep, and even those that did not make such a confusion nevertheless continued to utilize the term *sleep* as a metaphor for hypnosis. And so down to the present, where modern writers and therapists either continue to view hypnosis as a form of sleep or, at the very least, seem to fall into the same semantic trap. Countless texts discuss hypnosis as being quite different from sleep, yet continue to suggest the use of the term in induction procedures, thereby perpetuating the confusion in the patient's mind. We find this approach hard to justify in terms of modern theory and practice, and we consider that any references which seem to link sleep and hypnosis are best avoided. More than that, the therapist should go out of his way to emphasize that there will be nothing like sleepiness or a clouding of consciousness in hypnosis.

The most obvious difference between the two is revealed in the self-report data from people after experiencing each. Then there is the evidence from electroencephalographic (EEG) studies. For years now, researchers have been measuring the electrical activity of the cortex and, by studying the results, have identified a number of electrocortical patterns that can be correlated with states from sleep to alert, waking activity. Of special interest to sleep and hypnosis researchers is the low-frequency (8–13 Hz), high-amplitude alpha pattern. This is easiest to obtain when people close their eyes and take up a relaxed attitude; requests to perform difficult calculations or to engage in phobic imagery will break up the alpha pattern which, under such conditions, will be succeeded by the high-frequency (>13 Hz) and lower-amplitude beta pattern. The point to note here is that the alpha activity also disappears when the subject becomes drowsy and sleepy but it is maintained in hypnosis. Yet another difference is in the delta waves (0.5–4 Hz), which appear in Stage 4 sleep but do not appear in hypnosis (Evans, 1972). Finally, the EEG theta pattern (4–7 Hz), which is readily demonstrated in the hypnotized subject, is not correlated with any of the stages of sleep.

The therapist who wishes to challenge the mistaken notion that hypnosis is a form of sleep can present these findings in an abbreviated form and then go on to state: "Many people, especially those who have observed a stage hypnotist performing, think of hypnosis as being an unconscious or sleep state. In fact, it is anything but sleep, for if you were asleep, you would be unable to hear me and, consequently, be unable to respond to any suggestions that I gave and therefore therapy could not be carried out. It *is*, however, a state of awareness and relaxation, in which you are not only able to hear everything I say, but also other sounds around you. These sounds will not disturb you, but rather they will blend into the background and you will become less aware of them as you become more involved in this pleasant relaxed state." This appeal to logic is usually sufficient to lead to acceptance of hypnosis as being a conscious, non-sleep state, but it may need a few repetitions before the patient is fully convinced of the basic differences between the two. We have gone on at some length about the need for the therapist to bear down hard on the hypnosis–sleep distinction. The reason for this emphasis is that when patients practice self-hypnosis exercises at home they may think it something of an accomplishment when they fall asleep in the process. Since the home use of self-hypnosis should be a part of any hypnobehavioral program, patients must grasp the purpose of self- or heterohypnosis—which is the development of cognitive skills. This cannot be done if the person drifts off to sleep instead of carrying through the exercises to completion.

Myth: Hypnosis Impairs Memory

Another misconception associated with hypnosis concerns its supposed automatic production of an amnesic state. A great many people seeking hypnotic treatment in a clinical situation do so anticipating that they will be unable to recall the events that occurred in hypnosis, i.e., they expect to experience "spontaneous" amnesia. This idea may be based upon the behavior of subjects who participate in stage shows who often appear to be amnesic for the events of the hypnosis episode.

Unlike the questions of the relationship of sleep and hypnosis, the one about amnesia is not as easily settled. It is a fact that people may not recall all of the events which transpired in hypnosis. Whether or not this failure of recall should be given the label "amnesia" is not clear. A certain amount of forgetting is natural after any situation and can be explained in terms of the laws of memory and retrieval. Any forgetting over and above this (i.e., "hypnotic amnesia") has been attributed to one of a number of possible causes.

A popular view (Orne, 1966) is that posthypnotic amnesia occurs as the result of implicit or explicit suggestions given to the person or held by him before he enters the clinic or experimental laboratory. There is little doubt that many people who have had no direct experience with hypnosis nevertheless believe that amnesia is one of the outcomes intrinsic to hypnosis. In a bid to assess the extent of this belief, London (1961) surveyed 645 students from the University of Illinois. The students were asked their response to the statement: "People usually forget what happens in a trance as soon as they wake from it." London's (1961) results indicated that "a large majority of the respondents obviously feel that spontaneous amnesia is intrinsic to the experience of hypnosis and a large majority feel that some form of amnesia is to be expected as a result of hypnosis" (p. 157). What London did not try to prove was that these attitudes actually do influence posthypnotic recall. If the expectancy hypothesis is correct, then spontaneous amnesia should be a common occurrence. The clinical evidence suggests otherwise, and a recent study by Ashford and Hammer (1978) showed no experimental support for the expectancy account of posthypnotic amnesia.

A second and simpler explanation asserts that there is no forgetting (over and above normal loss) but only compliance on the subject's part. This is the argument used by the role-playing theorists of
hypnosis to explain all hypnotic phenomena. Later (see chapter 2)
we present our reasons for rejecting this theory of hypnosis but for
now we can note one clear-cut finding that is anomalous in terms of
the role-playing theory. Put simply, many subjects believe that amnesia is an expected outcome of hypnosis. Therefore, from the role-
playing account it could be predicted that reports of spontaneous
amnesia should be high whereas, in fact, they are relatively rare.

A third hypothesis invokes notions of "state dependent" effects
to explain posthypnotic amnesia. Retrieval is a function of the similarity between the cues present in the first situation and those available in the recall attempt. It is assumed that some of the relevant
cues arise from within the body as well as from the external environment. Since hypnotic subjects acquire this information under
one set of circumstances (the "disengagement" from external cues
giving prominence to internal cues) and attempt to retrieve it
under another and different set (less relaxed, in greater contact
with external cues), amnesia results (Overton, 1966). An implication
of this account is that better subjects (and subjects in "deeper"
hypnosis) should produce more disengagement and thus a greater
disparity and less overlap between the two sets of cues and, along
with that, a greater likelihood of spontaneous amnesia. The cues in
question can be spatial or temporal (Evans, 1980), and complex
effects of changes in "state" and the temporal sequencing promise
to make the final resolution of this problem a task for future generations of researchers.

Whatever the truth of the matter, it is necessary to discuss with
all patients their impression of whether they expect to experience
posthypnotic amnesia, and it is advisable for the therapist to raise
the issue in the following way: "Some people believe that when you
come out of hypnosis, you should be unable to remember what has
been said, or what you did in the hypnotic state. You may not have
given much thought to this before, but what do *you* think you may
experience? Do you expect, for instance, to be able to remember
everything, part of what happened, or nothing at all?" This approach allows the patient every opportunity to ventilate his thoughts
so that these can be fully discussed and erroneous ideas corrected.
The clinician should indicate his belief that spontaneous amnesia is
not common but that if it does occur there are methods of dealing

with it, and that the patient will not be "left in the dark" as to what occurred. The "repression" in this instance would be viewed as an adaptive strategy that could allow the patient to "try out" or "experiment" with such memories, realizing, at some level, that he would not need to deal with these out of hypnosis unless ready and able to do so (Evans, personal communication; see also the behavioral treatment of repression in Stampfl and Levis' 1967 theory of implosion). Some critics might object to the foregoing as borrowing excessively from controversial Freudian notions. While the present authors do not use suggestive amnesia in this way, the validity of these ideas about hypnosis and amnesia has yet to be established.

Myth: Hypnosis Requires Immobility

We have all too often come across patients who, though highly susceptible as measured by the standard assessment techniques, fail to enter hypnosis or to profit from the experience. This can be especially puzzling in a person who seems to have few if any anxieties about hypnosis and, indeed, who may be eager to participate in the experience. It has been more perplexing still in patients who do not articulate the real source of the difficulty, which is, simply, that they were overly concerned with acting out to the last physical detail what they believed to be the role of the hypnotic subject or patient. These people, and they are a significant minority, believe that a very solemn attitude must attend the induction of hypnosis. The careful, very restrained physical behavior of a devout churchgoer at a funeral service comes close to describing their feeling about what is the ideal behavior of the good hypnotic subject.

By analogy, hypnosis, as they see it, is to be entered into only by those who pay the strictest attention to the ritual. Just as one would refrain from laughing, scratching, coughing, or stretching during the religious service, so one must be "serious" about hypnosis. Note that one does not need to be told that energetic exertions and lighthearted humor is not to be shown in church. In like manner, this patient does not need to be told how to behave during hypnosis. He "knows" that he must not engage in any behavior not explicitly requested by the therapist, nor in any behavior that does not conform to what he believes the therapist expects of him. Such patients have told us that "I wanted to scratch my ear, and I knew that I shouldn't and yet I couldn't keep my mind off the urge." People may also worry about the impulse to laugh. Hypnosis is, as they see it, vulnerable to destruction if an easy lighthearted feeling emerges. They may complain afterward that "I was afraid that I'd giggle all the time; I barely managed to keep a straight face." We can only conjecture about the source of this myth about hypnosis. It may come from the way people seem to behave in stage hypnosis, showing a rapt attention to the hypnotist and acting as though they are carved in stone.

Whatever its source, it is, fortunately, an easy belief to counter and one that must be discussed and corrected. When patients hold these beliefs, they can become so preoccupied with keeping rigidly to the formula posture that they succeed only in becoming excessively tense and watchful. Until this is changed, we can say simply that hypnosis is not possible.

The patient should be told before the induction that he may from time to time feel like yawning, scratching, laughing, or in some way rearranging his position at any point during the proceedings. It is important to indicate that, while these experiences may not rise during the induction of hypnosis, if they do, they are quite acceptable and present absolutely no problems. Hypnosis is not, as they have previously been led to believe, a "spell" which will be punctured by an unrequested movement or twitch. Patients can be put further at ease about such concerns if they are told something such as the following: "Many people worry about changing their position in the chair (couch), coughing, speaking, or laughing, since they feel that this may 'ruin' hypnosis. However, such is not the case, and you should feel comfortable about doing any of these things if you feel the need. Now I realize that with these words, I may not have done away with your concerns, and you may still feel that the value of what we will be doing will be lessened if you are in any way active during the proceedings. But do let those concerns go as quickly as possible, since it is the concerns and not the readjustments of your hands and legs that will detract from the experience."

What we are saying here is that movements by themselves (twitches, scratches, yawns) are not important *unless* they are part of a larger action sequence. When this is the case, and when they are harnessed to a motive or goal that entails the subject making outcome decisions, then they are inimical to the disengagement conditions (see chapter 2) which must be satisfied for the successful use of hypnotic procedures.

Myth: Hypnosis Means Trying Hard

While practitioners do encounter those who come to therapy with a passive "you-cure-me-and-I'll-go-along-with-whatever-you-suggest" attitude, there are others who realize, or who have been told, that their active participation in behavior-change strategies is an essential precondition for a successful outcome. Some therapists reinforce this, unwisely we feel, by asserting that "all hypnosis is self-hypnosis." Patients are told that the responsibility for success or failure, therefore, rests solely with them.

While it is desirable as a general rule to have a patient who is motivated to change and who takes an active role in the planning and implementation of therapy, there is a disingenuous quality about the claim that "you are doing it all yourself." If it is the case that a person's hypnotizability is unmodifiable, then, in one sense, it *is* true that "all hypnosis is self-hypnosis." But if by this is also meant that the therapist can also be indifferent to his own performance or the reactions of the patient, then the statement is fundamentally incorrect. For even if an ability is inborn, stable, and unmodifiable (as some believe to be true of hypnosis), it certainly does *not* follow that the assistance—at least initially—of the expert "teacher" is of no consequence in bringing these potentials to fruition.

The approach that "it is all up to you," in addition to absolving the therapist of close and careful concern with the techniques and processes of hypnosis, can also, and more importantly, inculcate an effortful, striving attitude in the patient that carries with it concern over the likelihood of "failure." The "trying too hard" attitude is one of the most persistent and may require the therapist to reiterate repeatedly before and during the induction the importance of an easygoing, noncritical attitude.

Myth: Hypnotic Treatment Effects Are Transient/Permanent

Hypnosis and behavior therapy have both been charged with being too rapid and incisive to be deeply and permanently effective. This is more of a therapist-propagated belief and is the natural partner to its seemingly opposite belief, found more in patients, that hypnosis will effect sudden, dramatic, long-term transformations in any and all spheres of life.

Both of these beliefs rest on a serious misconception about the goals and methods of behavior therapy (and, hence, hypnobehavioral therapy). When properly used, behavior therapy methods, which can include hypnosis, equip the person to deal with his social and intrapersonal worlds more effectively. They do not aim to do things *to* the patient or only *within* the patient.

All patients who come to therapy hold some hope that hypnosis will be the "magic bullet" that will immediately improve their lives and solve their problems. The practitioner must deal gently but firmly with this belief, which if unchecked can grow into undesirable dependency or unrealistic disappointment.

This can present quite a challenge to the therapist. If he moves too forcefully he can detract from positive placebo effects (Lazarus, 1976) and set up the image of an uncaring, technical practitioner. While this may not be a bother in patients who have strong personal resources and mild and circumscribed problems, with the seriously anxious it can vitiate the effects of otherwise effective techniques (Andrews, 1966). We have found the best posture to be one which lays equal emphasis on the *initial* support the person can expect in hypnobehavioral therapy and the long-term growth of self-suffi-ciency. The technique of self-hypnosis can be an invaluable transi-tion tool (as well as a self-control technique skill of the first impor-tance) in bringing home this lesson.

Myth: Hypnosis Is Dangerous

Mesmer and Bernheim both postulated the operator-oriented con-cept of hypnosis, in which the hypnotist exerted his power over the subject. This approach to hypnosis persisted into the nineteenth cen-tury and was capitalized upon by such writers as George du Maurier. In du Maurier's novel *Trilby,* the heroine was an artist's model who was under the influence of a hypnotist called Svengali. Through the use of hypnotism, Trilby became a great singer, but her singing ability waned when Svengali died. Novels such as this have done much to contribute to the persistence of many of the undesirable views of hypnosis. To this day, patients still express concern about being "under someone else's control," or "being made to talk about things" which they are fearful of disclosing. Also, many patients feel that they may have "skeletons in the mind's cupboard" and, under-standably, are uncomfortable about the thought of disclosing these.

In more recent time, the issue of whether hypnosis is dangerous has become important from a medico-legal standpoint. If it could be unequivocally shown that through hypnosis one is able to control a subject to the extent that he can be induced to perform a crime or an amoral act, then the potential consequences of this could be disturbing and serious. The consideration of whether a hypnotized subject can be controlled and coerced to act contrary to his will is an important one. It is not surprising, therefore, that a great deal of experimental work, and also literature, should be devoted to this issue. Not unexpectedly, factions have become crystallized into two entirely opposing viewpoints. First, the school of thought represented by Watkins (1972) believes that subjects may be induced through hypnosis to commit antisocial acts. The contrasting attitude was succinctly expressed by Orne (1972): "Both the patient and the hypnotherapist are best served by the recognition that both the induction and maintenance of hypnosis involve a cooperative enterprise which may facilitate vivid and meaningful subjective experiences for the patient, but where in an ultimate sense, *the patient always remains in control*" (p. 115, our emphasis).

Another danger anticipated by most patients is that in hypnosis they will drift out of range of their own *or* the therapist's ability to recall them: "What happens if I go under and you can't get me back?" is the way one patient put it. There are patients who do not become "dehypnotized" or "reengaged" at the instant the termination procedure is completed (see chapter 4), but we have never seen nor heard of a person who took longer than a few minutes to "come out" of hypnosis. The patient can be told that most people worry over this but that he can be given absolute reassurance on this issue. Worries about "letting go," revealing awful secrets, or doing outlandish things in hypnosis are more easily dispelled by a clear account given beforehand about exactly what the practitioner and patient will be doing in hypnosis (for example, "On this first occasion I will not be asking you to do or say anything; all that I'd like you to do is just experience the suggestions and images I'll be giving to you. They will be. . . ."). With very anxious patients, a finger signal can be used to indicate excessive levels of anxiety ("If at any time you feel that you'd like to stop and talk some more about what we're doing or how hypnosis works just raise your right index finger and we'll go no further until you are ready again").

Myth: Hypnosis Can Uncover and Potentiate Psychological Disorders

Generations of novitiate hypnotists have been warned of the dangers of treating psychotic and prepsychotic patients in hypnosis—presumably because of the supposed intensification of the psychotic illness as a result of the dissociative process which is thought by some to be an integral part of hypnosis. However, Conn (1972), quoting Erickson, Kline, and Wolberg in support of his proposition, stated that "the psychotic process develops slowly over a period of years and . . . it is not 'precipitated' by one or more hypnotic experiences" (p. 70).

A more recent and detailed overview of this question has been made by Lavoie and Sabourin (1980), who, in assessing whether hypnosis may precipitate a psychotic state in a case of incipient psychosis, believe that "these dangers exist in a clinical situation, but they have not proved to be in any way particular to hypnosis" (p. 399). In short, the evidence does not reveal that hypnosis brings with it any *special* problems or dangers with psychotic patients (however, there is no persuasive evidence that hypnosis-assisted therapies are of any particular value in the management of psychotic problems).

A similar bit of clinical folklore has it that hypnosis is contraindicated in depressed subjects. The assumption is that the experience of hypnosis will incline the depressed patient toward suicidal thoughts and actions. The incidence of suicide is known to be much higher in depression than in any other problem (Beck, 1967), but there is no evidence that hypnosis in any way causes this already high risk to be increased still further. If a piecemeal attack is made on any one facet of a clinical syndrome without regard to the treatment of the overall problem, it can raise the possibility of sudden unintended and unexpected changes in other areas of the patient's functioning. In saying this we in no way imply the acceptance of the doctrine of symptom substitution but are merely calling attention to the complex ramifications of any treatment maneuver. Thus, and to state the obvious, using hypnosis in the treatment of depression would not obviate the need to sensible recourse to antidepressant medication.

A criticism with some validity that has been leveled at hypnosis over the years concerns its dangers in removing a symptom that serves as an indicator of underlying organic disease (for example, a headache that signifies the presence of a cerebral tumor). This situation, albeit rare, is likely to arise only when hypnosis is used by untrained and nonprofessional therapists. Its potential occurrence underlines the need for hypnosis to be performed only on patients who have been suitably evaluated, and only by therapists who are suitably qualified to do so. Another issue, closely related we believe, is the obvious need for therapists to work strictly within the confines of their professional training and field of competence.

Myth: Hypnosis Makes the Patient More Difficult to Live With

A concern sometimes voiced by patients, but usually more often by their relatives, is that following hypnosis the patient is more difficult to live with and not as pleasant to be around. These claims, though wrong in substance, cannot be dismissed as figments of the imagination. The whole thrust of contemporary practice in behavior therapy is to help the patient to be less reactive and more self-directive in his life. All of the well-known techniques, from hypnosis to rational-emotive therapy, are harnessed to these objectives (or should be). What behavior therapists have been late in admitting into their formulations is the impact of this training (for that is how "therapy" is now seen) on those who live with and/or interact with the patient. Assertion therapy is the paradigmatic instance of this. Many commentators have remarked upon the feelings of helplessness or the sense of being "pushed around" by others that anxious patients so often report (Alberti & Emmons, 1974; Lange & Jakubowski, 1976; Salter, 1949). Teaching the skills of responsible assertive behavior would seem to be an obvious goal in therapy and, indeed, the clinical benefits of assertion training have been widely recorded (Rimm & Masters, 1979, pp. 63–101). What is now coming to light in laboratory studies, however, is that the effects of assertion therapy may not all be pleasant and satisfying to the patient. Newly assertive individuals can be perceived by their peers as "lower on many measures of likeability, warmth, flexibility, and friendliness" (Kelley, Kern, Kirkley, Patterson, & Keane, 1980, p. 680). This problem is now being researched by students of assertion therapy, but we are confident that future work will reveal this to be the case for a variety of therapies, for the simple reason that when effective they all give the patient more independence and scope for change. This change for the better can, nevertheless, be stressful, at least in the short term, for those in the person's life. Because they are salient and "dramatic," assertion training and hypnosis may, mistakenly, be singled out and cited as *the* causes of the stress that calls for the (sometimes painful) readjustments of significant others. The upshot of this is that the therapist should consult with the most important of these people to prepare them for the changes they may have to make, as well as informing the patient of the mixed blessings of therapy.

A Final Word

Practitioners who pride themselves on holding a scientific orientation to therapy gravitate naturally to a position that emphasizes the importance of well-validated techniques. This can easily become the position which assumes the automatic operation of these techniques if they are applied correctly. It may seem that by introducing such nebulous matters as the patient's belief about his problems, and his feelings about the therapeutic techniques which are proposed to alleviate them, we confuse this issue unnecessarily. It is unfortunate that, up to the present, very little is known about the processes of expectancy, treatment credibility, and demand characteristics (nicely and humorously called the "Natural History of a Nuisance" in Bernstein and Nietzel's 1977 review). Our ignorance about their precise workings is a real burden because we are beginning to realize how central their role is in facilitating or undermining the value of our most cherished clinical techniques.

In this case, as in the rest of clinical practice, what holds for hypnosis also applies to other techniques. If patients do not find flooding (or, say, desensitization) to be a credible technique, then it will not work as well as it will in those patients who have a positive expectancy about it. It would not be too far from the truth to say that the need in clinical behavior therapy is not so much for the development of new techniques as for finding ways to systematically mobilize and understand positive expectancies about the ones already in our repertoire. This process begins with the correction of the myths and misconceptions which the patient holds about the techniques in question.

2

The Nature of Hypnosis: A Perspective

As the diameter in the circle of light lengthens, so too does the perimeter of darkness increase.

—Arabian proverb

The dictionary definition of hypnosis is that of "a sleeplike condition, psychically induced, usually by another person, in which the subject is in a state of altered consciousness and responds, with certain limitations, to the suggestions of the hypnotist" (*Webster's New World Dictionary*, 1970).

The definition lists the three stages or parts of hypnosis: the induction technique (the stimulus); the mental alterations (the organismic variable); and the heightened suggestibility (the response). Historically, interest in hypnosis has centered on the response of the person. The stimulus or induction side of hypnosis has not yielded to easy categorization. It would seem that a great variety of techniques can be used with nothing apparent in common save that they all lead to the hypnotic reaction. The intervening or organismic variables have only recently been subjected to experimental analysis. The response side of hypnosis has, from the beginning, been the basis for the interest in hypnosis. It is around the seemingly puzzling and dramatic behaviors that the disputes, storms, and dramas of hypnosis have swirled.

The responses, i.e., the hypnotic phenomena, can be divided into those which are spontaneous and those which are evoked. In actual practice, as Estabrooks (1957) correctly notes, "there is only one spontaneous phenomenon, namely, heightened suggestibility. The subject, left to himself, will do nothing, be completely inert. Everything [that occurs] is evoked, the result of suggestion" (p. 50).

Let us take a look at a few of the widely discussed hypnotic phenomena:

CASE 1.   A 28-year-old woman with a very low pain threshold—self-described as a "devout coward"—is able to have a long and arduous dental operation and reports feeling no pain or discomfort.

CASE 2.   A 45-year-old man is told during hypnosis that he is 15 years of age. He begins to recall—relive he says—a traumatic experience long since "forgotten."

CASE 3.   A 40-year-old woman is given the suggestion that following the termination of the hypnosis episode, the hypnotist will tell her that she looks very refreshed. At that point, she is told, she will leave the laboratory and go straight to the ladies washroom where she will splash some water on her face, dry it, and come straight back to the laboratory. The experimenter counts backward from 5 to 1 and tells the woman that "it is all over; you can open your eyes, sit up, take a nice stretch and relax." A few moments afterward, and in the middle of an easy conversational exchange, the experimenter remarks: "Yes, you do look very refreshed." The woman immediately gets to her feet and walks out of the room saying that she'll be back in a minute. Shortly afterward she returns, her makeup smeared across her face. She says, with a rueful grin, "that was a bloody silly thing for me to do." To the experimenter's question she replies, "It was silly of me to wash my face with this mascara on." When asked why she went, she replies, "because my face was dirty and I needed to wash it. Besides, I thought it would refresh me." This rationalization is delivered with force and conviction.

CASE 4.   A 26-year-old male graduate student is seated with his eyes closed, head to one side. A voice tells him that his arm will grow lighter and lighter. After a few minutes of these suggestions the man's arm begins to rise.

The overt responses performed by the subjects in these episodes are, by themselves, unremarkable. What makes them interesting and what has generated controversy and disagreement is the interpretations offered of them. The simplest explanation has been to view such responses, and all of hypnotic behavior, as some species of sham or deception. Hence, it would be said of the woman in the first example that she *claimed* to feel no pain while in fact experiencing all of the distress which people usually do when undergoing dental surgery without anesthesia. The behavior of the woman who gave the rationalization instead of the real reason for leaving the room upon hearing the cue word "refreshed" (Case 3) would be explained along the same lines; she only *pretended* to be unable to remember the instructions given to her. And it would be imagined that the man who reported the "involuntary" arm levitation *chose*, for some reason or other (perhaps to please the hypnotist, or to be a cooperative subject, or in the anticipation of social or material reward for "going along with" the hypnotist's wishes) to insist that the arm "came up of its own accord" when really he made the usual effort required to lift the arm into the air. In other words, all of these instances of hypnotic performance can be reduced to examples of voluntary compliance by the subject with the wishes of the experimenter or therapist. To put it another way, the subject is tacitly or directly giving a false and not a true report of his experience.

This explanation of hypnotic performance as a kind of hoax (to borrow the term used—but not accepted—by Orne, 1980) has a long history. In the middle of the last century W.S. Ward, a British physician, amputated the leg of a patient who went through the operation while in a "mesmeric trance" (this was before the discovery of reliable anesthetic procedures). Ward reported that the operation was a complete success due, in no small measure, to the fact that the patient had experienced no pain—and the patient signed a declaration to this effect. But when Ward presented his findings to the Royal Medical and Chirurgical Society in England in 1842:

> the Society refused to believe. Marshall Hall, the pioneer in the study of reflex action, urged that the patient must have been an imposter, and the note of the paper's having been read was stricken from the minutes of the Society. It was further urged that the method if correct (which, of course, it could not have been, the Society insisted implacably) was immoral, since pain is "a wise provision of nature, and patients ought to suffer pain while their surgeons are operating." (cited in Boring, 1950, p. 121)

The contrary view of hypnotic performance is found in the "group [which] seems convinced that hypnosis is a uniquely powerful state which results in almost magical abilities. They report that hypnotized individuals can perform feats of strength and have control of body and mind beyond the ken of the normal [i.e., unhypnotized] individual" (Orne, 1980, p. 33). This orientation is based on three assumptions: first, that there are *special* procedures of the hypnotic induction which, second, lead to a *special* state of neuropsychological functioning and, when established, make available to the operator and subject a *special* set of responses that are out of reach of the unhypnotized individual.

The two positions just outlined in brief, schematic form describe the most extreme forms of the categories into which efforts to explain hypnotic performance have polarized (Orne, 1980). They correspond, more or less, to the orientations that have been dubbed by Sutcliffe (1960) as the "skeptical" and "credulous."

A modern and forceful advocate of the skeptical position is T.X. Barber. He and his followers eschew terms like "hoax" and "fakery" but, as should be apparent from the following remarks, argue that the report of the "hypnotized" subject contains an element of concealment or deception. Thus, in discussing hypnotic analgesia, for example, Barber suggests that

> The motivation for the denial of pain is present in the clinical hypnotic situation. The physician who has invested time and energy hypnotizing the patient and suggesting that pain will be relieved expects and desires that his efforts will be successful, and by his words and manner communicates his desires and expectations to the patient. The patient, in turn, has often found a close relationship with the physician-hypnotist and would like to please him or at least not to disappoint him. Furthermore the patient is aware that if he states that he suffered, he is implying [that the physician has wasted his time . . . therefore] it may be difficult or disturbing for him to state directly to the physician-hypnotist that he experiences pain, and it may be less anxiety provoking to say that he did not suffer. (Barber, 1970, pp. 211–212)

Barber does not restrict this analysis only to the phenomenon of hypnotic analgesia but offers it as an explanation for the full range of all hypnotic phenomena.*

*More recently Barber (see Spanos & Barber, 1976) has shifted his ground somewhat and appears to be including intrapersonal (or cognitive) influences replacing his almost exclusive reliance upon antecedent events in attempting to understand hypnosis. While this concern with the person's subjective experience is, to our way of thinking, a

Although in this book we do not wish to identify with either the "special state" or "mere compliance" arguments, as set out above, we do find ourselves in agreement with those (for example, Bowers, 1977) who feel that the extreme skeptical position is an exercise in explaining away and not explaining hypnosis. It would be wrong, however, to list only the shortcomings of the skeptical position without making any mention of positive influences that have come out of this work.

Most generally, the presence of the skeptics on the scene has had a restraining influence on some of the most credulous (usually clinical) workers. At least that is our impression. Then, too, Barber has, with some justification, criticized the "vicious circularity" in the use of the word *trance* as an explanatory concept: the trance (plus suggestion) is cited as the cause of hypnotic performance and, in a quick turn around, the very performance explained via the trance is invoked a proof of its existence. It is possible to break out of this trap by getting independent evidence of "the trance"—apart from the behavior it is supposed to explain—or discovering behaviors that uniquely index the hypnotic state. Our aim in this chapter is to note the limitations of trance as an explanatory concept (see below) and yet to retain the interest in the inner, cognitive changes to which the word *trance* directs our attention. We find no serious reason to object to the word *trance*—except for the polemics from the past—when it is employed in a descriptive sense (cf. the two uses of the word *instinct*) or even as a construct. The fact that no one response has been found which indexes the trance, or hypnosis, is no more reason to deny the reality of hypnosis than is the absence of one response common to all instances of depression cause to rule out the existence of depressive disorders.

It is also true, as Barber (1966) has repeatedly argued, that there is no convincing evidence yet reported which sustains the claim that hypnotized subjects are able to transcend normal levels of performance over and above that shown by nonhypnotized subjects given task-motivating instructions. It is an undeniable fact that cooperative subjects requested to endure a painful stimulus for *x* seconds are able to do so. Furthermore, it is possible to have them go

---

welcome change, Barber continues to give the impression that it is mainly, if not only, the overt behavior that should concern the investigator. There is no question that the interpersonal transactions and the "laws of social psychology" comprise a vital part of the hypnotic episode. But to slight the experience of the hypnotic subject and to pass lightly over the central (brain, "mental," or cognitive) dimensions of hypnosis must limit seriously our grasp of the nature of hypnosis.

through the task without an outward show of pain and even to deny to an onlooker that they felt anything at all. But the fact that a carefully trained and fully cooperative unhypnotized subject may be able to mimic the overt behavior and to give the same verbal report as a deeply hypnotized subject does not allow us to assert that the same neuropsychological activities were at work in both. This is the logical error in arguing that similar response topographies prove the existence of identical processes. In failing to elicit and analyze the subject's report of his own experience, the Behaviorists were, in Bowers' (1977) apt phrase, "trying to catch 4 inch fish with a net which has 5 inch holes." If a subject is able to lift his arm at precisely the same rate as it came up when he was hypnotized and given suggestions of arm lightness, it is surely important to note his claims that "it may have looked the same to you but it didn't *feel* the same to me. I raised it as instructed (after hypnosis) but the first time it did it by itself." Our contention is that in failing to elicit the subject's self-report response an absolutely essential datum is lost. This is the most serious shortcoming of the voluntary compliance or role-playing* interpretations of hypnotic performance.

Finally, two lines of evidence attest to the shortcomings of the "mere compliance" explanations so long favored by the skeptics. There is the behavior of hypnotized patients during operations or who are suffering chronic pain. We find it implausible, to say the least, to imagine that unanesthetized patients can manage to pretend to an analgesia which is absent. For a nice response to this we offer the words of the Scottish surgeon James Esdaile to the charge that his patients were feigning analgesia when undergoing operations for the removal of scrotal tumors:

> I have *every month* more operations of this kind than take place in the native hospital in Calcutta a year, and more than I had for the six years previous. There must be some reason for this and I see only two ways

---

*There *are* forms of the role-playing explanation such as Sarbin's (1950) which suppose that the unhypnotized person can so thoroughly immerse himself in the role of "hypnotized subject" that he loses all notions of deception and concealment. When role-playing is looked at in this way, it is indeed difficult to maintain a clear conceptual separation between state and role-playing accounts (especially if it is argued that formal induction procedures are one though certainly not the only way to generate the hypnotic "state"—a position held by the present authors, among others). Unfortunately the term *role-playing* has also been used in a very different sense (for example, Sarbin & Coe, 1972) to refer to a conscious attempt to create an impression or to deliberately bring one's behavior into line with the implicit or direct requests of the operator. We agree with Orne (1980, p. 43) that care must be taken so as not to confuse the two meanings of role-playing.

of accounting for it: My patients, on returning home, either say to their friends similarly afflicted, "Wah brother! what a soft man the doctor Sahib is! He cut me to pieces for twenty minutes, and I made him believe that I did not feel it. Isn't it a capital joke? Do go and play him the same trick; you have only to laugh in your elbow." Or, they say to their brother sufferers,—"look at me; I have got rid of my burthen (of 20, 30, 40, 50, 60 or so lbs., as it may be), am restored to the use of body, and can again work for my bread: this, I assure you, the doctor Sahib did when I was asleep, and I knew nothing about it;—you will be equally lucky, I dare say; and I advise you to go and try; you need not be cut if you feel it." Which of these hypotheses best explains the facts my readers will decide for themselves. (Esdaile, 1957, pp. 218–219)

The other body of evidence comes from the behavior of subjects in real simulator studies. In these, simulating (faking) subjects are asked to behave as they imagine truly hypnotized persons would behave. It will be found that they exhibit some notable failures to parallel the behavior of deeply hypnotized subjects. As an example, a deeply hypnotized subject when asked to "hallucinate" a person in a (real) chair may report that he sees the person and yet, also, the back of the chair in which the person is "sitting." On the other hand, simulators, Orne (1980) notes, never demonstrate this "trance logic"—the ability to tolerate such incompatible responses as seeing the person and all of the chair, too. The ability of a hypnotized subject to accept the logical inconsistency of seeing a chair "through" the hallucinated person supports the assertion that "the 'essence' of hypnosis will be found in the subjective experiences of the S" (Orne, 1959).

Hypnosis: An Integrative Approach

The long-term history of hypnosis can be written as the dialectic between the special state and the voluntary "cooperative" explanations. Onlookers to this debate have tended toward the conclusion that these two explanations exhaust all of the plausible options. And, in one way of looking at it, this conclusion appears inescapable. The hypnotic subject is either going along with, i.e., "voluntarily" performing, the behaviors which he believes are expected of him, or another explanation is required. The deficiences and limitations of this account would seem to leave us with no option but to embrace the trance–special-state theory. This conclusion, however, is only logically correct. The central notion in the special-state theory is the

hypnotic trance which mediates the effect of the induction procedures. But on close inspection this trance turns out to be a general,
global term for a whole range of central or cognitive changes.
Calling all of these by the term *trance* is also an instance of explaining away instead of explaining hypnosis.

Another source of dissatisfaction with the trance–special-state
theory (and there are a number of varieties) is the view of "normal"
or nonhypnotic behavior implied therein. The central, but unrec-
ognized, premise is that outside of hypnosis a kind of "naive realism"
prevails. Thus we see all supra-threshold stimuli that impinge on the
retinae, feel all painful stimuli that impact the "pain receptors,"
smell all powerful scents that assault the olfactory receptors and, in
the main, function perceptually in such a way as to faithfully copy all
of the stimuli playing upon the sensorium. The view of the output
systems offers us yet another dichotomy between trance (hypnotic)
and normal (nonhypnotic) functioning. Most overt behaviors (walking, talking, looking) are classed as "voluntary," and these are modifiable in the "waking" condition; visceral-autonomic reactions (blood
pressure, blushing, heart rate, digestive changes) are given the status
of "involuntary" behaviors and can be modified in hypnosis but not
outside of it—that is to say, not in a deliberate manner for therapeutic purposes. The nature of central (cognitive, attentional) reactions
outside of the "trance" conditions is left unstated altogether. What
seems to be assumed here is that reason and thinking are controlled
by outer evidence and are directed toward the solution of objective
problems (those of a psychoanalytic orientation would assume the
very opposite—that thinking and all cognitive activities are under
the influence not of the demands of the external environment but,
invariably, of drives and wishes).

It bears repeating that we are not assuming that the traditional
trance–special-state supporters have made an attempt to articulate
clearly and precisely a picture of non-trance functioning. They
have not. It is for this very reason that they are most open to
critical attack. There is a nice irony here. The weakest point in the
special-state theory is just where it has not been challenged at all.
And there can be no mistake about it, this account of "normal,"
nonhypnotic, psychology simply cannot be harmonized with our
current knowledge of perceptual, cognitive, autonomic, and behavioral mechanisms.

The special-state explanation, then, creates two categories of
responding: non-trance and trance. Trance behavior is special only

because it appears to stand in dramatic contrast to the tacitly held perspective of non-trance functioning. If we alter our conceptions of the latter, then to the same degree we *must* change our views of the former. There is no room here to attempt even a summary of current research into perceptual, cognitive, autonomic, and behavioral processes and the relationship among them. Nonetheless, it is possible to detect a consensus around a number of broad generalizations. For our purposes the most important of these bear on the current perspectives on perception, memory, and involuntary activities of the autonomic system. Perception and memory are now accepted as activities by which we construct the world. Our perceptions and memories are complex central *acts* and not mere copies of the world or our experiences in it. The distinction between voluntary/involuntary and autonomic responses is no longer viable either. The deliberate alteration of "involuntary" responses has been amply demonstrated (for example, Benson, 1975). As Sarbin and Slagle (1972) put it, the question now is not whether symbolic processes can produce changes in biological processes—the answer is an unqualified yes. It is rather what conditions must we have in order to accomplish this most effectively?

We have just referred to a summary of experimental findings which stand as a strong counterargument to the thesis that hypnosis is special because only through it can "exceptional" phenomena be observed. Convincing though these findings of cognitive control over perceptions and the plasticity of autonomic reactions are, it is not necessary to go into the experimental laboratory to encounter them. We could borrow a page from Freud's position of abnormal behavior to help us. His book *The Psychology of Everyday Life* made us aware of the continuities between so-called normal and aberrant behavior. In the same way it might be helpful for us to begin our attempt at a perspective on hypnosis with the "hypnosis" of everyday life. Quite simply, all of the behaviors produced in hypnosis and in "waking" subjects in the laboratory can be matched by naturally occurring responses of a similar form and experience. Since we began our outline of the opposing views of hypnosis with the subject of pain, we will return to it here. Most of us have at one time or another sustained an injury in an athletic contest or during a moment of excitement without any sense of pain whatsoever. The same wound, if inflicted deliberately in a nonhypnotized and attentive person, would create immense discomfort. We say that we "didn't notice" the injury in the heat of the game (soldiers in battle not infrequently fail to realize that they have been shot until the battle subsides). It makes no sense to say that we really did feel the pain but in order to add to the vast fund of such stories we chose to deny what we felt. Positive and negative hallucinations are two more special "hypnotic phenomena" which are also associated with the trance state. The term *hallucination* with its connotation of pathology could equally, and perhaps better, be described as "nonveridical perception." Seeing things that are not there and failing to detect events that are present are by no means rare. As with the nonhypnotic analgesia, the importance of context, expectations, and the focus of attention are basic to these "hallucinations." The more "simple" ideomotor responses—body sway, arm heaviness, eye closure—can be elicited within and outside of hypnosis. To take but one more example, the absorption and dissociation of the hypnotized subject finds its everyday expression in the great detachment from the present environment when we are totally caught up in an exciting book or film. The list could be multiplied time and again.

Where have we come to in this discussion? The behaviors and experiences of hypnosis can be brought about outside of the formal induction situation. This is clearly the case, but dismissing both as some species of faking or role-playing is another matter. In both, continuities notwithstanding, we have striking departures from normal (i.e., statistical) functioning; we usually *do* feel painful stimuli and our constructions of the world usually *do* provide us with the basis for adaptive responding. Clinical improvements can be stimulated by *placebo* drugs, but the appropriate medication typically leads to a higher rate of change (for example, Neale & Oltmans, 1980). Common to these phenomena within or outside of hypnosis is a disengagement or dissociation from our usual interaction with the environment. The value of hypnotic induction procedures is threefold: (1) it permits for the deliberate production of phenomena which, as we have seen, may also occur in everyday life situations; (2) it can be done so as to sustain these effects for a given duration and intensity; and (3) it can be done for experimental or therapeutic purposes.

In traditional accounts of hypnosis, the word *trance* is the name given to the central systems that subserve hypnotic behavior. With all of its limitations (for example, Spanos & Barber, 1976), trance does at least direct our thinking to the processes as well as the techniques of hypnosis. The search for a more detailed understanding, however, requires us to go past the trance label to a study of the structure and function of these cognitive systems.

Hypnosis: Operations and Processes

The search begins with an account of what people actually do when they wish to hypnotize another. (The issue of self-hypnotic methods will be deferred for the moment; a full discussion of self-hypnosis can be found in chapter 7.) We will pay little attention to the terminology that workers from different schools use to describe their methods. Actually, there is, once these differences are put aside, a surprising commonality in procedure among hypnotists. Where they *do* diverge is in the uses to which hypnosis is put once the induction is complete. These turn upon differences in the conceptions of a particular problem and are covered in later chapters. Our strategy at this, preliminary, stage will be to focus on the hypnosis episode itself. Specifically, our aim will be to dissect the episode into its components and to give the psychological effect of each in turn. These, we will argue, can be measured along a psychological space of six dimensions (see Figure 2.1).

1). Anxiety Reduction

Practitioners, irrespective of their individual approach to hypnosis, recognize that a patient may experience difficulties in achieving a satisfactory hypnotic induction because of excessive anxiety. These anxieties may stem from any of a number of the widespread misunderstandings about hypnosis (see chapter 1) or the particular uses to which it will be put on a given occasion. The therapist must take the necessary steps to counteract any anxiety based on these misunderstandings, or any other causes. This is done through the presentation of accurate information about hypnosis and the giving of reassurance about the effects of hypnosis. If correctly done, the effect will be to reduce the subject's sense of threat. Here, as with all of the areas to follow, it will be more accurate and more useful to conceptualize these changes as occurring along a continuum or dimension. The one under discussion here could be labeled: Amount of Defensive Anticipation. If we, arbitrarily, assign the higher levels to the left side and the lower levels to the right side of these dimensions, then the aim will always be to help the patient to move as far as possible toward the right end of the spectrum. Before we leave this first step, the correction of misconceptions and the alleviation of the patient's anxiety, it is worth noting that this is an essential though often neglected step in any induction procedure.

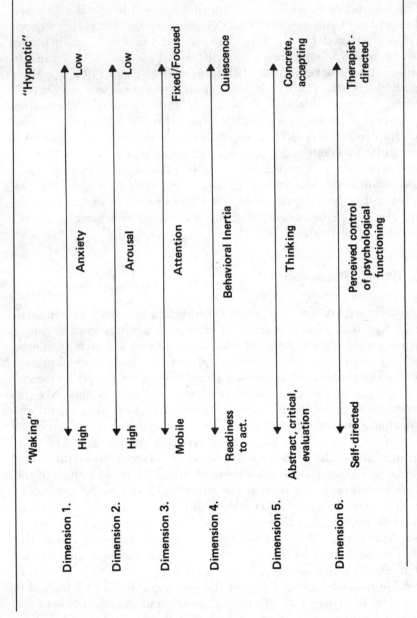

Figure 2.1 The components of hypnotic disengagement.

2. Reduction in Arousal

The next step in all standard induction procedures is for the patient to sit back or lie down in a comfortable position. This may be accompanied by a request for the patient to keep his gaze upon one particular object or, as is more usually the case, to begin by closing his eyes. At the same time the therapist usually, and advisedly, takes care to reduce to a minimum the level of noise, bright lights, or other intense distracting stimuli. The effect of these instructions and arrangements is to reduce the stimulus-input arising from the external environment and from within the patient's own body. These are the conditions favorable to a decrease in arousal. Arousal ("activation" and the Russian "orienting reflex" are roughly synonymous terms) is a word with multiple meanings (Duffy, 1962). It can refer to the level of activity in a variety of physiological systems or, at the psychological level, it can refer to the sensitivity to environmental stimulation and the readiness to engage in activity. The reduction of arousal is thought to be an indispensable event in the production of hypnosis, and practitioners invariably take the necessary steps to bring this about. Arousal is generally regarded as a scale ranging from coma at the lowest level to alertness, anxiety, and finally terror at the highest scale (Eysenck, Arnold, & Meili, 1975). At the lower levels, the patient's awareness of his inner and outer worlds fades, as does his generalized readiness to act upon the environment. Steps taken to reduce arousal also facilitate anxiety reduction (Dimension 1) and evoke desirable changes in the other dimensions; the dimensions of hypnosis are not independent of one another, and positive interactions are the rule.

3. Focused Attention

A third procedural commonality is the instruction the patient is given to listen closely to the words of the therapist. All other sensations or thoughts are to be ignored. Therapists usually avoid telling the patient *not* to attend to these events (there is no surer way to focus a person's attention on X than to tell him "don't think about X"). This is implicit in the request to "listen to my voice."

These directions call upon the patient to give up the otherwise automatic scanning of his world for intrusive stimuli arising either from the environment or from the person's covert self-statements and imagery. These changes are the source of the sharp "sensory gradients" which maintain the activity and integrity of those cognitive processes essential for directed critical thinking (Suedfeld, 1980). In short, on this dimension we are talking about reductions in the *variety* of input as opposed to the sheer amount or intensity of stimulation. Therapists show an intuitive awareness of this relationship when they use a monotonous, unchanging, and slowed-down style of delivery.

This dimension of the hypnotic process could be labeled at the left (and less hypnotic) end as Mobile Attention, and at the other (right) end, Focused Attention. Thus, the aim in *all* hypnotic induction procedures is to help the person fix or focus his attention. How he manages to do this may not be important—as long as the end result is that the attention is fixed upon one thing (Suedfeld, 1980). What we wish to stress here is the necessity for sustaining the attention against *intrusive,* irrelevant cognitions. In later chapters we will return to this question in our discussion of self-hypnosis and meditation, where we will see that the presence of the hypnotist is not essential for hypnosis. In practice, however, most people will need some assistance with an outside focus of attention (such as the voice of the hypnotizer) lest they return, without realizing it, to the restless scanning of the untrained and unfocused attention (Carrington, 1978).

4. Behavioral Inertia

A time-honored part of every induction procedure is the use of words like "sleep," "relax," or "heaviness." The purpose of these words is not in fact to induce sleep, which is very different from hypnosis (see chapter 1). We would reiterate that striving to achieve any outcome or end-state is undesirable in the production of hypnotic effects, and yet people are told they should try to sleep or relax. Why then are these suggestions used so often by therapists of all orientations? The answer, we would suggest, is to elicit the behavioral reactions which are associated with these cue words: quiescence and behavioral inertia. The dimension in question could be labeled Behavioral Inactivity, but this would fail to capture the most salient aspect of the changes to which we refer, viz. the *readiness* to engage in a goal-oriented sequence of behavior or thinking. In other words, the suggestions are aimed at helping the patient lose his predisposition to *self*-directed lines of thought and behavior—an important prerequisite in the achievement of the hypnotic "state." In emphasizing goal-directed cognitive-behavioral activity, we are distinguishing this notion from simple behavioral lethargy on the one hand, or random twitches or postural adjustments on the other.

5. Uncritical Thinking

In everything which he says and does, the therapist attempts to convey to the patient an attitude of acceptance to all of the suggestions and directions contained within the induction procedure. If the patient is told that his eyelids will grow heavier and heavier, and that his right arm will grow lighter, it is implied that he is not to subject these words to logical scrutiny nor is he to evaluate the reality status of the suggestions. Interestingly, in other clinical procedures (viz. autogenic training), the patient is urged to "passively repeat" the formulae and to put aside the sort of directed, rational thinking associated with an outer problem-solving orientation. This may account for the reported hypnotic-like reactions to autogenic training, and also to meditation (Carrington, 1978).

6. Transfer of Control

As the induction proceeds, the therapist will change his pattern of suggestions. Initially, he will draw attention to ongoing processes ("as you breathe in . . . and out, you can hear my voice very clearly"). Next, he incorporates suggestions of simple motor movements ("your eyes are becoming heavy . . . heavier . . . soon they will close"). Finally, the suggestions are followed by more demanding ones in the behavioral and cognitive spheres ("your arm is growing lighter . . . before too long it will float up from the arm of the chair, by itself, with no effort on your part" or "you will feel no sensations in your left arm, which is growing quite numb"). The objective is to establish the therapist's words and behavior as the effective stimuli for a host of changes *which are experienced by the patient as lying outside of his voluntary control*. The effective use of suggestions during the induction gives the reactions that occur in the patient a strong sense of inevitability and irresistibility. The particular reactions that occur are less important than the patient's perception of the source of these behaviors. The ordinary sense of control that the patient has over his own behavior is lessened, and the control that the therapist appears to exert is correspondingly increased. Success in moving the patient from the "self-direction" to therapist control hinges upon the timing and sequencing of the therapist's suggestion. This occurs across three stages, and the transition from one stage to the next must be gradual and imperceptible. This requires the therapist to "make himself into a sophisticated biofeedback mechanism" (Bandler & Grinder, 1975, p. 16). In stage one, the patient comes to accept the therapist's account of his experience as accurate. In stage two, the therapist employs a carefully contrived ambiguity which leaves the patient with two competing "explanations" for the segment of behavior to which the therapist refers ("my eyes are closing because they are tired—that is only to be expected—after all I have had them wide open for so long," as opposed to "my eyes are closing because the therapist said they were tired and he said that they would close"). The transition is completed in stage three, where the patient's experience is that the behaviors have, to him, no other cause but the therapist's word and activities. The guiding notion behind the changes in this most important dimension "is not whether the logic of the (therapist's) statements is valid, but simply whether they constitute a successful link between the subject's ongoing behavior and what the subject experiences next " (Bandler & Grinder, 1975, p. 19).

The Hypnotic "Trance"

In a provocative and important book written in 1965, Eysenck and Rachman criticized the S-R model in behavior therapy. Their main complaint was the failure of behavior therapy to give any systematic place in its schemes to "the recognition of the existence of an organism intervening between stimulus and response" (p. 15). They made a strong case for an S-O-R model ("O" for organism) and the study of these central or organismic changes, which take place between the reception of the environmental stimulus and the occurrence of the overt response. At the time, their call was not heeded (nor was Skinner's insistence in 1953 that "private events" played an important role in the control of behavior). In recent years, however, we have seen the acceptance and vindication of their position. Cognitive psychology and the study of cognitive processes have widened the scope of behavior therapy. Nowadays, the leading texts (for example, Rimm & Masters, 1979) have chapters on cognitive techniques side by side with those dealing with aversion therapy, contingency management, flooding, and so on. Along with the general acceptance of the proposition that cognitive psychology has a legitimate place within a liberalized behavior therapy has come a renewed interest in hypnosis. One of the main barriers to the full acceptance of hypnosis has been the use of "trance" as an explanation for the state from which hypnosis phenomena spring. It gives no clarity to our understanding of hypnosis, and thus requires the use of techniques on a cut-and-try basis or the adoption of methods merely because of traditional usage.

This is an unsatisfactory state of affairs. In addition to the rote or too "clinical" (in the pejorative sense of the word) use of hypnosis, the trance explanation stands as an obstacle in the way of a full integration of hypnosis with the broader fields of psychology and physiology. The need for a more precise specification of the processes of hypnosis requires no further emphasis. As a step toward this goal we began our search with the actual induction procedures employed by therapists and researchers. We noted that there is what might be called the standard set of procedures. These appear again and again regardless of the experimental issue nominated by the researcher, or the clinical problem confronting the patient and the therapist.

According to our account of hypnosis, the results of employing these procedures can be summarized as follows. In a successful induction the patient will move through a psychological space which can be defined in terms of six dimensions (Figure 2.1). In the perspective offered here, hypnotic reactivity is a function of conditions which lead to:

1. A reduction in anxiety
2. A reduction in arousal
3. A fixed, as opposed to a mobile or labile, attention leading to a reduction in the patterning of sensory input and a restriction in the number of sharp sensory gradients
4. The production of behavioral immobility or inertia
5. A shift in cognitive functioning toward concrete thinking and away from critical reflection
6. A transfer of perceived control over the person's reactions such that they appear less voluntary and more under the control of the words of the hypnotist.

To summarize in plain words, if we want to be sure of hypnotizing someone, we first eliminate anxieties—whether or not due to misconceptions about hypnosis (Dimension 1). Having done this, we must ensure that there is an absolute minimum in the way of bright

lights, loud noise, or other intense stimuli. The goal in doing this is
to bring down arousal levels (Dimension 2). Soon after beginning the
induction, the patient is asked to listen closely to the voice of the
hypnotist and to leave aside all other concerns. The result is a focused attention, which replaces the quickly shifting attention of our
everyday lives (Dimension 3). There is evidence that it is the single-
pointed thinking and the consequent lessening of variety and change
that are essential in hypnosis, and not the way in which this is
achieved. Having the person silently repeat an expression or word
over and over again can facilitate attentional focusing as well as can
the more traditional directions to "listen to my voice." Next, in
everything the hypnotist says and does he transmits the message that
the patient will find it easier and more enjoyable to sit quietly and do
nothing. The patient can be brought to behavioral inertia through
advice to "sleep," to "relax," or, as we prefer, through direct suggestions of behavioral inertia ("you *could* move if you *wished* to . . . but it
would be *so* hard, *so* much of an effort . . . better to just rest . . .").
This fourth dimension embraces cognitive activities as well as overt
behavior, and the raised threshold for activity extends to include
independent thinking. Thinking can also be rated as to how evaluative and goal-directed or uncritical and concrete it is. Hypnotic procedures, implicitly at least, aim for the latter. The patient is instructed to
just go along with the therapist's words instead of assessing the logic
or reality status of them (Dimension 5). Finally, the hypnotist works to
establish a shift in the person's perceived sense of control. The hypnotist does this by the careful placement of his suggestions for a given
reaction just before it is to occur. If there is no other apparent cause
for the targeted reaction, this leads to an increase in the sense of
hypnotist-direction as opposed to self-direction (Dimension 6). The
use of arm lowering can serve to illustrate this: when extended for a
period, a person's arm will grow tired and a host of related reactions
will occur. The arm will feel hotter, it will waver, and there will be a
slight tendency for it to lower during exhalation. If the hypnotist
gives these suggestions just as or before they occur naturally, he can,
as it were, "take the credit" for them in the eyes of the subject (a fuller
treatment of this is given in chapter 4).

   Our perspective bears a number of points in common with a
number of recent analyses of hypnosis, especially those offered by
Jaynes (1976), Shor (1969), Spiegel and Spiegel (1978), and Suedfeld
(1980). Shor (1969) begins with a description of the ordinary operations of cognitive processes, which are characterized by the mobiliza-
tion of a well-structured frame of reference as a background to

cognitive activities. It is through this frame of reference "which supports, interprets, and gives meaning to all experience" (Shor, 1969, p. 236) that we maintain our usual contact with the world. Shor refers to this as the *generalized reality orientation*. It is through this orientation that we are able to exhibit an awareness of surroundings, the employment of intellectual skills and critical capacities, and the ability and inclination to act in a varied and independent manner. This generalized reality orientation can be contrasted with hypnosis which, he says, is a complex of two fundamental processes: orientation to a small range of preoccupations and "the relative fading of the generalized reality orientation into functional non-awareness" (p. 243) usually brought about by the elimination of competing sensory input and the reduction in behavioral striving. A very similar position has been presented by Spiegel and Spiegel (1978): "[Hypnosis] is characterized by an ability to sustain in response to a signal a state of attentive, receptive, intense focal concentration with diminished peripheral awareness . . . [and] the trance state is a form of intense focal concentration which maximizes involvement with one sensory percept at a time" (pp. 22, 23). Suedfeld (1980) in comparing the similarities of hypnosis to "sensory deprivation" notes that in both, "Attention to distracting stimuli is minimized [and] contact with the external world is maintained only through the therapist . . . [and] . . . as a consequence the subject's ability to concentrate on the therapeutic input is magnified" (p. 290).

What, though, does our account as well as these others say about hypnotic reactions in everyday life or the hypnosis of the stage entertainer? Is it not the case, as Estabrooks (1957) pointed out long ago, "given the account of hypnosis which stresses focal attention, quiet surroundings, [and] a relaxed and passive attitude, [that] the stage hypnotist breaks every condition" (p. 34) supposedly essential for the production of "trance"? Do the results of stage hypnosis or the many reports of "spontaneous" hypnosis call for a different analysis from the one offered in this book? We think not. It is possible, in all of these accounts, to resolve this apparent paradox if what is perhaps the one essential condition for hypnosis is met: a large distance between the main, relevant idea or suggestion and all competing ones. In stage hypnosis, or in conditions of great fear or excitement, "one strong preoccupation mentally towers over all others. . . . Hypnosis achieves the same relative effect at low dynamic intensities" (Shor, 1969, p. 235). In other words, the procedures of standard inductions undercut all other events so as to leave the suggested idea without effective competitors. It hardly needs saying that techniques which work at lower dynamic intensities are essential if the therapist is to escape the burden of creating "intense emotional excitement in association with one dominant event" (Shor, 1969) each and every time he wishes to use hypnosis.

Left out of our account thus far is the phenomenon of "posthypnotic suggestion." As the words indicate, this refers to the extension of the therapist's suggestion past the temporal boundaries of the hypnosis episode. It should be immediately apparent what the problem is here: by insisting that a certain configuration of central or cognitive changes must come into being (through formal induction or spontaneously) before hypnosis is possible, a specific and testable claim is made. To put it succinctly: no "trance," no hypnotic phenomena. There is no well-controlled experiment to settle the issue, but we have seen too many subjects and patients carry out posthypnotic requests on signal to accept this hypothesis. Such people do not seem to be behaving under conditions of low arousal or reduction in sensory gradients and, obviously, do not exhibit behavioral quiescence. We agree with Shor (1969) that "when the generalized reality-orientation fades, special orientations or special tasks can be made to persist beyond the bounds of awareness and/or remain nonconsciously directive of further activities, *even when the generalized reality-orientation is again mobilized*"(p. 245).

This still tells us very little about the inner workings of posthypnotic phenomena. What is conspicuously absent is a detailed account of how posthypnotic suggestions are established and function later on cue. From the rudimentary understanding that we have of these phenomena, they seem to be strongest and most durable when they operate out of awareness, and appear to be more impervious to detection and reversal. Western workers (with the exception of the psychoanalysts) have largely neglected the role of awareness in behavioral control. The Russians (for example, Platonov, 1959) have done a great deal of work on this very question. Their evidence (especially with interoceptive conditioning preparations where the CS and UCS are delivered to the viscera) has led them to assert the fundamental importance of awareness in the modifiability of behavior. When patients are unable to recall the origins of the impulse to react in a particular way to a certain cue, they add their own "explanations"— usually in a most convinced and convincing way—and continue to act in accordance with the instructions unless they become aware of the origins. These are clinical impressions shared by many practitioners; all the same it must be conceded that our knowledge about the mechanisms of posthypnotic suggestions is very sketchy.

To this point, we have not touched upon the matter of "rapport" in hypnosis. Some writers make this the central issue (Haley, 1963; Meares, 1960) and the conventional clinical wisdom is that rapport between therapist and patient is the *sine qua non* of hypnosis. The justification for insisting on the need for good rapport is that there can be no success with hypnotic induction procedures without it. Although the term *good rapport* has still to be defined in a clear and satisfactory manner, it is difficult to resist the idea that it deserves the importance accorded to it in traditional clinical hypnosis texts. Despite the intuitive appeal of this notion, there is virtually no evidence for it. Accomplished stage hypnotists can elicit genuine hypnotic phenomena within a minute or two after meeting their subjects for the first time. Admittedly, stage hypnotists select only the most hypnotizable. Estabrook (1957), in an analysis of their brief but effective screening procedures, estimates that they work with only the most hypnotizable 20 percent of the population. Perhaps good rapport, whatever it is, counts most for the less hypnotizable. This assertion, however, although less sweeping than the usual ones made about rapport, runs into difficulties as well. In experimental psychology laboratories, researchers typically give no more than a very concise briefing to their subjects before they embark on the standard induction procedures. The uniformity of results from many such experiments testifies indirectly to the indifference of these results to conditions of "rapport." The procedures employed and the assessment of hypnotizability, on the other hand, are crucial. Orne reviewed the literature as well as his own experiences and had no hesitation in coming to the conclusion that "the induction of hypnosis does not require an intense interpersonal relationship nor even an intense wish on the part of the subject to be hypnotized" (Orne, 1980). This is a position which we wholly support.

Our views on the issue of rapport may be summarized as follows: first, the most effective use of hypnosis requires a more specific understanding of the relevant cognitive processes mediating these effects than is given by the term *trance*. Second, hypnosis is for the most part a potentiator of or an adjunct to other procedures. It is not, by itself, a treatment. The use of hypnosis, then, cannot be considered apart from the wider therapeutic context. One important component of this is the relationship between the therapist and the patient. Nowadays, behavioral therapists are attuned to the importance of the therapeutic relationship (DeVoge & Beck, 1976) and have provided evidence that an incompatibility of outlook or negative feelings between therapist and patient raises the probability of noncompliance with the therapeutic contract and premature defection from therapy, among other problems. All of this leads us to the obvious conclusion that good rapport, or as we prefer to call it, a good relationship, will facilitate the effective use of hypnosis—as indeed it will any other clinical technique.

Summary

In our presentation of hypnosis we have attempted to stand aside from the long-standing quarrels and theoretical debates that have marked the history of hypnosis. From an empirical examination, hypnosis has been revealed to be a state or condition marked by low arousal, reductions in patterned input, focal attention, and lowered awareness of peripheral events. These input or sensory changes are accompanied by the inhibition of self-initiated behavioral and cognitive programs and a corresponding decrease in critical thinking, together with a reduction in goal-oriented striving. Under these conditions, the alterations in psychophysiological responding, i.e., hypnotic phenomena, can be observed when suggestions are given in the correct manner.

Hypnotic responding can be elicited or produced in one of three ways. The best known of these is the formal hypnotic induction. Another is "spontaneously" through internal impetus (for example, daydreaming, intense absorption with a particular concern), or external pressures (great excitement and/or sustained focus upon one aspect of the environment). The third way is through self-induced procedures (self-hypnosis).

We have argued that the same cognitive processes are involved in all three. Hypnosis cannot therefore be identified solely with the formal induction procedures and considered a special phenomenon, unique and set apart from all other areas of psychological study. To the contrary, the continuity of suggestibility and hypnosis or hypnotizability seems clear. There is no absolute dividing line between them. The value of formal induction procedures lies, first, in making these alterations in functioning available when desired; second, in allowing them to be sustained as long as is needed; and third, in making them suit the purposes of the therapeutic team (practitioner and patient).

Before we close this chapter we should note that the formal induction of hypnosis depends on more than the use of a certain set of procedures in the assurance that the hoped-for changes will be brought into being. There are marked differences in the extent to which different people—or the same people at different times—will respond to hypnotic inductions. These individual differences will form the basis of the discussion of hypnosis and assessment which will be taken up in the following chapter. The model of hypnosis that we have presented does not say in quantitative terms exactly how much change must occur on these six dimensions—an important question for research investigation—but it does help to identify the ways in which "good" and "poor" subjects might differ.

3

Hypnosis: Assessment and Modification

Contradiction is not a sign of falsity, nor absence of contradiction a sign of truth.

—Blaise Pascal, *Pascal's Pensées*

"Can this patient be hypnotized?" This is the question which must be asked, and one for which an answer must be obtained as soon as the practitioner envisages a role for hypnosis as an adjunct to therapy. It might strike the reader as strange that we should take the trouble to state what, for some, is after all only the obvious: some individuals can be hypnotized and others not and the practitioner must be able to tell the former from the latter. But had this question been put to the early pioneers of hypnosis, it would have occasioned only surprise for a reaction. These men (Mesmer, de Puységur, and their followers) sought to explain the essence of hypnosis in the powers of the operator. If hypnosis were to be proven genuine with one person, then it stood to reason that it would be so with all. They had no doubts on either count and they gave no attention to the possibility of individual differences in hypnotizability. No doubt they were helped to this outlook by the self-selection of those individuals who presented themselves for mesmerism (Bowers, 1977). Such people would hold the highest hopes and expectancies for success. These could play a vital part in the impact of mesmeric treatments. Then, too, these men were advocates and evangelists of hypnosis—conditions not exactly favorable to disinterested analysis. Whatever the reasons, Mesmer and the others did not record any failures to hypnotize, and their true successors, the stage hypnotists, also claim a 100 percent success record. If we add to this the belief that has wide currency in some clinical circles that there are no insusceptible patients but only resistant or nonresistant ones, then altogether it might seem that with the right preparation and the correct techniques a hypnotic outcome is a foregone conclusion. The reader who examines our perspective of hypnosis (see below) may believe that we, too, subscribe to this conviction. For in this formulation or perspective we lay emphasis upon the optimal environmental conditions and the central or underlying changes correlated with these conditions. We did not enter individual differences in "trance" capacity into our formulation. It is now time to broaden this perspective so as to include the issue of hypnotic susceptibility.

The Reliability of Hypnotic Techniques

Are hypnotic techniques, when correctly used, universally effective? The short answer is: "no." When conventional hypnotic procedures are applied in the standard way, some individuals will respond and others will not. This *seeming* unreliability was one of the factors that caused Freud to turn from hypnosis to free association in the uncovering processes of psychoanalysis (another was the strong and unexpected sexual attraction that one young woman blurted out to Freud at the conclusion of one hypnosis episode). The "unreliability" of hypnotic reactions subsequently was perhaps one of the reasons for surgeons to give up on the use of hypnosis when chemical agents for anesthetizing became available. Today the criticism of unreliability can still be heard in orthodox medical, psychological, and dental circles. There is no evading this charge, and those stage hypnotists and clinicians who argue to the contrary are wrong: not all individuals react to the same degree, and the case for the existence of really substantial individual differences in hypnotizability is proven. Nevertheless, it is possible to make too much of these facts. It should be recognized that there are no other medical or behavioral techniques that are universally effective. Token economies do not help all hospitalized schizophrenics (Ayllon & Azrin, 1968), and some patients do not respond to major tranquilizers (Neale & Oltmans, 1980).

There are reports of people getting worse as the direct result of behavior treatments for phobic anxiety (Marshall, Gauthier, & Gordon, 1979) and the popular cognitive therapies for depression work with some, but not all, depressives (Beck, Rush, Shaw, & Emery, 1979). These are but a few examples of the many we could have chosen. The point we are trying to make is this: the claim that hypnosis (or any other technique) is a tool of unreliable effect and thus of no value can be upheld only by evidence that this variability is capricious and unpredictable. *In fact this is not the case.* First, the differences between individuals in hypnotizability can be measured and are reliable. Moreover, these differences are sustained over long periods of time. Second, evidence is now accumulating which favors the proposition that it is possible to modify—and specifically to increase—an individual's level of hypnotic reactivity. To return to the question with which we opened this chapter—"Can this patient be hypnotized?"—the answer must be: "perhaps." And in answer to the question "Why does one want to know?," at least two replies can be given. First, the measurement is of the person's potential to react to suggestions given in hypnosis, and second, there is evidence that levels of hypnotizability are positively and significantly correlated to treatment outcome whether or not hypnosis is actually used in therapy (Evans, 1982, personal communication). In promoting the value of assessment we are also mindful of the risks that may come with the patient's failure to "pass" a given item. To avoid the possibility of generalized and negative expectations arising out of such experiences, the therapist must take the appropriate steps to put the patient at ease about such matters (see chapter 4). The practitioner can proceed to a more determinate reaction only after the necessary assessment procedures have been completed. In the first section of this chapter, we will review the facts and methods of assessment in hypnosis. The second section will be devoted to the contentious issue of the modification of hypnotizability.

Concerning the Measurement of Hypnosis

The first task in any assessment procedure is to decide what to measure. Through the years the behaviors which have been taken to constitute the domain of hypnosis have changed. In Mesmer's time, hypnosis was defined as a procedure that invariably produced a convulsion. Conceptually, the assessment task was a simple one: the measurement of the duration and/or intensity of the "crisis" or convulsion (in practice there was little in the way of formal assessment). When the prevailing view of hypnosis changed from magnetism to somnambulism, the index of hypnosis was sleep walking and amnesia; convulsions were no more to be seen. With successive changes in the theory of hypnosis have come expectations that certain behaviors and not others will appear. Once transmitted to the subjects and patients, these expectancies are routinely transformed into *the* hypnotic behaviors. From this a conclusion that seems warranted is that there are no hypnotic behaviors as such and that hypnosis is indeed a condition of "heightened suggestibility." The suggestions can be delivered directly or, as in the examples just cited, indirectly and tacitly. It therefore makes little sense to set up a behavior of a particular topography as unique and carrying the stamp of "hypnotic phenomenon."

The answer to the assessment problem in hypnosis has been solved, as it were, through the selection of those suggestions and related responses which contemporary researchers agree make up an adequate subset of the most widely studied hypnotic behaviors (these include body sway, arm levitation, and perceptual distortions). These are presented one at a time and, very simply, those who "pass" more of the items are considered to be more "susceptible" than those who pass fewer. Not all of the items are of the same level of difficulty. It is typical for the more difficult items to be presented later and the easier ones first. If a number of such suggestions are grouped together and presented in the same manner and order to a large number of randomly selected subjects, a small percentage will respond to all of the items, even the most difficult, and a small number will not respond to any, regardless of how easy. Most of the people tested in this way will demonstrate a moderate level of hypnotizability, i.e., they will pass some but not all of the items.

The logic behind these scales (the most widely used of which will be discussed below) breaks with the earlier approach in which hypnosis was said to be a number of discrete and different states—hypnoses if you will. It is assumed that these scales are tapping a continuous ability factor the extent of which varies from one person to the next.

Distribution of Hypnotizability

What is the distribution of hypnotizability in the general population? The results from a large number of early studies were reviewed and summarized by Hilgard and his co-workers (Hilgard, Weitzenhoffer,

Landes, & Moore, 1961). Of the 19,534 subjects assessed in these studies, the following distribution was obtained:

1. Unhypnotizable—9 percent
2. Mildly hypnotizable, "drowsy"—29 percent
3. Moderately hypnotizable, "hypotaxic"—36 percent
4. Deeply hypnotizable, "somnambulistic"—26 percent

These data were gathered from a large number of studies carried out under a variety of conditions and with different induction procedures. Therefore they cannot be considered definitive and must be treated with some caution. The data do give some idea of the interindividual differences in hypnotizability and they do show a respectable amount of agreement with modern studies (Bowers, 1977). With these results before us, we can return again to the opening question and give a more definite answer. "Can this patient be hypnotized?" The best answer is: very probably, and the likelihood is that 91 percent of subjects are hypnotizable to some degree.

Can we really say this with such confidence? We can indeed, but only if we have evidence for the stability of hypnotizability. Otherwise the "deep" subject of category 4 above, as measured on Monday, could turn out to be one of the unhypnotizable when next encountered on Tuesday. This state of affairs would still allow us to make statistical generalizations (at any one time nine out of ten individuals will give evidence of at least mild hypnotizability). Generalizations of this sort might be of some theoretical interest but have no clinical utility. The clinical practitioner wishes to make predictions about a certain patient, not a whole population at an instant in time.

Hypnotic Stability

How, then, has stability been measured and demonstrated? There are two ways in which this can be carried out. The first way is for a particular test to be administered and then repeated, either at a short or a longer interval of time after the initial test. When the two measurement occasions are close together, the correlation is known as a reliability coefficient. Low correlations mean that either (1) the measurement device is a poor one, or (2) the thing being measured changes from day to day. From a low correlation we cannot be sure which is correct. Fortunately the results (for example, Hilgard, 1965) have been very impressive and clear cut. Correlation coefficients in the vicinity of .90 have been reported between the results of the two test occasions. This indicates that hypnosis shows short-term stability.

Long-term stability was investigated by Morgan, Johnson, and Hilgard (1974). They tested 85 students and retested them ten years later. What is more, Morgan et al. used a different measurement scale in a parallel form of the Stanford Scale and a different person to administer the second test. Despite these differences and the great lapse of time, the correlation between the two occasions was .60: "the hypnotic susceptibility score, for most Ss, did not change more than a point or two in spite of different [operators] and a different testing situation" (Morgan et al., 1974, p. 251). An interesting sidelight of this study was that in the midst of this impressive stability some changes *were* observed. "Motor challenge items" ("you'll be unable to move your arm") showed improvement over the intervening years, while cognitive items (amnesia and hallucination) declined somewhat. The changes in opposite directions balanced out, leaving the overall scores quite similar from first to second measurement occasions.

One inference that can be drawn from these changes is that the domain of hypnosis contains distinct subareas. Hilgard (1965) carried out a factor analysis of the Stanford Hypnotic Susceptibility Scale: Form A (SHSS:A) (Weitzenhoffer & Hilgard, 1959) to investigate this point. He reported that three (unrotated) factors accounted for about 70 percent of the total variance. These were called: (1) "challenge" items, which are thought to involve loss of voluntary control over certain behaviors (for example, inability to raise the arm)—53 percent of the variance; (2) the "direct suggestion motor" items (for example, hand lowering)—10 percent of the variance; and (3) the "cognitive items" (for example, hallucination and posthypnotic suggestion)—6 percent of the variance. Since the Stanford Hypnotic Susceptibility Scale: Form B (SHSS:B) (Weitzenhoffer & Hilgard, 1959) and the Harvard Group Scale of Hypnotic Susceptibility (HGSHS) (Shor & Orne, 1962) are very closely related, and the intercorrelations between them are very high, the factorial structure of these tests must bear a close resemblance to that reported by Hilgard (1965) for the SHSS:A.

There are two points about these facts which invite comment. First, there is the suggestion of different hypnotic phenomena and processes and, second, the possible clinical significance if such differences can be proven. We cannot report any data that settle these questions. From our clinical experience, however, we hold the view that hypnosis is a unitary phenomenon, i.e., a collection of measurable changes which are perceived as a unitary experience by the subject and are manifested in a number of dimensions or channels. (Hypnosis, then, is not to be identified with any one of these changes on any *one* of these dimensions any more than, say, one sign or symptom of a psychiatric syndrome is to be called *the* disorder.)

Measurement Concerns

Another and more serious clinical concern is the psychological effect of the choice we make. Certain items may be more appropriate by the criterion of efficiency but on other grounds one "appropriate" item may be preferable to another. As an example, consider the items on the Stanford and Harvard scales which impose motor or cognitive dysfunctions ("you will not be able to: raise your arm; say your name; nod your head; recall the tasks on the test"). If the suggestions are effective they can put the person at risk of feelings of helplessness and anxiety. We have seen this happen, and if there is any doubt that the person can tolerate these experiences, such "disability" items are to be avoided. This injunction holds especially for patients, like agoraphobics, who are prone to sudden panic attacks.

To sum up the main points of our discussion, the effects of hypnotic induction procedures are known to be variable from person to person. Some uncertainty of effect is a problem with all clinical procedures and necessitates the development of measurement strategies that give the clinician predictive power: who will and who probably will not respond to this standard procedure? If anything, we are further ahead in the rigorous assessment of hypnotizability than of other psychological and medical techniques. The existence of widely used and proven assessment devices changes "unreliability" to a variability that can be predicted.

Measurement and Therapeutic Outcome

Before we examine the specific tests and scales of hypnotizability, the reader might wonder about the need for hypnosis assessment. Is it necessary? Does it serve any purposes? The answers, without hesitation, are "yes" to both questions. For a start, to those who adopt the model of the scientist-practitioner (Kanfer & Phillips, 1970), there is no in-principle distinction to be drawn between scientific

treatment. In other words, phobic patients may spontaneously exhibit the same kind of mental functioning that is involved in responding to hypnotic induction procedures, and Frankel suggests that the capacity for spontaneous trance-like occurrences may be related to the origin of phobic symptoms.

Spiegel (1974) has also drawn attention to the clinical significance of hypnotizability. It is the Spiegels' claim that the Hypnotic Induction Profile (Spiegel & Spiegel, 1978) may aid in the identification of persons with relatively severe psychopathology (Stern, Spiegel, & Nee, 1978). If true, this would suggest that there are common features between hypnotizability and certain psychopathological disorders, a point that Spiegel (1974) has recognized when discussing the highly hypnotizable patient (the Grade 5 Syndrome). Spiegel's views are in line with those of Frankel (1974), and point to the highly hypnotizable patient who has a propensity for phobic symptoms, being more responsive to suggestive influences arising from his immediate environment, and thus is at a greater risk of developing severe psychopathology than a patient with low hypnotic susceptibility. The findings of these two workers suggest, therefore, that an individual's hypnotic capacity *may* be related to his propensity to develop certain clinical disorders (for example, see again, Foenander et al., 1980).

The Measurement of Hypnotizability

The best known and most commonly employed tests arc the Stanford Hypnotic Susceptibility Scales, Forms A and B (SHSS:A and SHSS:B) (Weitzenhoffer & Hilgard, 1959). These were developed at Stanford University. The tests are to be administered to one individual at a time. The tests contain 12 items and each is scored on a pass/fail basis: 1 point for each "pass"; 0 for each "fail." All items are weighted equally but they are not of equal difficulty. The tasks are:

1. *Postural sway.* The suggestion is given when the subject's eyes are closed: he will fall forward (or backward). A pass: compliance with the suggestion.
2. *Eye closure.* The suggestion, in this case, is given with the eyes open: his eyes are very heavy and he will be unable to keep them open. A pass: compliance.
3. *Hand lowering.* The subject is given a suggestion when he has one arm extended outward and parallel to the ground:

his arm is growing heavier and heavier. A pass: if the hand falls at least six inches by the end of ten seconds.

4. *Arm immobilization.* The suggestion: his arm is so heavy that he will be unable to lift it. Then he is asked to try this. A pass: failure to lift the arm by more than one inch in ten seconds.

5. *Finger lock.* The suggestion, given with fingers interlocked: he will be unable to separate the fingers of one hand from the other on request to do so. A pass: failure to separate the fingers or to separate them only slightly at the end of ten seconds.

6. *Arm rigidity.* This suggestion is given with the arm extended: the subject is asked to make his arm as rigid as possible and told that he cannot bend it. A pass: failure to bend the arm more than two inches in ten seconds.

7. *Moving hands together.* The suggestion: the subject is asked to extend his arms, separate them by about 12 inches with palms facing inward. A magnetic force pulling the hands together is then suggested. A pass: movement of the hands to within six or fewer inches apart in ten seconds.

8. *Verbal inhibition.* The suggestion: the subject is told that he will be unable to say his name aloud. A pass: failure to enunciate the name upon request in ten seconds.

9. *Fly hallucination.* The suggestion: a fly is buzzing about his face and body. A pass: acknowledgment of the "fly's" presence (such as by twitching of the face, or waving the hallucinated fly away).

10. *Eye catalepsy.* The suggestion, given when the subject's eyes are shut: his eyes have been glued shut and he will be unable to open them when asked to do so. A pass: failure to open the eyes after ten seconds.

11. *Posthypnotic suggestion.* The suggestion: when the hypnosis test is completed, he will want to change chairs upon a given signal from the operator. A pass: behavioral response to the suggestion.

12. *Hypnotic amnesia.* The suggestion: the subject will be unable to recall the items of the test. A pass: recall of three or fewer tasks.

Although there are no sharp boundary markers dividing the highly hypnotizable from those who are in the moderate or low range, it is traditional to identify those who pass eight or more items as highly hypnotizable. Those who pass four or fewer items are considered to be low hypnotizable subjects and, by exclusion, the ones in the middle are moderately hypnotizable. As we have pointed out above and stress in chapter 4, the individual score on a particular test at any given time may be an underreflection of a subject's hypnotic skills. Thus, to give an example, the anxious or highly distractable patient may, under better circumstances, show a considerable improvement when measured on two or more occasions by one of the standard assessment procedures. Note that it is the *total* number of items passed, and not which particular types of items, which determines the assessment of hypnotizability. In addition to the SHSS:A and B there is another Stanford Scale, the SHSS:C (Weitzenhoffer & Hilgard, 1962). This is a 12-item individually administered scale which is loaded with more of the "difficult" items than is the SHSS:A or B Forms (for example, a suggestion that the subject will be unable to smell a source of household ammonia held under his nose). The intercorrelations of these tests, especially of SHSS:A and B, which are essentially equivalent forms of the same test, are very high. That, along with their excellent psychometric properties, has led to them being used as the basis for other tests of hypnotizability.

Clinical Hypnotizability Scales

The Stanford Scales Forms A and B (Weitzenhoffer & Hilgard, 1959) and Form C (Weitzenhoffer & Hilgard, 1962) and the Harvard Group Scale of Hypnotic Susceptibility (HGSHS) (Shor & Orne, 1962) are considered by most practitioners to be too protracted for clinical purposes. For clinical usage, two shorter forms have been developed. The first of these (derived from the SHSS:A) is the Stanford Hypnotic Clinical Scale for Adults (SHCS: Adult). The value of this scale as a measurement device in the clinical setting arises from the following: It is short enough not to tire the patient (taking approximately 20 minutes to administer), can be used for those patients who have restricted physical mobility, and taps the processes most likely to be used in therapy, such as imagery and age regression (Morgan & Hilgard, 1975). The scale tests for five items of hypnotic responsiveness: moving hands together in response to suggestion, hypnotic dreams, age regression, posthypnotic suggestion, and amnesia. The items are scored on a 0–5 scale, and high susceptibility is indicated in patients who pass four or five items; medium susceptibility patients score on two or three items; and the patient who achieves a score of zero or one is considered to be a low susceptible subject. It has the further advantage of containing none of the "helplessness" items (as we have termed them).

Another clinical assessment scale is the Hypnotic Induction Profile (HIP) (Spiegel & Spiegel, 1978). This relatively rapid (ten minutes) measuring scale has the advantage that it can be integrated into the clinical diagnostic interview more easily than a more prolonged scale. The HIP arises from a consideration of hypnosis as being "a subtle perceptual alteration involving a capacity for attentive, responsive concentration which is inherent in the person" (Spiegel & Spiegel, 1978, p. 39). This measurement scale not only was devised to assess hypnotizability but is also claimed to test for the presence of severe psychopathology in the patient. The HIP involves two measurement scores. First, the profile score "which is a statement of the relationship between a person's potential for trance and his ability to experience and maintain it" (Spiegel & Spiegel, 1978, p. 41). It is a qualitative score and embodies the eye-roll sign, control differential (a posthypnotic measure of the difference in control between the person's "hynotized" and "non-hypnotized" arms), and arm levitation occurring in response to a signal. The second measurement is the induction score. This measures the patient's ability to maintain the trance experience. The five items which comprise the induction score, and which "rate the degree to which the subject can attentively focus" (Spiegel & Spiegel, 1978, p. 41) are: dissociation, signaled arm levitation, control differential, cut-off (termination of the "postceremonial trance response"), and float ("a postexperiential self-report measure of the amount of bouyancy that the subject remembers experiencing in the trance") (Spiegel & Spiegel, 1978, p. 35).

There is considerable controversy as to the efficacy of the HIP as an accurate measurement device of hypnotizability (the reader is referred to recent discussions on the issue; see Bowers, 1981; Frischholz, Spiegel, Tryon, & Fisher, 1981; Hilgard, 1981a, b; Orne, Hilgard, Spiegel, Spiegel, Crawford, Evans, Orne, & Frischholz, 1979). The most that can be said at the moment is that the validity of the scale is still in question.

The Modification of Hypnotizability: General Considerations

We began this chapter with the first question to be asked by a practitioner if he hopes to use hypnosis in his therapy program: "Can this patient be hypnotized?" This led us naturally to the issue of the measurement and assessment of hypnotizability. In our dealing with these issues, we came to a number of well-supported conclusions. Hypnosis can be measured reliably, and the scores obtained show great stability over time and repeated assessments. In reply to our own question, then, if you want to know whether the patient can be hypnotized, test him and find out. So, inevitably a second question arises once we have obtained an answer to the first: "If he cannot be hypnotized or if his score places him in the low hypnotizable range, can anything be done about it?" In other words, "is a person's hypnotizability modifiable?"

We believe that it is. Others would disagree and subscribe instead to London's (1967) view that "susceptibility is a very stable personality trait [and] extremely resistant to change" (p. 72). Which position is the correct one? At a quick glance the defenders of the modifiability hypothesis (for example, Diamond, 1977; Wallace, 1979) may seem to have an unanswerable case. There are many studies, most of recent origin, which report varying and often significant degrees of success in modifying hypnotizability. The methods used have been diverse and include sensory deprivation (Sanders & Reyher, 1969; also see Suedfeld, 1980), biofeedback procedures (Wickramasekera, 1973), and steps taken to instill an untroubled and favorable attitude toward the hypnotist and hypnosis (Tart, 1967).

Do these reports settle the matter? Has the plasticity of hypnotizability been clearly established? Wallace (1979) believes that they do and that it has. He writes. "Although at one time hypnotic susceptibility was believed to be a nonmodifiable or stable trait . . . no longer is it believed to be" (p. 20). We, too, are of the opinion that hypnotizability is modifiable (for the reasons outlined below), although it must be admitted that existing research findings give no more than equivocal support to the modifiability position. Critical commentaries claiming nonmodifiability have yet to be answered and overturned by supporters of this position. The authors of these commentaries have been at some pains to show that none of the studies in the modification literature is free of serious methodological problems (see below for a brief mention of these. For a fuller discussion the reader is directed to Perry, 1977; and Perry, Gelfand, & Marcovitch, 1979). Until the time when clear-cut evidence becomes available, the best that can be said for the modifiability position is that the case is not yet proven.

Practitioners who have had extensive experience with hypnosis in the clinic might wonder at this conclusion. After all, it is common to find that many patients improve in their hypnotic performance on the second occasion on which hypnotic induction is utilized. This improvement may be revealed in the greater ease and speed of entering hypnosis or the number of items "passed" on a standardized test. Such improvements, though readily demonstrated, have not brought about an end to the debate. One might imagine that they should. Is it not as simple as this: individual A receives a score of, say, 2 on the first administration of the SHSS:A and, say, 4 when tested again a week later? That surely is an improvement? Since clinicians and experimenters alike have observed such increases, it might be asked: what justification is there for continuing to deny what has been amply demonstrated?

The point at issue, though, is not the *existence* of data showing an increase in hypnosis scores; it is the interpretation of this improvement that the critics are questioning. Confront the fixed-trait theorists with these data and their reply would be to question the adequacy of the first score as a good index of hypnotizability. The distinction they are raising, and it is an important one, is that between hypnotic performance and hypnotizability. The former is a function of the latter but it is also influenced by factors extrinsic to the processes of hypnosis. An analogy could be drawn from the field of intelligence. A bright individual who is uncomfortable with the person administering the intelligence test or who is unsophisticated about test-taking and is uncertain of what is expected of him could score in the below-average range. If he were to be retested later in the week under more supportive conditions and given a clear explanation of why the test situation is arranged as it is, then he might register a big increase in this intelligence score. What conclusion could we draw from this change? It would be incorrect to deduce that our manipulation led to an increase in his intelligence. It would be permissible, and in this case more appropriate, to say that we had rearranged the conditions so as to remove some of the barriers to the person expressing his true level of ability.

To illustrate now the same interpretive problem in hypnosis research, consider the data linking increases in hypnotic performance to prior training in biofeedback (Wickramasekera, 1973) or the use of sensory deprivation (Sanders & Reyher, 1969). Sensory deprivation is known to have an inhibitory effect on goal-directed, reality-oriented thinking (Suedfeld, 1980; Zubek, 1969). We would predict on the basis of Dimension 5 that it should lead to a modification of hypnotizability—at least on that occasion (and for longer if the person acquired more proficiency in disengagement and subduing the processes of critical review). Relaxation, whether achieved through biofeedback or Jacobson's technique (see Appendix A), reduces physiological arousal or "noise" (Wickramasekera, 1973) and should also, therefore, increase hypnotizability (Dimensions 1 and 2). Findings of this sort are nicely consistent with the model of hypnosis that we have presented in these pages. They are also consistent with a "fixed-trait" model of hypnosis. The improvements would then be viewed as only apparent and due to initial subcapacity scores increasing to later "true" scores with the removal of one or more situational impediments.

To be powerfully convincing, improvements should be demonstrated after a sufficient number of pre-tests have been carried out to indicate that the subject's scores had achieved stability (cf. the notion of "plateau hypnotizability"; Shor, Orne, & O'Connell, 1962). Then we would be on safer grounds attributing further increase in hypnotic performance to the manipulations employed (meditation, relaxation, sensory deprivation, etc.) and going on from there to argue for the modification of hypnotizability. Even then, a certain amount of caution would be indicated. We would also need to be able to rule out mere (outer) compliance by subjects trying to "help" the experimenter. Subjects may correctly surmise the experimenter's hypothesis and give the behaviors they believe to be required of them (without undergoing the crucial affective changes). The possibility of such utterly spurious data contaminating the experiment is by no means rare, as any student of demand influences can attest (Orne, 1959, 1962).

Until such well-controlled studies are at hand, the best that we can do is to point to the many results in line with our hypothesis (see Diamond, 1977) while noting that there are not any which prove that hypnotizability is modifiable. Our reasons for continuing to hold with the modifiability hypothesis are conceptual as well as evidential (which, as we have stressed, is of an equivocal kind). In our model, hypnosis is a word that refers to a variety of central and peripheral modifications away from usual functioning (or, to state the case more cautiously, however many pathways into hypnosis there are, one of them is defined by the collection of changes on our six dimensions). Assuming that people can be taught how to increase the extent and duration of these changes, it would seem appropriate, then, to arrive at the conclusion that hypnotizability is modifiable. This assumption gets indirect, though impressive, support from many clinical and experimental studies showing that with proper training people can learn to modify levels of arousal (Borkovec

& Sides, 1979; Paul, 1969), control attentional systems through meditation (Benson, 1975; Carrington, 1978; Ornstein, 1977), and improve imagery skills (Strosahl & Ascough, 1981).

Of all of the changes involved in hypnosis, the one we see as most important is the ability to acquire and sustain a focused attention. The Spiegels (1978) say, and we agree, that hypnosis "is characterized by an ability to sustain in response to a signal a state of *attentive,* receptive, intense *focal concentration* with a diminished peripheral awareness" (p. 22, emphases added). Why do we say this? Well, quite simply, if the person is not able to keep free of intrusive thoughts, then the chances of "deep" or full hypnotic involvement are thereby reduced.

From this perspective the question which we have put twice in the last few pages, "Can hypnotizability be modified?," is better restated more specifically as "Can individuals learn to acquire attentional control (or, generally, learn the skills to make the requisite changes in the area of deficit)?" The data that bear on this question have been gathered by researchers studying the techniques of meditation aimed at teaching people to focus the attention and to keep it free of intrusive cognitions. We review the relevant studies in chapter 6. To summarize here, it has been shown that those who have had long-standing difficulties with attentional control are able to improve this deficiency and with it the freedom from intrusive (i.e., task-irrelevant) cognitions.

By way of reviewing the direction of our argument, we have said that hypnosis refers to a number of alterations in a range of cognitive and affective systems. Evidence (much of it gathered by those with no stake in the modifiability hypothesis or, for that matter, any interest whatsoever in hypnosis) suggests that the experimental subject or clinical patient can be helped toward the acquisition of considerable control of the activities of these systems. Therefore, we conclude in favor of the proposition that hypnotizability can be modified (again, a proposition that we acknowledge has yet to be proven).

A fact that we have left out of the discussion must now be faced: the stability of hypnotizability. Can we reconcile our position to the well-documented inter- and intrasubject reliability of hypnosis scores (reported in a number of excellent studies—see Bowers, 1977, for an admirably clear treatment of this literature)? In our view, yes. What we are saying is that if a person is *adequately* tested at time *A* and scores at or below level *X*, then unless he takes definite steps to improve his skills and the degree of control over, say, arousal or attention, then he should do no better when reassessed at time *B*. Therefore, we see no logical incompatibility between the facts of stability and the possibility of modifiability. To put it somewhat differently, the stability of *any* behavior or response pattern is a logically separate matter from its modifiability. There are many regularities or stabilities in our behavior which are *habitual*. Others are anchored in immutable predispositions. Which best describes hypnosis has yet to be decided. The role of individual differences can also be admitted into this picture. It is entirely conceivable that some people may profit more quickly from and require less "remedial" training than others to get to a certain level of control. (In pointing out the use of techniques like meditation and relaxation in the alteration of "susceptibility" we have not meant to imply that this is their only or main use. They are self-control techniques of proven value in their own right.) Differences of this sort may be traced to the kind of upbringing a person has had, his current environment, and/or his genetic makeup (Morgan, 1973; Rawlings, 1977).

All of the above comments apply to the dimensions of disengagement (1 to 5 in our model). What about Dimension 6, and the mechanisms which contribute to the "transfer of control"? In a sense, the skills associated with an increase in hypnotizability would, in this case, lie with the experimenter or clinician (or patient if it is self-hypnosis). His job is to gradually lead the patient or subject from the perception of the self-direction of behavior to that of "nonvoluntary" or "effortless" execution of the suggested changes ("I didn't lift my arm; it felt as though somehow it was lifted for me"). What follows is a frankly speculative version of how the processes of operant and classical conditioning may operate in a successful hypnotic induction to effect this transfer of control.

An Hypothesis about the Mechanisms of Dimension 6

The work we will consider here deals with those experiments in which direct attempts were made to bring hypnotic behavior under therapist control. We have given this a place in our perspective as the sixth dimension. The number 6 was used to indicate its place in the sequencing of the various steps of the hypnotic induction and not its relative importance—which can hardly be overstated. Once a position sufficiently to the right (see Figure 2.1, chapter 2) on the first five dimensions has been achieved, we can say that the person has disengaged from his normal hold upon the environment (and vice versa) and is ready to enter upon the second and final phase of hypnosis, the transfer of control to the therapist. To repeat, what we are talking about here is the individual's feelings about the control of behavior. When we act or think in a given way in a particular context, past learning and current contingencies of reinforcement play a large part in what we "choose" to do. This is the reality of psychological control. Coexisting with this is the individual's deep and ineradicable sense of being the author of his own behavior. He sees his thoughts and actions as devised by him (to maximize reward and minimize punishment). This is reversed in hypnosis, where the individual comes to feel that his experience and behavior come to him *via* the suggestions of the hypnotist. Now it is clear that the situation at the start of hypnosis is one in which the words of the hypnotist do not have the desired effect (at least not immediately). How, then, do they come to acquire this control?

Two methods have been studied as a means of establishing control by stimuli that would otherwise be ineffective (one example of which is the hypnotist's voice giving suggestions prematurely or in the wrong way). The two varieties are operant and classical conditioning. Operant conditioning can be effected by the use of reinforcement to strengthen behavior and the stimuli antecedent to that behavior over which we wish to acquire control. The basic principles of operant conditioning are easily stated but difficult to apply and require the practitioner to be sensitive to the need for *immediate* reinforcements to successive approximations of the desired behavior (Rachlin, 1970). Put into nontechnical language, the practitioner must not wait for the appearance of the desired behavior in its final form before dispensing the reinforcer. Faster and more effective results are obtained if reinforcers are first given when any behavior even remotely resembling the hoped-for end-product is observed. Then reinforcement is withheld until behavior somewhat closer still in appearance to the final product is exhibited, and so on until this "shaping" process is successfully completed. In hypnosis, if arm levitation is the target behavior, the therapist's reinforcement ("yes, good, that's right, it's starting to come up . . .") has to be tailored to the individual's reactions *as they occur* and not according to some standard timetable. When used in this way, large and durable increases in hypnotizability have been reported (Sachs & Anderson, 1967). Operant, or feedback, techniques operate on behavior *once it has occurred,* even if only in minimal form. What can the practitioner do "to get this behavior out into the open" in the first place so that reinforcement procedures can then act to strengthen them further still?

The techniques for establishing stimuli as effective *elicitors* of behavior (and cognitions) has been the chief interest of those who study classical conditioning. This work began with the experiments of Ivan Pavlov (1927). He was interested in the very same question which we are considering here under Dimension 6: the development of stimulus control. Pavlov began with an ineffective stimulus which he wanted to render effective. In the most famous experiment, Pavlov trained dogs to salivate to a neutral stimulus, a pure tone of 1000 Hz. He accomplished this by carrying out a number of tone-food pairing trials. The end result was that the dogs salivated to the tone, which preceded the food by a few seconds (as well as when the food was actually given to them).

First, then, there must be close temporal contiguity between the first presented (and initially ineffective) stimulus (CS) and the second stimulus, which naturally causes the desired responses (UCS). Second, the quieter the environment and the more attentive the subject, the faster the rate of classical conditioning. Recently, a third and crucial condition has been revealed. The target stimulus (Pavlov's tone or the hypnotist's words) must not be accompanied by a better predictor of the UCS (food in Pavlov's study). Suppose instead of beginning training with the tone–food pairings we had begun with another CS, a light. This would have established the light as a good conditioned stimulus for salivation. Had we *then* presented light plus tone and followed it with food, the tone would not have acquired any conditioned strength. We could say that the light "blocked" (Kamin, 1969) the transfer of control to the tone. Applying these findings to hypnosis, the therapist would want to present his stimulus (for example, the suggestions for arm levitation) just before the occurrence of a stimulus that would naturally have the effect of causing this response, to some degree at least. Furthermore, he would wish to present this stimulus in the absence of any other "better explanation" for its elicitation. Clinicians attempt to accomplish this by giving suggestions for a response just prior to a bodily reaction that would ordinarily elicit this response. Thus, the astute clinician is careful to give suggestions for arm lightness as the person is breathing *in*—when our arm will rest a little more lightly upon the leg than, say, during exhalation. These carefully placed suggestions have the best chance of working if the person it *unaware* that when breathing in, the weight of the hand on the leg decreases. Experimental validation of this comes from studies in which hidden sources of air or light were employed just after suggestions that the subject (with eyes closed) would feel a breeze or begin to notice a growing lightness (Diamond, 1977). Although this was not done, the present account predicts that if the experimenter has used sources of stimulation known to the individual, this increase in hypnotizability would not have been obtained. Had this been the case, the condition of temporal contiguity of therapist's words (CS) and air or light source (UCS) would have been satisfied but the other criterion would not have been met—the person would "know why" he felt the breeze. Readers who are knowledgeable about conditioning will detect a cognitive flavor to our account of conditioning. The work of Kamin, especially, has helped to free classical conditioning from its earlier mechanistic stage. In the cognitive account, it is imagined that when a particular event—salivation, arm levitation—occurs, the individual begins a search for the best predictor or cause of this reaction. Once the *apparent* cause is found, the search is terminated. The message for the use of suggestions is: be careful to locate these just before the reactions are going to occur anyway, but be sure the patient has only your suggestion as the "cause." Last, the patient or subject acquires a kind of learning set so that earlier success makes later ones more likely. The discussion just presented leaves open the means by which transfer of control (Dimension 6) occurs in self-hypnosis where there is no outside agency. Unfortunately, self-hypnosis is just beginning to receive systematic examination in the laboratory. The most that we can offer at this stage is the speculation that the impact of verbal stimuli is not essentially different when self-delivered as compared to the effects of such stimuli originating in the environment (Meichenbaum, 1976; Salter, 1941). This is an issue which we shall take up again in the chapter on self-hypnosis (see chapter 7).

Summary

Our position is that hypnotizability can be modified, though this must remain an hypothesis until evidence of the sort we have discussed is brought forward. For those whose chief interest is in compiling evidence for use in the dispute between the fixed-entity theorists and their opponents, just to have proven demonstrations of modifiability in the record may be sufficient. The clinical practitioner will want to know more. He will naturally be interested to know that there are ways to lift a person's hypnotic performance from the low susceptible to the moderate-to-high range. That fact in itself, though, does not say why biofeedback, meditation, sensory deprivation, or operant procedures help to increase hypnotizability. Knowing that hypnotizability is modifiable does not give the clinician a rule that will tell him beforehand which techniques to try, on which people to use them, or how they are to be used.

The answers to these questions have already been suggested, but we shall ask still another to make the direction of our argument quite clear. Should not an explanation devised to organize the facts of the modification of hypnotizability be identical with one used to reveal the processes underlying standard induction procedures? We would answer this strongly in the affirmative. To get to the end-state of hypnosis, the individual must be helped to disengage from his usual, active, goal-oriented contact with his environment (Dimensions 1–5) so that the therapeutic suggestions delivered have the desired impact (Dimension 6). The atmosphere evoked via standard induction procedures is sufficient for most people to undergo these changes. Some people, the highly hypnotizable, are so adept at attentional focusing, giving up critical review of their performance or that of others, and all of the other skills of "trance," that they can achieve hypnosis quickly or under conditions that for most would be impossible. Stage hypnotists and experimental researchers are eager to work with those people who have these cognitive skills. Others, though, are much less able to show flexibility on one or more of these dimensions. They remain "refractory subjects" until their specific deficits are corrected. The person who is unable to sustain his attention for any length of time may benefit from pre-induction training in meditation (see chapter 6), while another with a different difficulty, such as holding onto critical and self-directed thinking, would require extra assistance to "supplement" the standard induction with sensory deprivation (Suedfeld, 1980) or, perhaps, pleasant music (Diamond, 1977) or some other technique to inhibit cognitions of the logical–realistic variety.

To conclude, the fractionation of the hypnotic trance into its components helps to make clear the workings of the standard procedures of induction—and the extraordinary ones used to increase hypnotizability. The same perspective can be applied to clarify the processes of termination, which is a retracing of the movements along these six dimensions: increasing the intensity and variety of stimulation, asking the person to think of what is going on all around him, and so on for all the remaining dimensions. The six dimensions of psychological activity that are implicated in hypnosis are not independent, and changes on one increase the probability of changes in the same direction (toward hypnosis or toward termination) on the others. Ultimately, it may be possible to identify additional dimensions or, as is more likely, the six we have identified may be collapsed into a smaller number. What can be said with authority is that hypnosis is not a single response or one single thing. The term *trance* should be used only if it is understood that it is an economical way of covering all of the changes that constitute "being hypnotized."

We shall close this chapter with a quotation from Mark Twain. He said, of women swearing: "They know the words but not the music." This chapter and the preceding one have been about the music; the next chapter, which sets out the techniques of hypnosis, gives the words. To know the score, as it were, these chapters must be taken together as a unit.

4

Hypnosis: Preparation, Procedures, and Problems

The tone of a voice impresses the wisest among us, and can change a speech into an impromptu poem.

—Blaise Pascal, *Pascal's Pensées*

In the course of preparing this chapter, the authors reviewed a large number of the major texts and articles on the procedures of hypnosis. It would be difficult to summarize in a chapter, or even a book for that matter, the enormous number of hypnosis techniques proposed by the experimental and clinical practitioners in these many sources. The newcomer to the field could be forgiven for feeling overwhelmed by the plethora of recommendations and the sheer number of techniques available. The novitiate hypnotist may even be confused by the apparent contradiction in the use of some techniques, such as the use of arm levitation or arm lowering as an induction procedure. Indeed, it is fair to say that a searching evaluation of hypnotic techniques points to the fact that, quite often, the manner in which a particular procedure is employed is simply a measure of the ingenuity of the practitioner. Behind this bewildering diversity though, the operation of a few simple principles can be discerned:

1. Suggestions are presented in such a way that the patient experiences a gradual transition from the active to the disengaged mode of behavior. In a small number of induction procedures (for example, the rapid technique described later in this chapter), this principle does not entirely hold true. It must be emphasized, however, that the great majority of techniques used in the clinical situation provide for a stepwise shift of behavioral responses toward hypnotic disengagement.

2. The particular approach employed should be one that is acceptable to that patient. Two contrasting approaches can be identified in the literature. They have been termed the "permissive," wherein the clinician's role is one of facilitator and guide, and "authoritarian," wherein the clinician functions as the strong director of proceedings and the patient takes a more passive role. It will be found that most patients prefer a permissive approach to hypnotic induction, for this allows the individual to proceed at his own pace, and in this way he is more readily able to associate his particular hypnotic experiences with the therapist's suggestions. An authoritarian approach is rarely called for in the clinical situation and we eschew its use, for it may be misinterpreted, especially by the patient who fears a loss of control in hypnosis. We have already stated that the fear of loss of control in hypnosis is one of the most prevailing of all misconceptions (see chapter 1). In those patients who still retain these views (in spite of prehypnosis discussions with the clinician), an authoritarian approach is quite likely to produce some measure of resistance to induction. However, for a dentist who uses hypnosis in a clinic, such authoritarian and dramatic approaches may suit his purposes perfectly adequately. The clinical practitioner, on the other hand, will almost certainly wish to help the person acquire skills of self-direction (i.e., self-hypnosis), and thus will wish to avoid a sharp discontinuity between home and office practice.

3. An important issue when deciding upon the use of a particular technique is the need to select one that is suitable in all respects for that person. This would seem to be stating the obvious, and yet in our experience, therapists *do* fall into the habit of using favored techniques in a somewhat rigid and stereotyped manner for all patients. This approach may be satisfactory for the majority of patients, but occasionally the situation will arise (for example, in a highly anxious individual) in which the patient fails to respond to a set approach.

Management of this problem involves the clinician phrasing his suggestions in such a way that the "change in direction" of his approach is a subtle and imperceptible one. For example, if after ten minutes or so of arm lightness and levitation suggestion, the patient gives no visible sign of responding in the desired direction, the therapist can change to suggestions of arm *heaviness:* "All right, now see if you notice feelings of heaviness in your right arm [if that was the one used in lightness suggestions]. Each time you breathe out, notice the sensations of heaviness growing in your right arm, as though pulling it down *through* the arm of the chair." In this way, the patient is less likely to interpret his lack of response as a failure experience. Indeed, it is axiomatic when inducing hypnosis to convey to the patient that whatever he experiences is an acceptable and anticipated response. Failure of a person to respond to some particular aspect of an induction procedure will pose no problems provided the therapist is alert to it and is prepared to deftly manipulate suggestions so that a "successful" outcome is achieved. As another example of this approach, consider a highly anxious patient, who characteristically has an excessively mobile attention. Such a person may experience difficulty in responding to suggestions of eye closure when fixating a distant (or even near) point. In this case, the therapist can defuse this potential failure situation as follows: "You seem to be having some difficulty in letting your eyes close . . . this may happen when you feel very tense . . . but don't be concerned . . . just close your eyes now . . . and in a little while, you will feel the tension getting less and less . . . you will feel more comfortable and relaxed with your eyes closed . . . more able to enjoy this relaxation experience." One final point to be noted here is that the therapist must never leave a failure situation unresolved by simply moving on to another technique. If, instead, the patient is reassured that his responses are anticipated and not unusual, little difficulty will be encountered in subsequent induction and deepening procedures.

4. We have discussed elsewhere (see chapter 7) that self-hypnosis is an essential part of the patient's therapeutic program. In this regard, it is helpful to use procedures in heterohypnosis which the individual can apply to the induction of self-hypnosis. The value of this approach is twofold: first, the patient acquires familiarity with the techniques through experiencing them as part of heterohypnosis, and, second, their effectiveness can be reinforced through suggestions given in hypnosis (i.e., as a posthypnotic response). Indeed, we adopt the rule of setting aside part of one session so that the patient can induce self-hypnosis in the presence of the therapist. In this way, the patient's difficulties and doubts can be discussed and resolved *before* he attempts self-hypnosis on his own.

These general principles relating to hypnotic induction point to the fact that the therapist must be constantly vigilant to cues provided by the patient. (When training our students in their first induction, we ask them to memorize whatever general routine they wish to employ but *not* to sit next to the subject paying attention only to the printed induction sheet—from which they would like to read, if we allowed them to do so.)

It is not our intention here to encompass the exhaustive list of induction techniques that are employed. Instead, we have chosen to discuss some of those which, in our experience of treating many thousands of patients, have proved to be of value in inducing hypnosis for a wide variety of conditions and which also satisfy the principles outlined above.

The First Induction

Before the therapist and patient set forth on a hypnobehavioral program of anxiety management, there must be a clear understanding of how the tactics of hypnosis are to be structured. In broad outline, the strategies of hypnotic induction and anxiety reduction are clear enough but there is no proof that either or both will not fail in application. Indeed, this become a likely possibility when the therapist does not take the time to search out and accommodate his techniques to the idiosyncratic reactions of his patients. In later chapters we will look at this in connection with the use of systematic desensitization, flooding, and cognitive treatments. Right now we have the prior issue of the patient's introduction to hypnosis to consider.

As a tactic we recommend a maximum of 20 minutes for the first induction attempt, regardless of whether this consists of a more formal assessment or the use of one of the induction procedures outlined in this chapter. The purposes served by a specific time-limited period are: first, that it gives predictability—the patient knows that this is an exploration and not an open-ended marathon; second, by deliberately calling it an exploration, the patient is implicitly instructed that it is his reactions that count and that modifications of technique will be made in light of these; and, third, the therapist is reminded of the importance of uncovering potential problems before they become serious obstructions to clinical progress.

As a preparation for induction, the therapist should first go through the list of common myths and misconceptions. The wisest course is to spend at least a minute or two on each of these (see chapter 1) whether or not the patient appears at ease about hypnosis. Rarely do people ask for clarification on points of uncertainty, and it is just as unusual for the patient to initiate a request for the therapist to correct worries based on misinformation about hypnosis. Accordingly, we operate by this rule: *assume that every patient has the full complement of anxieties and misconceptions and each of these must be dealt with before the first induction.*

Before starting the first induction, and all others for that matter, the therapist should deliver a special reminder to the patient that he should allow himself to go along with things and not to fall into the trap of trying for a good outcome:

> "Don't forget, hypnosis is first of all an experience. If you *try* to 'do well,' you will only do the very opposite. What I'm saying is that the only way to 'fail' is to try to succeed. This is something that most people find difficult to accept. Possibly that is because in our everyday lives, success is associated with striving and making the big effort. If we want to push a stalled car up an incline or if we wish to memorize all of the dates of the battle of World War I, *then* we would have to exert ourselves. Otherwise the car would remain in the middle of the intersection where it stalled and the dates would remain in the history book. In situations like these we *do* get a payoff if we put everything into the job. Hypnosis is different, though. It is an *experience*. In this regard, hypnosis is more like listening to your favorite music than it is to being in a swimming race or mowing the lawn or pushing an automobile off to the side of the road. For instance, if you were to come home at the end of a difficult day, sit down and relax, and put on your favorite record, you'd think it pretty strange if someone said,'Hey, are you sure that you are trying hard enough to enjoy that music; you'll never succeed unless you do.' To enjoy the music you'd only have to sit back and go along with it, experience it. And now if you haven't any more questions we will begin. We'll put aside the next 20 minutes or so for the first experiment with hypnosis. All that I'll be doing is mentioning some scenes for you to see in your mind's eye and giving some pleasant suggestions for feeling relaxed and at ease. Afterward we'll have a talk about what *your* experiences were like; no two people find it exactly alike. I'll ask you afterward to tell me what it was like for you. OK, let's begin now."

Afterward the therapist should be sure to elicit information from the patient in these major areas:

Recall

Can the patient recall unaided (a) the suggestions given by the therapist and (b) his own responses to them. The failure to recall is certainly not common, especially when no suggestions for amnesia are explicitly or tacitly delivered and when in addition the patient is given every encouragement to recall the material. But if it does occur, it can be a cause of great concern to the patient. Unless the therapist makes a probe here *first*, he may not discover the patient's inability to remember most of the content of the hypnotic session. As a consequence, these patients may subsequently refuse to try hypnosis or any other similar procedure. Those who do continue despite the recall problems can harbor unnecessary worries during and after each session. For these people it is imperative that the therapist first become aware of the amnesia and then do what is needed to combat it and/or put the patient at ease about it.

The failure to recall after hypnosis may be taken as a sign that the imagery and other cognitive activities elicited during hypnosis were excessively troubling and even overwhelming to the patient. One way to view this is, in Freudian terms, as an instance of the lifting of repression in hypnosis and its reinstatement afterward. Our preference is to admit the possibility of cognitive avoidance which, however, we see as governed by the same rules as behavioral avoidance. On the surface this may appear to be a restatement of the psychoanalytic position dressed up in behavioral terminology. We would argue, though, that there are important differences to be noted between the two. In the behavioral model, avoidance, whether cognitive or overt, is countered by exposure therapies (see chapter 9). The dynamic account of repression, on the other hand, turns the clinician's head away from exposure therapies and orients him toward an exploration of the putative psychodynamic mechanisms and the use of free association, dream analysis, and transference to influence them (see chapter 8 for our account of the non-Freudian unconscious).

Idiosyncratic Reactions

During hypnosis and with other cognitive techniques (for example, Weitzman, 1967), the patient's imaginal reactions may stray far from the ones suggested by the therapist. Lightness suggested in the right arm may be experienced in the left, and a beach scene may be constructed in place of the country hideaway sketched out by the therapist. Through careful questioning, the therapist should be able to glean the clues for these alterations. More often than not they will turn out to be as straightforward as a dislike of some aspect of the therapist's scene and a preference for the patient's own. Not a great deal needs to be said about the obvious value of using imagery and suggestions that are constructed expressly for a given patient. Some suggestions may trigger anxiety in the patient (for example, "just let go" in the patient who feels he has only a tenuous grip on his feelings, or the suggestion "you are getting heavier and heavier" given to the patient who is very sensitive about his obesity).

Even patients whose responses are entirely in line with those intended by the therapist may be unhappy and distressed after the first induction simply because hypnosis was not what they expected. They ask questions like: "But was I *really* hypnotized?" This reveals the belief that if some sort of a strange and dreamy stupor is absent from the experience, then the therapist must record a "failure to hypnotize." In fact, as we tell our patients, most people do *not* go through an altered state of consciousness in hypnosis. The reader might wonder why we have troubled to list this "problem" at all. It might well be asked if it matters for the subject to hold the conviction that he has been hypnotized. Our answer to that is "no"; the technique and the critical cognitive processes are doubtless the same in either case. Where there is such a sharp divergence between the patient's expectancy of hypnosis and his own experience with it, however, the doubts he retains may seriously undermine his willingness to continue with the therapeutic program. To dispel the person's doubts, the question that must be put by the therapist is: "Did you *lift* your arm (lower your arm, close your eyes, etc.) or did you have the feeling that, somehow, *it was being* lifted for you?" Where there appears to be any remaining doubt, have the person lift his arm right then and there: "Go ahead and raise your arm in the way it came up before. Does it feel the same or different?" The therapist's aim here is to make apparent to the person the difference in the experience of self-initiated versus suggested arm levitation (or whatever the target response used). To finish off this section, we have tried to underscore the value of the careful postinduction search for the patient's specific reactions to the techniques and suggestions associated with hypnosis. The general message which must be transmitted to the patient, whatever the specific concern, is "There is no wrong way of reacting to hypnosis; your experience is what it is and that is 'right.' "

Perseverative Reactions

The formal termination of hypnosis occurs with the count backward
from five to one, the request to "open your eyes and sit up" or some
such explicit and clearly delivered cue which signals the end of hypnosis. People seldom have difficulty in understanding what is expected of them and usually comply immediately by opening their
eyes, sitting up, or showing an outer conformity to the directions of
the hypnotist. Furthermore, in their return to clear awareness and
verbal fluency, the therapist may be satisfied that all of the effects of
the induction have been completely reversed. While these appearances may be a reliable gauge of reality, the therapist should, nonetheless, take care to ensure that the patient has in fact regained full
contact with his environment and that the reengagement process has
been completed. Behavioral compliance and verbal fluency by themselves do not tell the whole story. The therapist should be attuned to
the extent of any disturbances in the precision of motor coordination and skilled performance. We have encountered these so often
(we are not referring to a severe form of ataxia but to subtle
changes), that as a routine matter we leave a few minutes between
the termination of hypnosis and the patient's departure from the
clinic. When circumstances require the patients to leave immediately,
we caution them against driving an automobile or using machinery
for a few minutes at least. (The same problems and, thus, the same
advice can be tendered after the person emerges from other disengagement techniques which produce hypnotic-like effects such as
meditation, autogenic training, and sensory deprivation.) One way to
facilitate reengagement and shorten the disability period is to conclude the termination ceremony by asking the patient to make some
reasonably energetic movement just after the eyes have reopened:
"Take a big stretch now . . . yes, that's fine. Take another and while
you're doing that open and close your hands into fists. . . ."

Less common but still a problem is the prolongation of responses after the termination of hypnosis, such as heaviness of limbs,
paresthesias in the limbs, or "dreaminess." The patient should be
reassured that within ten minutes or so these should disappear. If
they do not, and the patient is troubled by them, then rehypnosis
with careful suggestions to reverse the effects may be indicated.

Very occasionally, either during or after hypnosis, sudden and
strong emotional responses ("abreactions") may emerge which have
no obvious relationship to the content of the therapist's activities.
These disinhibitory episodes are marked by rapid breathing, auto-

nomic hyperactivity, tearfulness, and, at times, disorientation. The therapist may be alarmed by these responses and move precipitously to terminate hypnosis and "wake up the patient." This is to be avoided, as is any effort to get the patient to explain what is happening right there and then. The first step to take is to give firm but quiet support and reassurance. This should be coupled with requests to breathe easily and slowly—control of the hyperventilation will invariably limit the abreaction. Once the spontaneous abreaction has been controlled, the therapist should aim to deepen hypnosis. A deepening approach that we have found valuable in this situation is to count slowly (and in time with the patient's breathing) from 1 to 20. The patient is told that as the therapist counts, "Each number will be like a stepping-stone, taking you into a deeper and deeper state of relaxation."

Induction Techniques

Arm Levitation

One of the most widely used techniques for inducing hypnosis is arm levitation. There are a number of reasons for its utility as an induction procedure. The first is that it can be used as a measure of hypnotic responsiveness (Hilgard, 1978/79). The importance of this from the therapist's standpoint is obvious, but the patient's attitude to becoming aware of his arm levitating is not to be lightly dismissed—especially in one who is critical and evaluative and who needs to be shown that "something unusual is happening to him." Notice, too, that it undercuts the patient's attempt to give a "logical" explanation for the occurrence of the suggested reaction. For example, if in eye closure or arm lowering techniques, either of these reactions occurs then the patient has two "explanations" to bring to bear: "my eyes are closing/my arm is descending because, after all, my eyes must close after a while" or "there is a limit to how long I can hold my arm upright against the pull of gravity" on the one hand, or "this is happening because he said it will" on the other. By contrast, arm levitation is not susceptible to these commonsense "explanations."

Another cogent reason for the use of this procedure relates to a person's imaginative ability. Since imaginative capacity is correlated with hypnotic susceptibility (Sutcliffe, Perry, & Sheehan, 1970), it can be anticipated that the greater majority of low hypnotizable patients will experience some difficulties in using techniques that call upon the use of imagery. Thus, in this group of individuals, arm levitation may prove to be the technique *par excellence*. Finally, this induction procedure is of special value to the excessively tense, anxious patient who has difficulty in focusing attention on imaginative induction processes.

The technique we employ is a variation of that described by Wolberg (1948):

> "I want you to place your left [or right] hand in a position so that the fingers are lightly touching your thigh . . . that's it, just touching. Feel the sensation of the cloth of your dress [trousers] against the fingertips as they lightly touch the material. Now, fix your gaze on some point on your hand . . . it may be a spot, or the knuckle of one of your fingers . . . or a ring . . . and as you concentrate on that spot . . . so you may notice certain sensations in the fingers and hand . . . perhaps tingling . . . or a feeling of restlessness in one or more fingers . . . or again, you may feel a sense of warmth coming through the hand . . . just enjoy whatever sensation you are experiencing . . . keep looking closely at the spot all the time."

A point to be noted here is that having the patient focus his attention on a sensation rather than on the hand itself reduces the likelihood of his "trying" to comply with the following therapist's suggestions of arm levitation:

> ". . . and as you do so, you will notice another interesting sensation . . . the hand is becoming much lighter . . . light and buoyant . . . just like a helium-filled balloon . . . that's good . . . you can no longer feel it touching your leg . . . it's floating . . . floating . . . getting lighter all the time . . . and each time you breathe in, it seems to get lighter . . . weightless . . . floating of its own accord."

It must be realized that what we are proposing here is a way in which suggestions may be sequenced, rather than a definitive approach. The therapist will, of course, use terms and phrases that are familiar to *him* and, furthermore, must be prepared to continually repeat these suggestions until the desired response (for example, arm levitation) is achieved. The timing of the suggestions is also of some importance. For example, suggestions of arm lightness are more likely to be effective if they coincide with the patient's inhalation. This potentiating effect of breathing may be further aided by the therapist synchronizing his breathing with that of the patient. In this way, the therapist delivers the suggestions (for example, lightness, deepness, or relaxation) with maximum effectiveness.

"As the arm floats gently upward . . . it feels even lighter and more buoyant . . . you are feeling so much more relaxed now . . . more and more relaxed all through your body . . . you feel a sense of ease all through you . . . and as the arm floats gently upward . . . you feel it being drawn closer . . . and closer to your face . . . as though there is a magnet acting on it . . . drawing your arm and hand to your face . . . and as it gets closer . . . your eyes feel *so* tired . . . the eyelids feel heavy and limp . . . feeling *so* heavy that they want to close."

At this point, the patient may spontaneously close his eyes. If this response does not occur, however, then the therapist should continue with further suggestions of eyelid closure:

". . . that's fine . . . you feel so much more relaxed now . . . your eyelids are so heavy . . . like lead shutters . . . wanting to close . . . heavier and heavier . . . and when the hand touches your face . . . your eyes will close . . . easily and completely . . . that's fine . . . you feel so relaxed and comfortable . . . feel that deep relaxation all through your body . . . it is so comfortable . . . to relax . . . and enjoy this experience . . . to feel as though you have no cares or worries now . . . just feel that sense of ease . . . all through you."

A response like arm levitation can be useful in promoting in the patient, and indicating to the therapist, the process and stage of disengagement. Such a response, however, if allowed to persist unduly within the hypnosis episode, may cause the patient consternation and even worry (for example, the patient may wonder, "Will I ever retrieve the normal sensation in my arm"?). If this occurs, then it will stimulate anxiety and critical review by the patient—processes which are at odds with the ones necessary for sustained and deepened disengagement. What we are emphasizing here is different from the standard and appropriate advice to take the necessary steps before the termination of hypnosis so as to reverse all of the induction (as opposed to therapeutic) suggestions given:

"And now . . . notice that as I count from one to five, how the
ordinary feeling of weight will return to the hand and arm . . .
so that it sinks gently downward onto your lap . . . and as it sinks
downward . . . you will experience an even deeper sense of relaxation . . . becoming deeper all the time. Ready . . . one . . .
two . . . three . . . four . . . five . . . that's fine . . . your hand is
now resting so comfortably on your lap . . . and you feel extremely relaxed . . . and at ease."

An Indirect Eye-Fixation Technique

This technique, first described by Adler and Secunda (1947), is a
useful alternative to the more conventional eye-fixation methods
which rely on the subject focusing on a near or distant focal point.
Here, the patient is asked to rest his elbow comfortably on the arm
of the chair, hold his hand about 18 inches from his face, and form
his thumb and forefinger into the shape of a letter "u" placed on its
side. We have discussed elsewhere (see chapters 2 and 6) that one
necessary prerequisite for disengagement is the attainment of a focused attention. Indeed, the therapist's aim in all induction procedures is to utilize those which will lead to a progressive narrowing of
a person's attentional processes. For this reason, the patient should
be directed to separate his finger and thumb by no more than one
inch because of the obvious difficulties he may experience in focusing on a wider space, and this should be demonstrated by the therapist. The following suggestions are then given:

"As you fix your gaze on the *space* between the finger and
thumb, you will gradually become more and more relaxed . . .
so relaxed that the finger and thumb, too, will relax . . . and will
start to move toward each other . . . slowly at first . . . but they
will move closer and closer together . . . and as you feel this
happening . . . so your eyelids are becoming limp and heavy . . .
heavier . . . like lead shutters . . . they feel so heavy . . . heavy
and relaxed . . . they just feel as though they want to close. . . ."

Eye closure is frequently achieved at this point, especially in
those patients who are familiar with this technique. It will be noted,
too, that the therapist phrases his suggestions in such a way that
there is an imperceptible change in emphasis from anticipated responses to those which are actually occurring. If there is a delay in

eye closure, the therapist will continue with further suggestions of lid heaviness:

> "That's fine . . . continue to concentrate on that space . . . and as the finger and thumb get closer . . . so your eyelids are feeling *so* heavy . . . heavy and relaxed . . . as heavy as lead . . . wanting to close . . . as the finger and thumb come into contact . . . that's the signal for your eyes to close . . . fine . . . feel that deep relaxation all through you."

We have observed that the majority of patients readily respond to suggestions of movement of the digits toward each other. The success of this induction technique appears to stem from: (1) the patient experiencing a sense of surprise that his finger and thumb actually move together; (2) a narrowing of the focus of attention as the space between the digits narrows; and (3) the facilitation of eye closure arising from the implicit suggestions being conveyed by the movement of the thumb and finger toward each other. This technique is eminently suitable for the induction of hypnosis in most patients, especially for the novitiate hypnotist who feels unsure of his ability to produce eye closure with more conventional eye-fixation procedures.

This technique when used in the manner described above may not be advisable for patients who are very tense and worry about, or feel embarrassed by, hand tremor. In such cases the patient should be asked to rest his hand on the arm of the chair with the thumb and forefinger in the same "u" shape.

Imagery Techniques

It is curious, but nevertheless true, that many patients still present for hypnotic treatment anticipating that they are going to be hypnotized by means of a swinging pendulum or some such external device. This underscores the continuing influence of the stage hypnotist. A patient with such attitudes may, understandably, be apprehensive about the use of an eye-fixation technique because of what he interprets as its stage connotations. An alternative approach, and one that does away with eye fixation, is the use of imagery. These procedures are of particular value in patients who have a high imaginative sensibility.

Imaginal induction techniques may take two forms: (1) a de-

tailed scene as depicted by the therapist, or (2) one in which the
patient visualizes a scene of his own choice. In both instances, the
therapist should first ask the patient about *his* preferences regarding
a scene in which he could imagine himself being relaxed and peaceful. This may seem an obvious question to put, and yet it is one that
is frequently omitted. Failure to select a scene appropriate for that
patient may lead the therapist into portraying one with unpleasant
connotations for that person (some fair-skinned people, for example, dislike visualizing a beach scene because they immediately
associate it with having been sunburned in that situation).

> "I want you to sit [lie] back and close your eyes . . . that's it . . . feel
> comfortable . . . adjust your position if you wish . . . until you feel
> at ease . . . good, now I want you to imagine that you are lying
> back on a beautiful beach . . . it is very secluded and peaceful . . .
> the sun feels pleasantly warm . . . there is a warm, gentle breeze
> blowing over your body . . . enveloping you in a comfortable
> way . . . you feel the sand warm against your body . . . soothing
> you . . . relaxing you all over . . . you let the sand gently trickle
> through your fingers . . . it is all *so* peaceful . . . you can hear the
> surf gently breaking onto the beach . . . making you feel . . . even
> more relaxed . . . hear the surf coming in . . . and going out . . .
> you relax deeper all the time . . . you may even smell the sea
> air . . . and recall pleasant memories of times spent . . . relaxing
> in this way . . . it feels good."

Notice that in this scene, abstract and generalized expressions
are avoided in favor of concrete and detailed accounts of the stimulus situation. Suggestions like: "You will feel better and better"; or
"The further on we go, the happier and more at ease you will feel"
do not contain any reference to the "adequate stimuli" for the suggested reactions. Imagery techniques can be used to good effect only
when the practitioner understands the need to present the (symbolic) stimuli that *elicit* these reactions.

The phraseology used by the therapist should be patterned on
the preinduction discussion of what the patient likes to experience
and should be so presented that it induces feelings of relaxation and
calmness. The more hypnotizable subject is able to hallucinate
sounds and smells, and the use of olfactory cues (invoked by past
memories) is a most effective way of inducing and deepening hypnosis in these patients.

The second way in which imagery can be used is to have the

patient visualize his own scene. The therapist may portray the scene in general terms, and then allow the patient to imagine it in greater detail. Two points should be noted when using this particular procedure. First, the patient must be allowed sufficient time to incorporate his own imagery into the hallucinated scene, and, second, he should be instructed to indicate by ideomotor signaling (for example, finger raising) when he feels a deep sense of relaxation. Pauses of up to six seconds can be programmed between each phrase from the practitioner. (In general it is not a bad idea to use a slow and measured delivery in most inductions. If there is one fault that most inexperienced practitioners display in hypnosis—and desensitization—it is filling up all of the time with their words. This can transmit a sense of rush and tension. Moreover, the therapist's constant talk can seriously interfere with the development and elaboration of imagery by the patient.)

> "I want you to sit [lie] back and close your eyes . . . that's it . . . feel perfectly comfortable . . . adjust your position if you wish . . . until you feel at ease . . . that's good . . . now I want you to imagine a pleasant scene in the countryside . . . one that you associate with feelings of relaxation . . . as soon as you can picture that scene in your mind's eye, your right forefinger will lift . . . that's good . . . relax back and enjoy it . . . lose yourself into that scene . . . become part of it . . . let your mind drift along with the sounds and sights all around you . . . and all the time . . . you are becoming more and more relaxed . . . so very relaxed . . . don't be hurried . . . spend as long as you wish in that scene . . . and when you really feel very relaxed . . . your right forefinger will lift to indicate this to me."

It must be realized that this procedure may take a good deal longer than a scene depicted by the therapist, and its success is dependent on the patient being able to achieve relaxation *at his own pace*.

Rapid Induction

The thrust of all our remarks in this chapter is obviously to question the need for or the desirability of speed in the induction of hypnosis. There are occasions, however, when rapid-induction techniques are called for. Some patients, try as they might, find it impossible to step aside from a critical scrutiny of the proceedings and lose themselves in hypnosis. A rapid-induction approach can work to "rush them past" these obstacles. Patients in pain may find the careful pacing of the usual induction procedures too arduous to wade through, and fast-acting techniques may be indicated for these persons.

The simplest method for shortening the time for the onset of hypnosis is to suggest during one episode that the patient will be hypnotized more quickly the next time hypnosis is attempted: "The next time when I say the word 'X' you will find it easier, much easier, to pay attention to what I'm saying; hypnosis will be faster. . . . " When successful, the time needed for subsequent inductions can be reduced by half *if all other conditions are optimal* (i.e., assuming no reappearance of anxiety, misunderstandings about hypnosis, and so forth). When they are less than ideal, it may be unwise to count on this facilitation through cuing and suggestion. Furthermore, with the less hypnotizable patient, the therapist may not get far enough in the first induction to establish a cue word as a facilitator for later inductions. Under these conditions the therapist may wish to consider the use of a fast-acting technique.

The rapid-induction technique presented below has a number of advantages as well as some shortcomings. In its favor is its speed of action and its effectiveness with the great majority of people. In an unselected sample of more than 50 clinical and experimental subjects, the target response, arm levitation, was achieved by 90 percent. The average time for a levitation response of four inches or more was about two minutes. The technique is simple to present and easy to apply. Essentially, it involves no more than rapid breathing by the patient with suggestions of hand lightness being given at the same time by the therapist. It differs from the conventional and widely used arm levitation in two important ways. First, the therapist adopts a much more insistent and forceful style, and, second, there are specific requests which the patient is told to follow:

> "In just a moment we'll begin hypnosis. First though, I'd like to tell you what I'll be asking you to do once we get started. Once I ask you to close your eyes, I'll then ask you to breathe very deeply and very quickly [the therapist then demonstrates going through a complete inhale–exhale cycle every two seconds or faster]. That's all you'll have to do. If I want you to breathe faster or deeper I'll let you know. All right, let's begin.
> "Breathe in, out . . . in, out . . . faster, in, out . . . in, out . . . in, out. [The therapist continues for at least 10 seconds directly pac-

ing the rate, rhythm, and depth of breathing and then begins to give suggestions of lightness in the arm, tingling in the fingers, and a general feeling of floating and disorientation, all of which are produced by hyperventilation.] Each time you breathe in, your (dominant) hand is being *pulled* up [always said just as inhalation begins] . . . pulled up and back . . . pulled up. . . . [If the patient's rate or depth of breathing slackens *or becomes irregular,* the therapist should return to the pacing for another five seconds.] Notice the tingling in your fingers, your *whole body* feeling light, lightness in your arm and especially your hand as you breathe in . . . your hand is pulled up off the chair." [Once this begins the therapist can give directions to slow the rate of breathing and at the same time to lighten the depth, very gradually, blending the initially dramatic demanding and "authoritarian" directions toward the slower-paced and more "permissive" suggestions of the popular arm levitation technique.]

Rapid-induction arm levitation is a powerful and effective technique mainly because it establishes an immediate focus of attention, a suspension of critical assessment, and allows the therapist to "predict" responses (lightness, tingling) which are byproducts of hyperventilation. At the same time the limitations of the technique must be kept firmly in mind. To begin, hyperventilation is *absolutely contraindicated* for agoraphobics, who can be catapulted into a panic attack by this rapid-breathing technique. Another area of concern, and one which is medically oriented, are the idiosyncratic reactions that some people can experience as the result of hyperventilation. Included among these are apprehension, chest tightness, a sense of suffocation, sweating, rapid heartbeat, muscular weakness, blurring of vision, paresthesia in the hands and face, and fainting. These effects are caused by a relative cerebral hypoxia occurring as the result of lowering the partial pressure of carbon dioxide in the blood stream (Pco_2). Highly anxious individuals are particularly susceptible to these effects, and it is in these individuals that the rapid-breathing technique may prove to be highly distressing.

Although we suggest that the rapid breathing be maintained for only a minute or so, nevertheless, in certain people, this may be sufficient to produce these hyperventilation side-effects. We have remarked elsewhere in this chapter that the therapist must never exit from a technique just because the patient is experiencing difficulties with it but, rather, should manipulate his suggestions so as to achieve a successful outcome. The one exception to this rule is when a patient experiences difficulties with the rapid-breathing technique. To continue with the procedure in the face of developing distressing symptoms would be unacceptable in any therapeutic situation. Certainly, the worst that could happen is that the patient would lapse into syncope, but the ultimate effects on the therapeutic relationship would be far more devastating.

The Direct-Stare Technique

It may seem strange that we have come this far in our list of induction procedures without mentioning the one that in the minds of many is *the* hypnotic technique—hypnosis through direct stare. Presentations of hypnosis in the popular media invariably portray the hypnotist staring directly into the eyes of the entranced patient. In many clinical texts, the use of direct stare is listed as a standard procedure. One of the most widely read of these (Meares, 1960) describes it as "not just a matter of historical interest [but] as a technique of real importance in modern hypnotherapy" (p. 191). Meares puts the value of the direct-stare technique in the power it has to overcome resistance in difficult patients. Our reservation about the use of eye stare does not come from any doubts about the power of the technique. We advise against it because of *how* and not how well it works: eye stare, as even its strongest advocates acknowledge, works through the establishment of a dominant and submissive relationship between therapist and patient (Meares, 1960). Moreover, there is a special problem with eye stare in anxious patients, where sustained eye contact can elicit alarm reactions of some considerable magnitude (Bowlby, 1975). Then too, it is difficult to reconcile the authoritarian relationship necessary for the "overpowering" (Meares, 1960) eye-stare technique with the major aim of behavior therapy, which is to assist the patient toward autonomy and self-control.

Hypnotic Relaxation
via Sensory Awareness

We have said a number of times that before he gives up on those individuals who show only a slight response to the induction procedures covered in this chapter, the therapist should make a clinical assessment of where the impediments to hypnotizability lie. Remedial procedures can then be brought into play to "free up" movement toward hypnosis on the relevant dimensions [assuming that the anxieties—Dimension1—have been dispelled beforehand and that the problem(s) are related to one or more of the remaining five dimensions]. Three commonly encountered difficulties are: excessive arousal, restless attention, and an excessively critical or "objective" attitude in the patient. Elsewhere in the book we have discussed the techniques of choice for the first two problems: progressive muscle relaxation (Appendix A) and meditation (chapter 6). To lessen the person's reliance upon independent (or evaluative or critical) thinking, the therapist must take care to directly and explicitly instruct the patient to give up his preoccupations with logical or realistic scrutiny. "Just let yourself react" is the message given to the patient. When it proves difficult for the patient to relinquish this critical review, a preinduction period of training in the toleration of fantasy and sensory experiences can help him past this barrier. The following procedure is designed to do just this. It takes less than ten minutes to administer, and at the conclusion the therapist should move straight on to the particular hypnosis induction procedure he wishes to employ.

The subject should be sitting in a comfortable chair, in either an upright or a reclining position. The various instructions will assume that the subject is seated in this fashion. The therapist should begin:

"Just sit comfortably in the chair and listen very closely to what I am going to be saying to you. I'm going to try a series of experiments with you. Each experiment will be in the form of a question. Each question is answerable by either "yes" or "no," but it will not be necessary for you to say "yes" or "no" out loud or even perhaps to yourself, because the answer to each question will become very clear as we proceed. Just remember to listen to the questions that I pose to you, and do not be bothered by the unusual nature of some of them. Let yourself react to each question. However you react is fine. There really is no right or wrong way. Let your own reaction to each question be your own answer to each question.

Is it possible for you to allow your eyes to close? [10 second pause]
If they are not yet closed you may close them now. [5 sec.]
Can you be aware at the point at which the back of your head comes in contact with the chair? [10 sec.]

Is it possible for you to imagine the space between your eyes? [10 sec.]

Is it possible for you to be aware how close your breath comes to the back of your eyes every time you inhale? [10 sec.]

Can you imagine that you are looking at something that is very far away? [10 sec.]

Is it possible for you to be aware of where your arms are in contact with the chair [5 sec.], and can you be aware of the points at which your arms lose contact with the chair? [10 sec.]

Is either your left or right foot resting on the floor and if either or both of them are, can you feel the floor beneath your foot? [10 sec.]

Can you imagine in your mind's eye a beautiful flower suspended a few feet in front of you? [10 sec.] Is it possible for you to close your lids of your inner eye so you can no longer see the flower? [10 sec.]

Is it possible for you to be aware of the space within your mouth? [10 sec.] And can you be aware of the position of your tongue within your mouth? [10 sec.]

Is it possible for you to feel even the slightest breeze against your cheek? [10 sec.]

Are you aware of one of your arms being heavier than the other? [10 sec.]

Is there a tingling or feeling of numbness in one of your hands? [10 sec.]

Are you aware of one of your arms being more relaxed than the other? [10 sec.]

Is it possible for you to notice any change in the temperature of your body? [10 sec.]

Is your left arm warmer than your right? [10 sec.]

Is it possible for you to feel like a rag doll? [10 sec.]

Can you be aware of your left forearm? [5 sec.] Can you feel any tightness in it? [10 sec.]

Can you feel yourself floating as if on a cloud? [5 sec.] Or are you feeling much too heavy for that? [10 sec.]

Can your arms feel very heavy, as if they were stuck in molasses? [10 sec.]

Is it possible for you to imagine once again that you are looking at something that is very far away? [10 sec.]

Is there a heaviness coming into your legs? [10 sec.]

Is it possible for you to imagine yourself floating in warm water? [10 sec.]

Can you feel the weight of your body in the chair? [10 sec.]
Can you allow yourself just to drift along lazily? [10 sec.]
Is it possible to feel your face getting very soft? [10 sec.]
Is it possible for you to imagine in your mind's eye another
  beautiful flower? [10 sec.] Can you notice what color the
  flower is if you see one? [10 sec.] Can you close the lids of
  your inner eye to no longer to see the flower? [10 sec.]
Is it possible to notice whether one of your arms is more heavy
  than the other [10 sec.], and can you notice whether one of
  your legs is heavier than the other? [10 sec.]"

Deepening Procedures*

We have discussed elsewhere (see chapter 3) that hypnotizability
is an index of a subject's ability to achieve his maximum level of
hypnosis, when tested under standard and optimal conditions. But it
is important, from a clinical standpoint, to draw a distinction between hypnotizability and the depth of hypnosis that a patient actually experiences under different and varying conditions, especially
since these two terms are often taken to be synonymous. Thus, a
patient's hypnotic capacity may measure as Grade 4 on the Hypnotic
Induction Profile (Spiegel & Spiegel, 1978) when tested in a quiet
room where no outside sounds or distractions intrude. On the other
hand, the same patient when treated in a busy Pain Clinic setting
may experience only a *depth* of hypnosis equivalent to Grade 2 or 3.
Here, such things as the intrusive noises of the clinic, or his raised
pain level, may seriously impede the disengagement process and
thereby prevent him reaching his maximum hypnotic potential.

From the evidence arising from existing clinical and experimental studies indicating that there is a relationship between hypnotizability and therapeutic outcome (see chapter 3), there is an obvious
need for the therapist to facilitate the process of hypnotic disengagement through the use of specific deepening techniques. This is not

*Both authors have misgivings about the use of the word *deepening* to indicate process
of increasing disengagement. In the spatial metaphor, we construe people in hypnosis
as moving *away* from their contact with the external environment, *away* from their
practical concerns, and *into* or *toward* hypnosis. A more serious objection to the deepening is the implied acceptance of hypnosis as a process of "going under," and the
implied picture of hypnosis as something that happens to one. We much prefer to
characterize hypnosis as we have, and not as deepening, because it draws the practitioner's attention to the skills of disengagement that are essential. With all of these
objections we, nevertheless, have decided to retain the word *deepening* because it has
attained such widespread use.

to say that deeper levels of hypnosis are necessarily dependent on the utilization of these techniques, for obviously this is not the case. One has only to witness the stage hypnotist in action to realize that other factors also play a role in the achievement of deep hypnosis (in this case, the authoritarian demands of the hypnotist and the expectations of the subject). Notwithstanding this, in the clinical setting the patient is more likely to achieve satisfactory hypnotic disengagement when one or more of these deepening procedures is employed.

Another, and related, issue is the variability of depth of hypnosis that patients experience—not only from one session to the next but even within the same session. This may be of some concern to the patient, who usually assumes that hypnotic depth will increase in a direct relationship to the number of times he is hypnotized. To some extent, these expectations are not entirely unfounded, for many patients experience, and comment upon, the progressive increase in depth of hypnosis for the first three or four inductions.

But just as they are aware of increasing depths of hypnosis, so too are they sensitive to a changing depth from one session to another, and may express this as: "I wasn't as deep today as last time." In saying this, the patient is really voicing a concern that he has failed in some way or has "not cooperated." These reports should be taken seriously, for they indicate that the patient is experiencing difficulties in modifying one or more of the dimensions of hypnotic disengagement, usually resulting from excessive arousal or very high levels of anxiety. Armed with this information, the therapist should take the necessary steps to diminish these particular factors when next treating the patient in hypnosis. Often this requires a change in induction and/or deepening techniques, and this further underscores a point which we have already raised—that a therapist must always adapt his hypnotic approach to suit the needs of the patient. Furthermore, when a patient expresses such concerns, he should be reassured that his response to induction is not a deliberate attempt on his part to forestall hypnosis, but is arising from his tension and anxiety.

A consideration of the merits of one deepening procedure compared with another is unlikely to be rewarding. What is more important is that the clinician be familiar and comfortable with their use and that those which he chooses are presented in such a way that hypnotic disengagement is ensured. The techniques we describe below are not meant to be an exhaustive list but are selected because of their proven ability to lead to hypnotic disengagement in the clinical situation.

A Relaxation Method

A great many patients who present for hypnotic treatment are tense, anxious, or highly strung individuals who, in spite of detailed prehypnosis discussion with the therapist, still possess a full complement of concerns about being hypnotized. Indeed, the anxiety and fears experienced by these patients may be so great as to effectively interfere with the therapist's efforts to deepen hypnosis. In such patients, it may be necessary to use a relaxation procedure so that anxiety is reduced to a level where hypnosis becomes possible. The therapist may either choose to use a progressive muscular relaxation technique before attempting hypnosis (see Appendix A), or incorporate relaxation as a deepening process. Although both procedures involve muscular relaxation, they differ from each other in one major respect. Progressive muscular relaxation occurs in response to specific motor activities performed by the patient (for example, tensing and then relaxing the limbs), while the relaxation technique described below emphasizes the (cognitive) stimuli associated with relaxation.

There are a multiplicity of ways in which relaxation can be induced in a patient. Some therapists, for example, prefer to start by having the patient relax one leg at a time, and then progress upward through the body. We favor commencing relaxation in the muscles around the eyes and face. It is far easier initially to relax small rather than large muscle groups and it is these muscles, rather than those from the lower body, which are so troublesome in tense patients (Malmo, 1975). Having achieved success in relaxing this area of the body, the patient then finds it easier to experience a similar response in the large muscles of the trunk and limbs.

The timing of the suggestions of relaxation is another important consideration. Patients exhibit a wide diversity in the time taken to relax particular muscles, and it is incumbent upon the therapist, therefore, to allow a sufficient period to elapse before proceeding to another part of the body. Only in this way will the patient achieve a satisfactory outcome from suggestions of relaxation. The method we employ is as follows:

> "I'm going to help you relax even more deeply now. Just go along with the things I suggest . . . and you will experience a much deeper sense of relaxation . . . you will enjoy the experience . . . just listen to what I say . . . and let things happen. Now feel this relaxation coming into the small muscles around the eyes . . .

they are feeling so relaxed that presently . . . the eyelids will feel heavy . . . very heavy . . . like lead shutters . . . almost too heavy to move . . . feeling as though they are glued together . . . and you feel this relaxation spreading outward . . . just as ripples spread out on a still pool when the water is disturbed . . . spreading out into the muscles of the face . . . so that your jaw feels relaxed and your lips part a little . . . into the forehead and scalp . . . the neck . . . notice how your head feels so heavy and relaxed . . . so comfortable against the back of the chair . . . the shoulders feel quite limp and relaxed . . . the arms are relaxing . . . heavy . . . loose and floppy by your side . . . from your shoulders right through to the tips of your fingers. Your back, too, is becoming more and more relaxed . . . sinking deeply into the chair . . . especially the small of your back . . . your muscles in your stomach and your chest are relaxing more and more . . . notice that each time you breathe out . . . you go deeper and deeper into this pleasant relaxed state . . . notice this, just let yourself be aware of this . . . don't try to do anything . . . and now your legs are gradually letting go of all the tension as well . . . all through your hips . . . your thighs . . . your knees . . . calf muscles . . . even the ankles and feet are relaxing. You feel as though all the tension within you . . . is flowing out through your toes . . . and being replaced by this very pleasant feeling of relaxation. As this grows you'll also become more aware of how fleeting and unimportant all of your thoughts are . . . aware of the quiet deep within you . . . the quiet."

A Breathing Method

Breathing plays a significant role in a variety of hypnobehavioral techniques. Meditation, autogenic training, yoga, and hypnosis all utilize a breathing procedure either in the induction process or in therapy. Although one would expect to find a similarity between the breathing process in each of these therapeutic techniques, such is not the case. In hypnosis, relaxation therapies, and meditation, the exhalation component is emphasized, while in the fourth exercise (control of respiration) of Schultz's autogenic training (Schultz & Luthe, 1969) there is no particular emphasis on either the exhalation or inhalation components ("I am breathing slowly and easily"—supplemented by "I breathe with no conscious effort"). In yoga, on the other hand, the expulsion of air from the lungs takes place in a series of sudden, strong rhythmical actions initiated through diaphragmatic movement. It is clear, then, that the manner in which a patient utilizes his breathing, either in induction or in therapy, is dependent on the therapist's phraseology and placement of suggestions. In other words, the therapist must be specific in his suggestions so that the patient is left in no doubt as to whether he should focus upon the exhalation or inhalation component. The emphasis on one or the other aspect of breathing will be determined by the sensations, emotions, and actions that the therapist wishes to produce in the patient:

> In general, long, slow, deep exhalations bring about relaxation with the accompanying sensations of sinking, widening, opening up, and softening; the feelings of comfort, heaviness, warmth, and moisture; the moods of patience and calmness. Inhalations evoke invigoration, tension, or levitation; and they are related to the feelings of lightness, coolness, and dryness, and to the moods of courage, determination and exhilaration. (Jencks, 1978, p. 169)

Thus, from the standpoint of deepening hypnosis, the practitioner should time suggestions of relaxation so that they coincide with the exhalation component.

The breathing technique is especially of value in those patients who, because of a high level of anxiety, find it difficult to "let go," and also for those who have a poor imaginative capacity. The procedure we favor is as follows:

> "I feel sure you would like to experience an even deeper sense of relaxation, and I'm going to tell you how you can achieve this through your breathing. In a moment, I am going to ask you take ten deep breaths. I want you to hold each breath for a moment, and then let it out slowly. As you breathe out each time, think of the word *relax*. With each breath, you will notice that you become more and more deeply relaxed; you will feel as though you are releasing all the tension from within your body with each breath. Now, go ahead and take those ten deep breaths, relaxing deeper with each one as you do so."

The Descending Steps Method

Imagery can be a most effective means of deepening hypnosis but is obviously dependent on the patient having a good imaginative capacity. Deepening imagery may be used in two ways: first, active imagery where the patient imagines himself performing a task (for example, walking on the beach) and, second, passive imagery in which the scene is the predominant figure and the subject plays a passive role (for example, gazing at a flower). The descending steps method incorporates both forms of imagery, and its effectiveness centers around its ability to change a number of dimensions leading to hypnotic disengagement. Thus, the arousal and anxiety factors are reduced by having the patient imagine himself in a tranquil scene, and the attentional processes are narrowed when he focuses on descending the steps in time with his breathing. Although we describe a technique involving a garden scene, it must be reemphasized that the therapist must use one that the patient finds acceptable and that is associated with feelings of relaxation and tranquility:

> "You are now feeling so relaxed . . . very relaxed indeed . . . and you can imagine things with such ease . . . almost as though you are there . . . experiencing them . . . and in a moment, you are going to picture a scene that will help you to relax even more deeply . . . you will enjoy this experience. When you are ready to start, let your left forefinger lift into the air . . . good . . . now, imagine that you are standing at the top of a flight of ten steps . . . looking down to a beautiful garden scene . . . that scene looks so peaceful . . . you may see a small courtyard leading out to the garden . . . shady and cool . . . with the sun filtering through the leaves of the trees . . . casting shadows on the ground . . . see the flowers and the lawns in the garden . . . perhaps a small stream flowing through one part . . . with the water gently flowing over the smooth stones . . . it is all so beautiful . . . and tranquil . . . and if you can visualize yourself standing at the top of the steps waiting to go down to that inviting scene, your left forefinger will lift into the air . . . good . . . in a moment, you are going to slowly descend each step . . . in time with your breathing out . . . and as you do so, you will count silently from ten back to one . . . let each step take you deeper . . . and deeper . . . into relaxation . . . and when you are in the garden and feel peaceful . . . tranquil . . . relaxed . . . again, your forefinger will lift a little to indicate this to me. Now, in your own time . . . picture yourself going down each step . . . in time with your breathing out . . . and as you go down each step, you will become so much more relaxed."

At this stage, hypnosis can be further deepened by having the subject "hallucinate" feelings of warmth, while, at the same time, the attentional focus is narrowed to an even greater degree when he visualizes the finer details in, say, a flower.

> "In this beautiful garden . . . the soft and lovely colors relax you so . . . make you feel calm . . . tranquil . . . the sun feels warm on your body . . . relaxing you still further . . . and then . . . you notice some flowers . . . they are your favorite flowers . . . you feel a sense of pleasure at seeing them . . . your left forefinger will lift a little as soon as you can picture them . . . that's fine . . . you want to look at them more closely . . . to smell their fragrance . . . and so you walk across to them . . . gazing intently . . . becoming so involved in one of the flowers . . . that you can see all the fine details of the petals and inner parts of the flower . . . nothing else seems to matter . . . just the flower in all its beauty . . . you may even be able to smell the fragrance . . . your left forefinger will lift if you can do so . . . good . . . and all the time, you are relaxing even more deeply . . . even more completely."

Two features should be noted at this point. First, the presence of an olfactory hallucination is an indication that the patient is experiencing a significant depth of hypnosis, and, second, the patient should be allowed to dwell upon the flower for a period of time without further interjections from the therapist. Short periods of silence, if correctly applied in deepening procedures, may in themselves have a significant effect on the disengagement process. To reiterate our earlier coments on this issue, novitiate therapists, in particular, seem to feel the need to keep up a constant flow of verbiage throughout induction and therapy in the mistaken belief that any periods of silence will work to the detriment of their efforts.

Fractionation Method

This procedure, first described by Vogt (1894–95), involves the patient being hypnotized and dehypnotized in a rapid and sequential manner. The theory underlying this technique is that each hypnotic experience renders the patient more suggestible to the next. Weitzenhoffer (1957) suggests that this response results from the perseveration of hypnosis for a short while after termination, and thus the rapid reinduction is potentiated by the carry-over effects of the previously induced hypnotic state. The principle advantages of using this procedure for deepening hypnosis are: first, it is a relatively rapid technique; second, it can be used in patients who demonstrate a poor imaginative responsiveness; and finally, in those individuals who express concern about their ability to be hypnotized (or having been hypnotized in a previous session), their response to suggestions of eye closure is usually sufficient to convince them that hypnosis has occurred.

The fractionation technique which we employ is as follows:

"You're now feeling so much more relaxed, but I'm going to help you to relax even more deeply. In a moment, I will count slowly from one to ten. At the count of five, your eyes will open but as I go on counting, the lids will become very heavy and relaxed; they will begin to blink; and as they blink they will feel even heavier—so heavy in fact that they will feel as though they just want to close. When you feel this happening, you should let them close and as they do so, you will become even more deeply relaxed. Now, I'm going to count to ten; at five your eyes will open but the lids will feel so heavy, so very, very heavy, that they will simply want to close. As they do, so you will go into a much deeper state of relaxation. Ready. One . . . two . . . three . . . four . . . five . . . that's good . . . six . . . seven . . . eight . . . nine . . . ten . . . deeply relaxed all through you. Now I'm going to count again to ten, and once more your eyes will open at the count of five. But this time, your eyelids will feel even heavier than before—so heavy in fact, that they will close almost at once. And when this happens, you will experience an even deeper sense of relaxation than you are feeling at this moment; a deeper sense of ease. Ready. One . . . two . . . three . . . four . . . five . . . that's it . . . six . . . seven . . . eight . . . nine . . . ten. So very deeply relaxed all over."

We have already noted (see chapter 3) that a desired response may be more readily achieved when a reinforcing stimulus (such as a suggestion or breathing) is provided in such a way that it stands in close temporal contiguity to the desired behavior. The importance of this principle can be noted in the fractionation procedure, for here, the disengagement count (one through five) should be timed to coincide with the patient's inhalation, and the reengagement count (six through ten) synchronized with the expiration phase.

Most patients readily respond to the technique just described, but occasionally a patient will fail to close his eyes following the disengagement process. This usually occurs in the more highly anxious individual and can prove disturbing for both the therapist and the patient. In such an instance, the following suggestions will invariably lead to eye closure (and reengagement):

> "I note that you are experiencing some difficulty in letting your eyes close. Don't be concerned about this, for it simply indicates that you didn't *really* believe that you could respond in the way that I suggest. In time, though, you will be able to, but just close your eyes now and let yourself relax a little more. That's it. Good. Again I am going to slowly count from one to ten, and once more the eyes will open at the count of five. Only this time, you will find that your eyelids feel *so* much heavier than before. So heavy in fact, that they will begin to blink; and as they blink, they will feel heavier and heavier and will close of their own accord. When this happens, you will become even more deeply relaxed."

The importance of persisting with a procedure as described above cannot be overstated, for many apparent "resistances" to induction and deepening suggestions arise, in fact, from the patient's fear that he cannot be hypnotized. When such difficulties are encountered, it is imperative that the therapist not leave the situation unresolved, for this only serves to potentiate the person's existing negative beliefs. This calls for the therapist to be alert to the likelihood of it happening, and also for him to deftly manipulate suggestions so that a potential failure experience is converted to one of success.

Nonverbal Techniques

The techniques we have discussed so far rely on verbal input from the therapist. The greatest preponderance of clinical and experimental techniques have looked into the semantic content of hypnotic techniques. Much less is known about the paralinguistic or nonverbal procedures. Paralinguistic factors include the rate of speech, intonation, and other nonsemantic items, and although there is little in the way of hard research data to justify firm recommendations, experienced clinicians agree that a quietly insistent mode of delivery with interspersed pauses seems to be useful and necessary to hypnotic induction.

Moving away from verbal deliveries altogether, researchers are now beginning to ask whether nonverbal, nonsemantic techniques may not have a place in hypnotic induction and therapy. In this regard, music would seem an obvious technique to employ. The selection of the piece of music to be played will usually be determined by the individual's idiosyncratic responses. Two pieces of music that are equal favorites in the patient's estimation, however, may not be equally desirable in the induction of hypnosis. To follow the line we developed earlier in this chapter concerning the use of imagery for relaxation and hypnosis, it is not merely a matter of selecting positive imagery but, more important, of avoiding that which has an exciting and arousing effect and, in preference, selecting positive tranquil images. So too with the search for the musical selections to be used in hypnosis, and in keeping with our perspective of hypnotic disengagement, the type of music should be such that it diminishes the person's anxiety and arousal, and leads to a narrowing of his attentional focus. Needless to say, the patient should be consulted about his musical predilection, but it must be emphasized that the final selection may not necessarily be his favorite piece of music but, rather, one that will lead to a quiet, stable equilibrium. Thus, the therapist must select music which avoids intense cognitive or affective reactions. Baroque chamber music (J.S. Bach and Vivaldi); concertos for lute and orchestra (Vivaldi, Kohaut, and Handel); or Canon in D Major (Pachelbel), for example, are works which have no harsh cadences and are capable of producing pleasant evocative imagery—irrespective of the musical sophistication of the patient.

Music is essentially used as a deepening procedure in hypnosis, although there are also impressive reports of its use as a form of therapy in its own right (Hamel, 1978). Following routine hypnotic induction, Walker and Diment (1979) suggest that the music (which may last from 10 to 25 minutes) be introduced in the following way:

> "In a little while I am going to play some tape-recorded music. I want you to listen to the music in a special way. While your body goes on relaxing more and more, automatically, I want you to let the music pick your mind up and carry it along. Let yourself become more and more absorbed in the experience of the music. Perhaps you will experience imagery in response to the music, perhaps not; whatever you experience will be *pleasant and absorbing*. Listen to the music and let it take you further and further into hypnosis. I will start the recorder in a moment. Just let the music carry you along, more and more absorbed, further and further into hypnosis. Listen for the music to begin. You

will be quite absorbed in it until it fades away and I begin to talk to you again. If random thoughts come to mind, you will simply not bother with them; you will let them slide away and refocus your mind on the music. Right, wait for the music to begin. . . ."

A point to be noted when using this technique is the need to incorporate a suggestion that the subject will not spontaneously enter hypnosis when listening to that particular piece of music, but will only do so in specific therapeutic situations. This is especially important when using it with a highly hypnotizable patient.

Termination

The clinical literature contains a smaller number of termination techniques than it does methods of induction, but there is still a great variety in use. As with the induction, the practitioner can make use of the one that best suits the patient and the kind of anxiety being treated. And, as with induction, the same principles apply—but in termination the aim, naturally, is to produce reengagement and not disengagement. The practitioner will structure his comments so as to gradually stimulate the patient's awareness of his surroundings and restore the sense of self-direction: "Notice the noises in the room and outside, how the chair feels against your back, the feelings in your hands and legs. Think of all that we have done since beginning hypnosis, and perhaps some of the comments you'd like to make when we finish." These requests call upon the patient to return to a more mobile attention; to give up the intense present-centeredness by having him recall what happened (the recent past) and what he'll soon be doing (the immediate future). The therapist gives only the most general guidance here ("all that we have done") and so the patient has to carry out a brief and self-initiated critical review of the proceedings—a style of thinking which is very much a part of the reengagement process. The therapist can then begin the final phase of termination. It is best if this is done in clear and direct instructions to the patient:

"In a moment I'm going to count backward from five to one. When I get to one you'll feel quite at ease, just as you felt before we began. When I get to one, you'll open your eyes and take a big stretch. Five . . . four . . . three—we're halfway there . . . two . . . *one* [said with force as the patient breathes in]. That's it, stretch, clench your fists, tightly, and now open them . . . sit up. How do you feel now? [The practitioner should check for any perseverative reactions.] Fine, now let's talk over the whole thing." [In this debriefing, the patient should be encouraged to talk about any departures from the suggestions proffered to him and *his* advice as to how improvements could be made.]

There is no need to spend an excessive amount of time on the termination procedure. Five minutes should be more than enough for most patients. On the other hand, we would advise against trying to complete the termination in less than one minute. It will do the patient no serious harm if he is told suddenly and abruptly "OK, now you can open your eyes," and no more than that. Most will find it unsettling and unpleasant, however, to open the eyes and begin a conversation while still disengaged. One final point that we wish to emphasize is that the termination *procedure* should not be confused with the termination *process*. For up to ten minutes (or, in the occasional instance, even longer) after the completion of a gradually paced termination procedure, the patient may still be in a "twilight" zone between full disengagement and the normal mode of engagement. This is particularly noticeable in the highly hypnotizable patient, who will often remain disoriented for five to ten minutes after the termination *procedure* has been completed. Another feature demonstrated by this group of patients is their great capacity for imaginative involvement and the literal nature of their responses. The therapist must bear these behavioral characteristics in mind when selecting termination procedures for these individuals. Thus, if the descending steps technique is used for deepening, it is advisable to have the patient imagine himself retracing these steps when exiting from hypnosis. Failure to do so may, in some cases, invoke feelings of distress that they have been "left in the scene" (garden, beach). To those unfamiliar with hypnosis, this may seem a far-fetched notion, but the authors can attest to the occurrence of this problem in highly hypnotizable patients.

5

Hypnosis in Children

Train up a child in the way he should go: and when he is old, he will not depart from it.

—Proverbs, xxii, 6

Over the last decade the amount of basic data on hypnosis has grown by orders of magnitude. In parallel with this there has been a sharp increase in the clinical uses of hypnosis. The development of this information and interest has been uneven across the areas of clinical practice and very little of this work has been devoted to hypnosis in children. As is to be expected in the absence of an adequate data base, extreme positions flourish and are defended with vigor. The practitioner interested in the application of hypnosis to children's disorders has to steer a sensible middle course between the two extremes of incautious application and outright rejection and must also be able to recognize the special problems of children's hypnosis. We agree with Gardner (1974, p. 29) that ". . . to be optimally successful as hypnotherapists, we must be able to experience the child that remains in us and resonate with our young patients at this level as well as from the level of our adult selves." It is obvious that the child, lacking developmental maturity, will approach hypnosis with a fundamentally different set of views from those of an adult. As right as these points may be, they still leave the clinician in need of the facts of hypnosis in children from both an assessment and an application point of view.

The more general requirements of "good rapport" and "effective therapist–child relationship" will be best met in those situations in which the correct procedures are used.

Hypnotizability in Children

To the misconceptions about (adult) hypnosis that are so prevalent we can add one that applies specifically to children, which is that children are not hypnotizable. In fact the opposite is true. Hypnotizability, or hypnotic susceptibility, climbs from age 5 to ages 9 through 12, after which it declines gradually up to age 32 (Morgan & Hilgard, 1973). After that there appears to be a sharp drop-off to age 40 and a rise thereafter. In view of the fact that children are such excellent hypnotic subjects, it is surprising that so few practitioners use this therapeutic approach. This underuse of hypnosis in children can be traced to, first, parental concerns about the risks of hypnosis and, second, uncertainty on the part of the therapist borne of inexperience. We shall return to these difficulties later.

Since the bulk of the evidence supports the view that children are indeed *more* hypnotizable than adults, it is worthwhile considering for a moment the features that may underlie this greater hypnotizability. Children spend much of their playtime in fantasy and in general exhibit a boundless imaginative capacity and the facility to become totally involved in whatever interests them—so much so that they effectively shut themselves off from outside distractions (Hilgard, 1974). These are many of the qualities that make up "hypnotic trance," as we have defined it on the six dimensions of hypnosis. Additional to this, children are curious about new ideas and are usually eager to explore new horizons—which suggests the value of getting the child to see hypnosis as an opportunity to try out a new adventure. Finally, unlike adults, who have usually developed their own misconceptions and conflicts about hypnosis, children are generally quite free of such encumbrances. When the practitioner recommends the inclusion of hypnosis in a therapy program it is the *parents* more than the child who need reassurance; it is their myths and misconceptions which take first place on the clinical agenda.

Children's Assessment Scales

The two assessment scales in wide use are the Children's Hypnotic Susceptibility Scale (CHSS) and the Stanford Hypnotic Clinical Scale for Children (SHCS:Child).

The CHSS was devised by Perry London (1963) and is based on the Stanford Hypnotic Susceptibility Scales for Adults (Weitzenhoffer & Hilgard, 1959, 1962), with certain items being rewritten so that they conform more to children's usage. The CHSS is a 22-item scale and is divided into two parts: the first contains the 12 items which form the SHSS: A and B (Weitzenhoffer & Hilgard, 1959). The second part of the scale incorporates ten items derived from the SHSS:C (Weitzenhoffer & Hilgard, 1962), included in which are tests for anesthesia, age regression, and auditory and visual hallucinations. One of the most interesting and, from a therapeutic point of view, valuable findings that has arisen out of the use of the CHSS is the inherent tendency that some children have to simulate—especially those in the 8 to 11 year age group (Cooper & London, 1979; London & Madsen, 1968). This is not to say that hypnosis should not be used for this age group of children, but the clinician has to be on guard against "behavioral" hypnosis. By that we mean simply that the simulator can show a convincing but merely outer compliance. Throughout this book, we have identified hypnosis with a number of cognitive changes. It is these as well as related behaviors that "make" hypnosis, not just the behavior itself.

A second scale, the Stanford Hypnotic Clinical Scale for Children (SHCS:Child) was constructed by Morgan and Hilgard (1979) as a means of testing hypnotic susceptibility in the clinical situation. It is a seven-item scale and is so devised that it fulfills four essential criteria: testing takes no more than 20 minutes, brevity being an essential feature when assessing an ill or disturbed child; every child experiences success in at least some of the items; the scale proves interesting for children; and finally, the scale has direct relevance to the clinical situation.

In this scale, a relaxation/eye closure induction is carried out by having the child concentrate on a face drawn on a thumbnail while at that same time being given suggestions of relaxation. Once eyelid closure occurs (failure to close the eyes calls for the use of a modified scale), then the following items are tested:

1. *Hand lowering.* The young patient is requested to hold his arm directly out in front of him, and is then told to imagine a heavy weight pushing it downward. Pass: hand lowers at least six inches at the end of ten seconds.
2. *Arm rigidity.* The patient is instructed to hold his arm out in front of him and imagine it is stiff and straight "like the branch of a tree." He is next requested to try to bend

it. Pass: if within ten seconds the arm bends no more than two inches.

3, 4.   *Visual and auditory hallucination (TV).* The patient's ability to hallucinate is tested by having him imagine his favorite TV program. Visual pass: if the child sees a program as though he was actually viewing it. Auditory pass: if the child reports sounds, words, and music.

5.   *Dream.* The capacity to dream is tested by asking the child to dream as he does at night. Pass: a report of experiences comparable to a dream.

6.   *Age regression.* This item is tested for by asking the patient to think back to a very special time when he was younger. At the same time, it is suggested that he is becoming younger and younger. Pass: The child gives appropriate answers to the therapist's questions, indicating that he had some experience of being there.

7.   *Posthypnotic response.* It is suggested to the child that he will take a deep breath and open his eyes, but on hearing a clap of hands, will close them again and return to just the way he is at present. Pass: compliance with suggestion.

A modified form of the SHCS:Child was also constructed, designed for use with very young children (below six years of age) and also for children who are very anxious and cannot relax. The modified form of the SHCS:Child differs from the standard scale in the following ways: Induction is achieved through the use of active fantasy; the child is permitted to keep his eyes open; suggestions of relaxation are avoided, and the posthypnotic suggestion is ommitted because of the implied reentering of a relaxed state.

In their study of the SHCS:Child, Morgan and Hilgard (1979) administered the scale to a sample of children from elementary and nursery schools. The subjects were assigned to one of two induction groups: a conventional relaxation/eye closure induction and one involving fantasy. The mean scores for the two induction groups were compared, and the findings have considerable clinical significance. For example, none of the three- to four-year-olds responded to relaxation suggestion, but when the same age group were given the active-imagination induction, over half passed between two and five items, and only one-quarter of the subjects scored zero on all tests. These findings point unequivocally to the fact that if a clinician wishes to hypnotize a younger child (say, below six years of age), he should utilize imagination and not relaxation/eye closure techniques.

Another issue that arose from the development of this scale is that "while for some purposes it appears desirable to have the eyes closed, and this is readily achieved with the older child, it is too difficult at the younger ages, *though hypnotic responses are achieved well with the eyes open*" (Morgan & Hilgard, 1979, p. 150; emphasis added). This is a point worth stressing in light of the almost universal belief that eye closure is a prerequisite for hypnosis. Inevitably, the question must be asked: "But how do I know that a young child with his eyes open *has* been hypnotized?" For that matter, the clinician may also wonder the same thing concerning the child before him with his eyes closed. The answer would seem to lie in experimental studies, and indeed Cooper and London (1976, p. 140), in studying the relationship between children's hypnotic susceptibility and EEG patterns, have shown that "Hypnotic susceptibility was found to be positively correlated with alpha duration in the Eyes Opened condition." A number of studies (Bakan & Svorad, 1969; London, Hart, & Leibovitz, 1968; Morgan, MacDonald, & Hilgard, 1974) have clearly demonstrated a moderate and positive correlation between alpha activity and hypnotizability in adults, and thus it can be seen that Cooper and London's (1976) work validates the clinical impression that young children are hypnotized even though they have their eyes open. But few practitioners will have or care to use such devices in everyday clinical practice, and the final decision as to whether a child is hypnotized must still rest on the therapist's observations of and judgment about behavioral signs (for example, slow breathing, infrequent movement) and, most important, through posthypnotic questioning.

Although many clinicians still question the need to assess hypnotizability in children, we emphatically believe that the same essential reasons hold true as in the assessment of adults (see chapter 3). Thus, measurement of hypnotizability gives a therapist valuable knowledge of a child's hypnotic "strengths," while at the same time providing the young patient with an insight into hypnosis before starting therapy (especially important in an anxious or phobic child). Furthermore, accurate evaluation of hypnotizability adds greater import to documented clinical reports.

Preparation

Here, as with hypnosis in adults, the therapist must spend a few moments, at least, introducing the basic ideas, procedures, and benefits of hypnosis. In this preliminary talk, he must emphasize how pleasant the experience can be and how the child and therapist *together* can have an easy and safe "look" at the things that bother him. This point is vitally important and deserves reiteration. Some of the most common and disturbing fears in children are those they exhibit when separated from support in novel or unpleasant situations (Bowlby, 1975; Ollendick, 1979). In all situations in which anxiety is elicited, feelings of anxiety about separation can act as a potent exacerbation of anxiety, whether or not this is the focal complaint. Thus, presenting hypnosis as requiring the cooperative work of two people, therapist and child, is not only to state the truth—it also can give important reassurance that the therapist will be "with" the child on the "journeys."

Another issue that deserves mention is the need to make sure that the child *really* understands the meanings of words that are commonplace in therapy. One assumes, for example, that an adult knows what the word *relax* means. On the other hand, few children (particularly those under the age of 12 years) seem to understand its meaning, and therefore it is important for the therapist to discuss and clarify it by not only talking of "floppy," "loose", and "being like a rag doll," but also to demonstrate it on himself and on the young patient. This is best done by first picking up his own arm and letting it drop limply down and then doing the same to the patient. A practical demonstration of this kind makes a much greater impression on the child than a verbal explanation.

Finally, it is always advisable to ask the child whether he would prefer to sit or lie down in therapy. Many children associate lying down with going to bed (and hence to sleep) and, for this reason, may be quite resistant to the idea. Accordingly, we generally prefer to use hypnosis in the sitting rather than the reclining position. It must be recognized, however, that many children, and especially the smaller ones, *do* prefer to lie down on a couch or even on the floor and the therapist should always accommodate their wishes.

Parental Expectations

Aside from the usual apprehensions and misconceptions about hypnosis (see chapter 1), parents may be especially prone to the hope or belief that hypnosis will, somehow, all by itself relieve the child of all of his anxieties. And all too often parents imagine that this will be done with almost magical ease and speed. Finally, parents will not infrequently identify the problem as lying "inside" the child, and thus imagine that they are mere onlookers as the therapist does therapeutic things to the child.

This last problem is in some respects the most serious one and will, if left unaltered, prove to be an insuperable barrier to therapeutic change. Parents must be helped to see that no problem can be located solely within the child. It is a truism that the child's interactions with his environment will be the determinants of the topography, frequency, and modifiability of his behavior. It is no less axiomatic that the child's parents constitute the most important part of this environment. It is beyond the scope of this chapter to go into the use of contingency management procedures for the analysis and elimination of problem behaviors. The interested therapist can consult one of a variety of good texts in the area (for example, Sulzer-Azaroff & Mayer, 1977). We would strongly suggest at this point only that the therapist give to the parents an overview of operant (contingency management) explanations and techniques. Patterson and Guillion (1968) have written a readable and extremely practical step-by-step guide to the use of these reinforcement procedures with children. The book is written in a programmed-text format and manages to convey the essential information in a nontechnical fashion. Irrespective of how it is done, the therapist's first job is to educate the parents to an appreciation of *their* role in the child's problem. Blame of course is out of the question and the therapist should not assign the cause of the child's difficulties to the parents' malevolent intentions or pathological inattention. But delivering a reinforcer after a (problem) behavior, whether intentionally or not, still operates to strengthen that behavior. Furthermore, the child's behavior may be a reflection of serious parental problems which call for attention in their own right. For example, separation fears in children are often most pronounced in those children who have an agoraphobic parent (Bowlby, 1975).

Even where parents have learned to appreciate the role of the child's environment in the genesis and persistence of his problems, they may nevertheless have excessively optimistic hopes about the speed or mode of change. Anxiety, phobic or otherwise, yields to a combination of the following: the acquisition of the requisite skills (self-control relaxation through to whatever behaviors are linked to the performance requirements and demands of the target situation), and imaginal and, where possible, direct exposure to the anxiety-eliciting environment (Goldfried & Davison, 1976).

Parents, therefore, can form the correct view of hypnosis only when they see it as a means whereby the child can learn to relax and a way of creating vivid and realistic, but safe, exposure to innocuous and yet frightening things. If parents can also acquire an appreciation of the need for integrating office-based therapies and their home application, then they can function to prompt and reinforce the child's efforts at self-direction. Reward for *daily* practice can be the difference between the child's compliance with the therapy program or his defection from it after spasmodic adherence. Again, the contingency management texts noted above contain a great deal of useful and practical guidance. Our purpose here is to state the general point: programs that begin and end in the therapist's office or clinic have a built-in bias toward failure and are, in light of what we know about the principles of behavior change, indefensible.

Before beginning induction proper, the therapist and the parents must decide whether the parents are to be absent or present during the explanation and application of hypnosis. We strongly suggest that the explanation phase—what hypnosis is and what it is not, how it can be of help to the child, and so on —be conducted with the child elsewhere. If the youngster's first contact with hypnosis is a collection of more or less unintelligible words passing between therapist and parents, then he will be more confused than informed about "what is to happen to him." Parents, too, will need to feel free to give their account of the child's problem without holding back for fear of upsetting or alarming the child. They may wish to give expression to whatever doubts or misgivings about hypnosis they hold.

During induction the parents should be out of the therapy room—if the child can tolerate this separation. The good contact, sometimes referred to as rapport, which is so essential to hypnosis with children, can be diluted or impeded by the presence of the parents. The child, instead of orienting himself to the therapist and his own reactions to the therapist's behavior, may begin to look for the parents' reaction. With those children who show very strong attachment concerns and separation distress (Bowlby, 1975), the absence of the parent may prove to be terribly disturbing. Under such conditions the parents' presence may be necessary—at least at the outset. If so, then the next best strategy is for the parents to sit out of direct sight of the child. Eventually, after a few initial checks on the parents' whereabouts the youngster will begin to pay greater attention to the therapist.

Duration of Hypnotic Episodes

Whereas adults are able to involve themselves in therapy for relatively long periods (say, 45 minutes), it must be recognized that children lack this attentional durability. Generally speaking, they have a short attention span and, consequently, hypnosis must be geared to take this into account. We would suggest that hypnotic sessions be prolonged for no more than 15 or 20 minutes, since any extension past this time only results in the child becoming restless and inattentive. In some younger or highly anxious children, we even adopt the policy of dividing the hypnotic session into two parts, each being of approximately ten minutes' duration. Following initial hypnosis and termination, the child's experiences are discussed with him. This provides the child with an opportunity to voice any fears or concerns, while at the same time providing the therapist with valuable feedback which he can use to advantage in the second session. Most children find it easier to deal with a short session in this way, and, furthermore, it seems to have a potentiating effect on the induction of subsequent hypnosis (similar to the fractionation procedure used in adults).

A brief duration, however, does not guarantee that the child's hypnotic reactions will be stable across that period. The depth of hypnosis a child will achieve may vary markedly within a hypnotic episode. This variability can also be recognized in adults, but there is no doubt children experience a more labile hypnotic state, and this will be more evident when the episode is prolonged. Since the clinical facts indicate that when a threshold of moderate levels of hypnotizability and/or depth of hypnosis are exceeded suggestions and imagery gain greater impact, the practitioner will need to be attuned to changes in depth of hypnosis. We recognize that this is easier to defend in theory than it is to carry out in practice. The child can be asked to rate how "floppy" or "floaty" he feels, but such questions may stimulate cognitive processes of calculation and self-scrutiny which are, by our reckoning, at odds with the processes of hypnosis (this problem holds for adults, too). The practioner may have to be satisfied with entirely peripheral measures (rate and depth of breathing, the number and kind of patient-initiated postural changes, etc.). These are imperfect measures of hypnosis, and it must be acknowledged that assessment of depth remains a problem without an ideal solution.

Hypnotic Induction Techniques in Children

In general terms, hypnotic induction procedures should aim at exploiting a child's inherent behavioral characteristics: his desire to explore new horizons, learn new skills, and indulge in boundless fantasy. For this reason, imaginal techniques obviously are eminently suitable for children, but it should not be thought that these are the only induction methods that can be used. We take Gardner's (1974) point that confining induction to the use of imaginal techniques only will minimize our rate of success, and in all cases the procedure used must fit the child rather than the reverse. We have chosen to describe below a number of methods that lend themselves to children's usage, but as in the case of adults, it must be recognized that the phraseology should be adapted to suit both the therapist and the child.

Before commencing induction, it is vital that the therapist ensure that the child fully understand the words and terminology, especially the word *imagine*. We stress this issue because it is a word which occurs with considerable frequency in children's induction techniques ("I want you to imagine that you are playing at the beach"). Unless the therapist clarifies its meaning *before* therapy commences, he is likely to assume, quite wrongly in many patients, that its meaning is understood by the young person. If, however, the child's hypnotic responsiveness has already been assessed by means of the SHCS:Child, the patient will already be familiar with the concept of imagination—another reason, we believe, for using an assessment scale before embarking on hypnosis in children.

The induction procedures that have been used can be grouped under two headings, imaginal techniques and eye-fixation techniques.

Imaginal Procedures

It has already been stated that children have a great capacity for imaginative involvement (Hilgard, 1970). Most children appear to have the ability to fantasize what is, for them, an unusual scene (floating on a cloud), although some do prefer to visualize scenes with which they are familiar (for example, beach, garden, or country situations). We cannot overstate the need to determine, beforehand, the type of imaginative scene that the child prefers to visualize. For the child whose imaginative sensibility is such that he enjoys the idea of floating on a soft woolly cloud, or floating in space like an astronaut, the type of imagery we employ is as follows:

"We were talking just now about how nice it would be to float along on a soft woolly cloud. Why not close your eyes, just as if you were resting . . . that's fine. See if you can picture yourself lying back on a soft woolly cloud . . . it will feel as though you are floating on a bed of cotton wool . . . notice how soft and comfortable it feels . . . so comfortable . . . so peaceful that the whole of your body feels as though you are floating . . . your arms are resting in the air and your head is resting on an air pillow . . . imagine that you are lying back in this cloud, gently floating along with it. . . . As soon as you feel this pleasant, comfortable feeling of floating, just nod your head . . . that's good . . . notice the clear blue sky all around you . . . the sun is shining and you feel very warm and peaceful . . . and you know, the cloud that you are floating on has a number . . . number ten . . . there are lots and lots of clouds . . . and in a moment you are going to float gently downward from cloud ten . . . you will feel as though you are floating from cloud to cloud . . . and all the time you will feel more relaxed . . . and comfortable . . . so peaceful . . . you are going to float to cloud nine, then to cloud eight, and so on until you reach cloud one . . . as you float from cloud to cloud, you will feel yourself becoming more relaxed and peaceful.

"Now, as I count slowly backward from ten to one, I should like you to see yourself and feel yourself slowly floating from cloud to cloud . . . and as soon as you feel yourself comfortably floating on that cloud, you will nod your head. Ready . . . picture now that you are floating . . . floating gently to cloud nine . . . relaxed and floppy . . . it feels good on that cloud . . . floating downward to cloud eight . . . peaceful, calm . . . you are now at cloud one, feel yourself sinking back in that soft, woolly cloud . . . every part of you feels peaceful and calm . . . and I want you to go on imagining that you are lying back in that cloud even as I talk to you. It feels so nice just to be calm and relaxed."

Another imaginative technique that can be employed is having the child visualize descending a flight of steps to a favored scene (a room full of toys; a beach).

"How would you like to imagine that you are going down to a
magic room, where there are all sorts of beautiful toys to play
with? Good . . . would you like to close your eyes, and in a moment, you are going to imagine yourself standing at the top of
ten stairs which will take you to this very beautiful room . . . as
soon as you can picture yourself standing at the top of those ten
stairs you will nod your head . . . good . . . now, I'm going to
count slowly from ten back to one, and as I do so I want you to
imagine that you are walking down each stair in time with my
counting . . . and as you go down each stair . . . you will become
more and more comfortable, peaceful and calm . . . until by the
time you get to the bottom of those stairs, you will feel very
peaceful and relaxed indeed.

"As soon as you reach the bottom of the stairs, and feel completely comfortable and relaxed, you will once again nod your
head. Ready? As I count, imagine yourself walking slowly down
each of these stairs . . . becoming so much more relaxed and
peaceful as you go down each one. Ten . . . nine . . . eight. . . .
Good. You are now in that very beautiful room . . . it is such a
peaceful room. . . . It is so quiet, isn't it? . . . You will probably
notice lots of toys and games that you like. . . . Nod your head if
you can see them. . . . Good. . . . You can probably see toys that
you have always wanted to play with. . . . Why not go ahead and
enjoy playing with them . . . you can even do this as I go on
talking to you. . . ."

The content of the aforementioned scene (playroom, toys), as
with all induction imagery, must be carefully assessed as to the
impact it has upon the child. If the imagery has the effect of
lowering the child's anxieties, producing a focused attention and a
sense of quiet and relaxation, then it should be retained. However,
any imagery, which, on an *a priori* basis, seems to be appropriate,
but which, nevertheless, stimulates the child's excitement (even if it
is pleasant in tone) should be discarded in favor of equally pleasant
but low-arousal imagery (Dimension 2; see chapter 2). To take
another example, most children slow the tempo of their activities
when eating or drinking. There is some evidence that eating something nice *or the imagination of that,* exerts a calming influence
(Jones, 1924; Wolpe, 1969) in most but not in all people. If it does,
then the practitioner can insert imaginal eating ("as you rest on the
cloud, propped up on a cloud pillow, you are slowly licking a tasty
ice cream cone") at any point during the induction or, later, during
imaginal contact with a phobic scene. The *content* of the induction

scenes is not what counts; it is the central effect(s) which is (are) produced by them which must be the final determinant of whether it is hypnotic or exciting.

A technique favored by a number of authors (for example, Ambrose, 1968; Falck, 1964) calls upon the child to imagine a television program. Before using this particular procedure, it is necessary for the therapist to ask the child about his favorite program, whether he has a color or black-and-white TV set, and details about the room in which the set is situated. The therapist then proceeds:

"How would you like to imagine you're watching your favorite program on TV—*The Brady Bunch* isn't it? Well, you can do this and learn to relax at the same time. I'm sure you will enjoy this, so why not close your eyes and imagine that you are at home, in your TV room. You can see your TV set in the corner near the window . . . as soon as you can picture it, just nod your head . . . good. . . . In a moment, I'm going to ask you to switch on that set, and as soon as you do so, your left pointer finger will lift into the air. That finger is the picture finger, and as long as you keep it raised you will always be able to see the picture. Now, go ahead and switch on the set . . . good. . . . I can see that the picture is on. But you will notice that you can't hear any sound yet . . . and its no good watching TV unless you can hear the sound. If you lift your right pointer finger, that will turn on the sound, and you will be able to hear it as long as that finger is raised . . . that's good. As you go on watching the show, you will become so very, very relaxed . . . you will feel peaceful . . . you may feel floaty . . . or heavy . . . that's OK . . . just enjoy it. You will hear me talking to you as you watch your TV program, but it won't seem to bother you. Just go ahead and enjoy your program and all the time, you will become so very relaxed."

The practitioner can also use the TV screen procedure for therapeutic purposes by asking the child to imagine that he is changing channels, and seeing some scene (for example, at school) associated with his difficulties. In this way, the therapist can incorporate therapeutic suggestions as part of the child's imagery.

Eye-Fixation Procedures

These methods differ from those used in adults only in the respect that they should be used in a way that captures the child's interest. The essential process here is the narrowing of the attentional focus, and the ways in which this can be achieved are obviously unlimited. Young children, in particular, are often fascinated by a therapist's watch (assuming that it is not of the digital variety), and this can be utilized to good effect as follows:

"You seem to be interested in my watch. . . . It's nice isn't it? . . . Why not hold it in your hand and see how that big hand keeps going around and around [indicating the sweep second hand]. Now, if you keep on looking at that hand going around . . . you are going to feel very relaxed . . . very comfortable . . . each time it goes around you will feel your eyelids getting heavier and heavier . . . heavier . . . and heavier . . . so heavy in fact that in a little while they will feel as though they just want to close . . . good . . . and now that your eyes are closed you feel even more relaxed and comfortable . . . feeling heavy like a piece of rock . . . it feels so nice to relax in this way."

An eye-fixation technique which is more suitable for an older age group of children (say, six to ten years) is an adaptation of the induction procedure used in the SHCS:Child. This technique is thought to be "especially useful with children who want some outward and visible sign that they have entered the trance state" (Gardner, 1981). Here, the therapist first draws a face on the child's thumbnail ("a clown's face") and the child is requested to rest his hand on his legs and to stare at the face. The procedure then continues:

"As you keep on looking at that clown's face, you may notice some different feelings coming into your hand . . . the fingers may become restless and move a little . . . the hand is becoming lighter and lighter . . . and all the time, you are feeling so much more relaxed . . . so relaxed that your eyelids are starting to feel very heavy . . . the hand is becoming even lighter . . . lighter . . . so light in fact, that it feels as though it wants to float . . . just like a balloon . . . there you see . . . it is starting to float."

We have already discussed elsewhere (see chapter 4) the importance of timing suggestions of lightness with the inhalation phase of breathing, and this same general principle applies to children. Conversely, suggestions of heaviness and relaxation should be associated with exhalation, for in this way, the therapist is able to maximize induction responses. Once hand levitation is secured, it becomes possible to utilize this to achieve eye closure and deepening of hypnosis:

"And as your hand floats upward ... it feels just like a balloon ... light and bouyant ... floating upward more and more ... and you'll feel it being drawn toward your face ... as if a string is pulling it ... gently moving closer and closer to your face ... and as it does so, your eyelids become very heavy ... very relaxed ... *so* relaxed that they may feel as though they want to close ... if they do, just let them close ... they will feel so comfortable and relaxed when they are closed ... and as the hand moves closer and closer to your face, so you will feel a nice relaxed feeling all through your body ... it will feel heavy ... floppy ... relaxed all over."

Usually, eye closure will occur spontaneously as the young patient's hand levitates. Occasionally, however, this does not happen, and in this event the therapist suggests eye closure when the hand comes in contact with the face. Following arm levitation it is, of course, necessary to return the arm to a resting position and normal sensation through the use of appropriate suggestions. These can be given in such a way that they facilitate the hypnotic response (for example, by stressing the involuntary nature of the reaction: "your arm is being pulled down by a very heavy weight").

The Dropped-Coin Technique

It has already been noted that, irrespective of the techniques used for achieving eye fixation and closure, the essential underlying mechanism is the same whether we are considering children or adults, i.e., to narrow the patient's attentional processes and thereby progressively eliminate distracting influences. We have also indicated that many of the procedures used with children are no more than variants of adult techniques, modified in a way that they will more readily capture a child's interest. The dropped-coin technique is an example of a method which has been widely used for the induction of hypnosis in adults (Tinkler, 1971), and which also lends itself to children's usage. Olness (1975) described the successful use of this induction method in the treatment of nocturnal enuresis in children. Her approach involved drawing a clown's face on a thumbnail; having the child hold that hand in front of his face; and then placing a coin between the forefinger and thumb of that hand. The young patient is told that as he concentrates on the thumbnail he will become very relaxed, and that the coin will become so heavy that it will slip down and fall. Further, at that point, his eyelids will feel so relaxed that they will close.

A point to be noted here is that the technique described by Olness favors the holding of the coin between the forefinger and thumb. The adduction force exerted by the thumb is the most powerful of all the digital muscle actions, and this may be of special importance when using this procedure in an anxious child. Here, the child's tension state may be of such magnitude that he holds on to the coin with a determined tenacity and thus will fail to release it even in spite of persuasive suggestions from the therapist. A way around this has been devised by the second author, who places the coin between the child's forefinger and middle finger. These two fingers have a relatively weak adduction action (compared with that of the thumb), and thus there is a greater likelihood of compliance to suggestions that the coin will drop as the young patient relaxes. The procedure we adopt takes the following form:

> "I'm going to help you relax today, and in order to do this, let's first of all draw a funny face on one of your thumbnails. Which one would you like to use? Good. Now I'm going to draw a clown's face on your nail so that you can stare at it all the time. I want you to hold your hand level with your face and to stare at the clown's face all the time. But as you do so, I am going to slip a small coin between your fingers . . . so. Just go on staring at that funny face on your thumbnail . . . and as you do, you will feel your eyelids becoming very relaxed . . . so very relaxed and heavy . . . and this feeling of relaxation will come all through your body . . . it feels so nice and comfortable . . . and the fingers too will relax a little more all the time, until in a little while . . . the coin will gently slip from your fingers. When that happens, that will be the signal for your eyes to relax completely and close . . . just keep staring at that thumbnail all the time . . . becoming more and more relaxed all the time." [The therapist should keep on repeating suggestions of relaxation until the coin slips away from the fingers and the eyelids close.]

Although children are recognized as being highly susceptible to hypnosis, it will frequently be found that the time taken to achieve eye closure is, on average, longer than for adults. This apparent paradox is presumably due to the fact that many children are reluctant to close their eyes because of the fears and beliefs that they harbor, or because (in the case of young children particularly) they have a need to keep track of their environment (Morgan & Hilgard, 1979). Thus, if the therapist elects to elicit eye closure (and as noted earlier, it may not always be appropriate or possible to do so), then he must also be prepared to spend an adequate amount of time to achieve this goal. This issue alone points to the dropped-coin technique being less than ideal for some young patients, since it relies heavily upon eye closure occurring in response to a cue, i.e., the dropping of the coin. Even using the modification described above, it has been our experience that many children will release the coin long before their eyes are ready to close. Such an occurrence will inevitably lead the young patient into having even more self-doubts about his ability to be hypnotized. This is best dealt with in the following manner:

> "That's fine, now that the coin has dropped down, you will feel even more relaxed . . . the eyelids will become even heavier . . . so heavy in fact, that they will want to close in a little while. Keep on staring at the clown's face . . . and you will feel yourself becoming more relaxed . . . heavier . . . the eyelids feel heavy . . . *so* very heavy. Just let them close now . . . and feel relaxed all through your body."

Other Induction Considerations

So far in this chapter we have described induction techniques which are specific for children—especially younger ones. In older children, however, the therapist can often utilize adult techniques, modifying their presentation where necessary to fit in with the child's level of understanding. Many children above the age of ten years, for example, prefer the eye-fixation technique outlined in chapter 4. This further points to the need for the clinician to be eclectic in his approach to induction—always selecting those techniques best suited to that particular individual.

It may seem strange to the reader that we have not, to this point, discussed deepening techniques in relation to children. Such procedures are indicated in the attainment of hypnotic disengagement in adults, but they are rarely, if ever, called for in children's hypnosis. This probably relates to the fact that, because of their superior hypnotic potential, they are readily able to achieve a state of hypnotic involvement or absorption (Tellegen & Atkinson, 1974) using induction procedures alone. At the same time it must also be recalled that children can show intraepisode variability, or lability, in hypnotic disengagement. So where a therapist feels the necessity for some form of deepening procedure, we advocate the use of counting. This technique, although very simple in format, is an effective way of deepening hypnosis:

> "I am going to count slowly to ten, and as I do so you will feel yourself relaxing even more than you are at this moment . . . becoming even more comfortable . . . even heavier and floppier. . . . Ready . . . one . . . you can feel your whole body becoming so heavy in the chair . . . two . . . heavier and heavier. . . ."

Home Practice: Self-hypnosis

The strength of any clinical technique for the modification of behavior is exactly proportional to the changes it can foster in the natural (i.e., nonclinical) environment. These changes are of two sorts: the ones directly relevant to the presenting problem and those which prepare the patient to engage in or refrain from certain key responses. The anxious person, to oversimplify a little, needs to learn how to keep from being over-tense and has to approach, stay in, and show competence while in the distressing environment.

The Technique

Although Gardner (1981) has differentiated between self-hypnosis (a self-induced procedure following heterohypnosis) and autohypnosis (a spontaneously induced hypnosis produced without therapist guidance), in practical terms (and abiding by Gardner's definition), most young patients use self-hypnosis for home practice. Thus, the technique suggested for use by the patient at home should be modeled upon that used by the therapist—a point we have already discussed in connection with adults (see chapter 4).

Children are particularly adept at using imagery, and for this reason we favor an imaginal technique for self-hypnotic induction. Many children feel, but rarely voice, certain concerns about using therapy on their own—in particular, whether they can do it themselves and whether they can exit from it when they so desire. It is important, therefore, that the therapist *assumes* that the child holds these fears, so that they can be openly discussed before therapy commences. Furthermore, it is a wise step to have the child induce and terminate hypnosis (by whatever selected procedure) in the presence of the therapist, but this should not be done until the young patient has experienced at least two sessions of heterohypnosis. Only in this way will the child feel reasonably comfortable and confident about using self-hypnosis at home.

A suggested approach is as follows:

"Since you have been coming to see me here, you have noticed how comfortable and relaxed you can become by doing the things that I suggest to you. And because you feel so relaxed, it seems to help you feel better each day, and much more able to deal with [specify the presenting problems]. Now, I'm going to show you how you can have these same pleasant feelings at home. It will be quite easy really for you to relax just as you do here. Simply do the things that we do here and let things happen. But before we start, I want you to tell me how you are going to use each of the stages. [The child describes the procedures and these are clarified by the clinician wherever appropriate.] That's good. Today, you are going to go through each of these steps so that you understand them and can then use them at home on your own.

"Now, rest back, close your eyes, and imagine that you are standing at the top of ten steps looking down to a beautiful beach. You are looking forward to playing and relaxing on the warm sand, and when you are ready, picture yourself going down each step in time with each occasion that you breathe out, and as you do so, you will count silently from ten back to one with each step that you go down. Once you are on the beach you can imagine playing in the sand; feel the warm sun on your body; feel as though you are really there. As soon as you feel very peaceful and relaxed on the beach, you will nod your head—so that I know that you are very comfortable. When you do this at home and get this nice, relaxed feeling, I want you then to think of some of the ways that you are learning to get rid of your problem."

Self-hypnosis plays a very real role in the elicitation and maintenance of these sought-after changes. To this end, the anxious child should be encouraged to practice self-relaxation every day in order to reinforce desired behavior (increased control over his problem), and he should also be encouraged to approach instead of avoid the situation in which he feels anxious and threatened. We ask older children to fill out a form—which we provide—and to indicate: (1) whether they did the exercise; (2) how tense or "floppy" they felt while doing it; and (3) how they felt when they took an imaginal trip into the anxiety situation. Next, the children should be encouraged to do daily live practice, if possible in the anxiety environment or one like it.

Role of Parents in Self-hypnosis

To help the child keep up with these homework assignments, the cooperation of the parents is essential. At this juncture we wish to take up the question of the parental behavior which is needed to encourage the necessary practice in self-control relaxation, imaginal, and *in vivo* exposure. If there is no parental cooperation then we have little hesitation in offering this pessimistic assessment: if the child's parents do not wish or are not able to cooperate, then little, if any, benefit will come out of any hypnobehavioral program regardless of how intelligently conceived.

Exceptions to this general rule center around those situations where there already exists a disturbed parent–child relationship, or where one or other parent is especially anxious about the child's problems. Here, the involvement of the parents is quite likely to precipitate a resistance on the part of the child to self-therapy, for he will view it as just another way of being coerced.

Another consideration with regard to parental involvement is whether parents should be present as the child does his home therapy. Gardner (1981) recommends the presence of parents while the child practices his self-hypnosis on the basis that they "provide assurance and encouragement [to children] as they enter and deepen the trance state." In order for the parents to be familiar with the child's being in hypnosis, she suggests that they should be present when the child is practicing the procedure in the therapist's office. The presence of the parents may be indicated in an anxious child, but overall, we tend to take a different view and believe that the parents' role should be that of encouraging the child to discuss his feelings and responses in self-hypnosis openly at home, and also of gently reminding him to use the technique. In this way, the young patient is able to gain the satisfaction of developing his own skills with hypnosis—a matter which may be of considerable importance to one who lacks self-esteem and self-confidence.

Resistance to Home Practice

No matter how detailed the explanation of the therapist concerning the need for regular use of self-therapy, some children will consistently fail to practice it. When this occurs, the child is invariably harboring a significant underlying concern. Often, for instance, he may doubt his abilities to use it on his own. These doubts can usually be allayed by discussion and having him repeatedly use the technique with the therapist or in the presence of a parent who has been informed of the child's fears. More often, resistance to self-therapy stems from more subtle factors. Thus, a child who has "a strong need for autonomy may resist the therapist's suggestion for regular use of self-hypnosis, perceiving the suggestion as one more external demand" (Gardner, 1981, p. 304). In short, it can be said that whenever resistance to home practice occurs, there is usually a sound underlying reason, and once elicited by the practitioner, it can be dealt with by discussion with the young patient and/or the parents. In the event of noncompliance thereafter, it is better to restrict treatment to the consulting room rather than convert the issue into one of major importance.

In this chapter we have had to place more reliance on our own views and to draw more heavily upon our own experience than was the case in our treatment of the nature of hypnosis, its modification, meditation, and all of the other topics. The reader may wonder whether the sparse literature on hypnosis in children does not, after all, indicate some serious obstacles to or limitations of hypnosis with children. We do not think this to be the case, and apart from the myths and misconceptions that can deter patient and practitioner from exploring its use, there is a more general explanation for the underuse of hypnosis in children. Quite simply, the "cognitive revolution" which came to behavior therapy over a decade ago has never really taken hold in the area of child behavior therapy. It is true that operant contingency management methods have been remarkably successful. But the practitioner should not overlook the requirement of an external manipulator of reinforcement which leaves the child dependent upon the behavioral engineer (or parent) who devises and runs these home-based programs. Critics have been quick to point out the advantages of cognitive therapies that can be used in a complementary way to these techniques and methods *in adults*. It is not clear to us why the full range of cognitive techniques cannot be investigated with children. Our final point, then, is that hypnosis in children can and should be used to assist or potentiate other clinical techniques.

6

Meditation: Its Relationship to Hypnosis

Close up his eyes, and draw the curtain close; And let us all to meditation.

—William Shakespeare, *King Henry VI, Part II*

We have said that a person's progress toward hypnosis, the extent or "depth" of hypnosis, and the reengagement (i.e., the termination of hypnosis) can be assessed through the psychophysiological changes on the six dimensions we have enumerated. In this chapter we will take up the question that arises from this analysis: Which of these changes has the status of being crucial or essential for hypnosis? The related, clinical, concern is: Can patients be taught to increase their degree of control over the relevant systems which subserve this change?

We surveyed the perspectives and definitions of hypnosis proposed by the major contemporary and earlier writers and discovered a solid consensus that a more focused as opposed to a more mobile (or scanning) attention is the indispensable ingredient in hypnosis. We see this clearly expressed in the Spiegels' (1978) definition of hypnosis, which because of its importance we requote here: the hypnotic "experience is characterized by an ability to sustain in response to a signal a state of attentive, receptive, intense focal concentration with diminished peripheral awareness" (p. 22). This is stressed in much the same way by Frankel. The object of hypnosis, he writes, "is to lead the subject—to redistribute his attention *so as to withdraw it from the general surroundings and focus it on a circumscribed area*" (Frankel, 1976, p. 22, emphasis added). Notice how similar these two specifications are to White's (1941) words in his classic paper. The operator must work "to reduce as far as possible the perceptual supports which might *serve to sustain a wider frame of reference*" (p. 502, emphasis added). Shor (1969) not only placed great emphasis on the control of attention (hypnosis requires the "focusing of one's attention on a small range of preoccupations") but goes further to insist that "suggestibility and hypersuggestibility are not conceptualized as the fundamental processes of hypnosis . . . *but as secondary* or derivative consequences of isolation" (p. 241, emphasis added). By isolation, or focusing, he refers to the attenuation of intrusive, task-irrelevant cognitions. Full imaginative involvement is possible, Shor (1969) says, "because the usual competitors for attention have been . . . quietened" (p. 235).

There is research support from within the area of hypnosis pointing to the importance of attentional control and the ability to maintain a psychological "tunnel vision." Tellegen and Atkinson (1974) found that high hypnotizability was positively related to "absorption" (and see Hilgard, 1970, p. 23). Outside of hypnosis, the value of imagery therapies (for example, covert sensitization, imaginal desensitization) has been demonstrated, and clinical researchers have begun to be interested in the means by which the integrity of imagery can be protected. This concept may also be pursued by asking which conditions are inimical to rich, vivid, absorbing imagery. It is known that imagery is "degraded when too much irrelevant material is injected" (Strosahl & Ascough, 1981, p. 427; also see Kosslyn, 1975), and this in turn will be influenced by minimizing the amount, variety, and rate of change of the covert or cognitive stimuli sampled. Said another way, attentional focusing, and the control necessary for this, must be present.

It is clear enough that there is a very wide measure of agreement on the central role of attentional focusing in hypnosis. We would add that the ability to tune out irrelevant and intrusive material is even more important in self-hypnosis. One major difference between heterohypnosis and self-hypnosis is the presence or absence, respectively, of an outside aid to attentional focusing (most notably the presence of the hypnotist and his words). We have seen many patients who score in the moderate or higher range when

tested with a clinical assessment scale but who perform as low hypnotizable subjects when using self-hypnosis. Invariably this occurs
because they are quite unable to keep their mind from wandering
once they sit down and close their eyes. This means that the therapeutic suggestions and images are drowned out or attenuated by the
internal cacophony produced as attention jumps from instant to instant for the whole period of self-therapy.

We come now to our second question. If attentional control is
as crucial as all seem to believe, and we believe that it is, what, if
anything, can be done to bring this goal within reach? In recent
years significant advances have been made in our understanding of
the neural substrates of attention (Ornstein, 1977; Pribram &
McGuiness, 1975). More important, "A growing body of data indicates that humans can acquire some degree of control over usually
autonomous psychobiological processes through a variety of procedures. . . . One of the oldest techniques for achieving such self-
regulation, particularly of attention, is meditation" (Davidson &
Goleman, 1977, p. 292). In view of this, it would seem appropriate
to examine the concepts, benefits, and techniques of meditation.

Meditation Conceptualized

Anyone conversant with the literature on meditation will be aware
that there are many different kinds of meditation. They include
such diverse practices as sitting quietly, usually with the eyes closed,
and silently repeating certain words or phrases, staring fixedly at a
specially selected figure or object, engaging in repetitive and stereotyped movements, or any combination of these. The well-known
meditation systems comprise a heterogeneous set of practices, and
judged in terms of their surface details there would seem to be
justification for always using the word *meditation* in its plural form.
But when scrutinized closely, commonalities among these seemingly
diverse practices can be detected. This has been nicely summarized
by Ornstein (1977). His survey revealed that behind the great variety
of procedures, a unity can be perceived:

> The common element in these diverse practices seems to be the active
> restriction of awareness to a single, unchanging process and the *with-*
> *drawal of attention* from ordinary thought. It does not seem to matter
> which actual physical practice is followed; whether one symbol or
> another is employed; whether the visual system is used or body move-

ments repeated; whether the awareness [i.e., attention] is focused on a limb or on a sound or on a word or on a prayer. This process might be considered an attempt to cycle the same subroutine in the nervous system. The instructions for meditation are always consistent with this surmise: one is instructed always to rid awareness of any thought save the object of meditation, to *shut oneself off from the main flow of ongoing external activity and to pay attention only to the object or process* of meditation. Almost any process or object seems usable and has probably been used. (Ornstein, 1977, pp. 171–172; emphases added)

In the emphasis given to disengagement, a continuing metaphor in this book, the elements of meditative practice converge with those of hypnosis. First, the meditator usually begins by closing his eyes. Whether eyes are closed or open, he arranges for the surroundings to be quiet, and he isolates himself from the demands of the social environment. The very same is true of most (nondramatic) hypnotic techniques. Second, the meditator will sit at rest or adopt some comfortable posture which promotes relaxation while at the same time preserving a degree of wakefulness. In most systems, a straight back and not a slouched position is deemed to be important. Less muscular effort is required, and with a straight back, the discomfort of constricted viscera is avoided (Hirai, 1975; Humphreys, 1935). In the Eastern writings, the reasons proposed for the attention to posture, and the insistence upon the need for a straight spine, come from the religious-vitalistic theory of physiology held by these meditators.

The third element, attentional focusing upon a simple repetitive word, phrase, or mental image (or in some systems of meditation, a brief cycle of movements done over and over), has already been discussed. At the same time, in hypnosis and meditation alike, the student is encouraged to adopt a disinterested and tolerant attitude toward intrusive cognitions and to gently dismiss and/or to let them pass from the center of awareness. (Specialists in the area will note we are talking about "concentrative" meditation; the other kind, "opening-up" meditation, to use Ornstein's terminology, will not be dealt with here. We have encountered serious difficulties in using the opening-up varieties and we do not recommend them for patient populations.)

A direct test of comparability of hypnosis and meditation was reported by Bärmark and Gaunitz (1979) of work they carried out at the University of Uppsala in Sweden. They, too, were impressed with the resemblance in application of hypnosis and meditation. As they noted:

Meditative techniques often involve a procedure which restricts the attention of the meditator . . . the stimulus used as the focus of attention is repeatedly presented in a monotonous manner . . . the attention is restricted to the silent repetition of a word—the *mantra*. The importance of adopting a passive, detached attitude toward the object of attention and toward the functional result to be achieved is especially emphasized. (p. 227)

In hypnosis the same encouragement toward a detached attitude coupled with instructions to focus the attention can be seen:

In heterohypnotic techniques, S is usually invited to focus his/her attention on suggestions of relaxation and concentration, which are monotonously repeated by the hypnotist . . . [and thus it can be concluded that] meditation and hypnotic relaxation may be considered as techniques for regulating the information from the environment, considerably lowering the intensity and variation of external stimuli. (Bärmark & Gaunitz, 1979, p. 227)

The results from this study revealed that the similarities between meditation and hypnosis extend beyond the common procedures, through to the physiological and psychological reactions measured in their subjects. The physiological changes, though of no startling magnitude, did, nevertheless, show up in the same direction across heart-rate, respiration-rate, and skin-temperature variables. In the main, the self-report data from the hypnotic subjects were very much like the experiences reported by the meditators. Bärmark and Gaunitz (1979) drew the following conclusions from their results: meditation and hypnosis are both phenomenologically altered states of consciousness which bear a marked resemblance to one another.

Reports along the same lines have come from our patients, with one interesting exception. There seems to be a lag between the onset times of the disengagement reactions in hypnosis compared with that of meditation. The hypnoidal responses in meditation are often not demonstrated until days or even weeks after starting a meditation program. This seems to be linked in part to the difficulties people experience in achieving and holding a focus of attention without the aid of an outside source—as is given by the therapist in hypnosis.

The chief difference between meditation and hypnosis is that specialists in meditation, Western as well as Eastern, have made the control of attention a number one priority. They recognize the great difficulties many people have in acquiring and maintaining a relaxed but focused attention. Accordingly, they have occupied themselves with a personal, clinical, and experimental study of the most effective meditation techniques to accomplish this. Some have described their researches as the investigation of meditation (LeShan, 1975); others (including the present authors) prefer the more neutral term "cognitive centering techniques" (see Carrington, 1978), while Benson (1975) has coined the expression "the relaxation response" to emphasize the effects of this training. As we see it, these are simply different ways of talking about the control of attention. If more than that is involved (as, for example, is claimed by Transcendental Meditation) then the control of attention is, at least, a common feature in all. Behavior therapists have long appreciated the many benefits that can be derived from training in progressive muscular relaxation (Goldfried & Davison, 1976; Jacobson, 1929; Paul, 1969). The acceptance of cognitive influences into behavior therapy has been accompanied by an interest in the control of attention and "mental calm." Thus, behavior therapists are, in increasing numbers, informing themselves about the techniques and uses of meditation. To date, those interested in hypnosis have held themselves aloof from this work. Beyond the use of some attention-getting technique and the inclusion of focused attention in most definitions of hypnosis (for example, Spiegel & Spiegel, 1978), hypnotists have done little or nothing to discover or to deliberately train their patients in the skills of attentional focusing. Too often the person who is deficient in these skills is written off as "insusceptible" and the matter is left at that. With the evidence before us favoring the possibilities for the modification of attentional styles through correct training, such a pessimistic or casual attitude is difficult to defend. Simple reasoning brings us to the conclusion that the practitioner who wishes to become expert at hypnosis should become proficient in the use of meditative (or "centering") techniques.

The Effects of Meditation

The initial interest in meditation centered on the ability of practiced lifelong meditators to control a wide variety of physiological reactions. The first published studies conducted with at least a degree of rigor indicated that the journalistic reports of yogis who could stop their heartbeats and survive for hours without any air were unfounded. Nevertheless, they did indicate very considerable control over supposedly involuntary reactions (Anand, Chhina, & Singh,

1961a, b; Wenger & Bagchi, 1961). Later research has made it abundantly clear that these changes could be produced, after a relatively short period, in Western subjects given "secular" training in meditation. Reductions in heart rate (Hoenig, 1968), oxygen consumption (see Carrington, 1978), and electrocortical changes [especially an increase in alpha activity of 8–13 Hz (see Benson, 1975, for a review of this work)] and decreases in the frequency of spontaneous G.S.R.s and the intensity of elicited G.S.R.s (Orme-Johnson, 1973) are changes usually taken to index a decline in anxiety (Marks, 1969).

Taken together, the physiological effects of meditation form into a configuration which resembles what W.R. Hess (1954), the Swiss Nobel Laureate in physiology, called the "tropotrophic response." These changes occur concurrently and in a coordinated manner probably under hypothalamic control and are opposite or antagonistic to the flight-or-fight responses associated with stress reactions. Hess, who studied this in animals, believed that the tropotrophic response functioned as a protective mechanism against overstress. These restorative processes in humans were called the "relaxation response" by Benson (1975), an expression which has gained widespread acceptance through Benson's best-selling book.

To sum up, meditation training can effect, sometimes in a matter of days, significant changes in a host of physiological systems. The pattern of these changes represents the existence of a hypometabolic state. This is the outcome in most, but certainly not all, of those who try meditation—a point to which we shall return when we look at the problems that can arise in meditation.

The psychological effects of meditation have received relatively little attention when compared with the enormous literature on the physiological effects. There is evidence that meditation increases performance on such diverse tasks as memorizing lists, thinking creatively, finding the solution to arithmetic problems, and discriminating pitch (Carrington, 1978). Clinicians will be more interested in the claims that long-term practice in meditation reduces the abuse of alcohol, tobacco, and other drugs (Carrington, 1978). On one finding there is widespread agreement: whatever the technique used and whatever the test applied, meditation reduces anxiety during its practice and afterward. Thus meditation (or, as we have put it earlier, neutral hypnosis) takes its place beside progressive muscular relaxation and biofeedback as a potent method of directly reducing anxiety and, indirectly, raising performance efficiency of skills which are impaired by high levels of anxiety.

What has not been established is that these benefits are unique to meditation. As far as is now known, other techniques and procedures such as progressive relaxation and biofeedback may do equally well in generating a hypometabolic state or the "relaxation response" (see Benson, 1975, pp. 70–71). And Carrington (1978, p. 58) points out that simply playing soft, pleasant music can elicit similar reactions.

There are, however, other criteria for judging the utility of the many counter-stress techniques and procedures. Compliance with practice schedules is one consideration. There is evidence that patients do not persist in biofeedback and progressive relaxation for as long as they do with meditation (Glueck & Stroebel, 1975). And that has certainly been our experience. Another criterion is the easy transferability to the nonclinical environment. Unlike biofeedback, which depends upon the use of an expensive and elaborate apparatus, and soft music, which may not be available at all times, meditation is "portable" and can be practiced anywhere—in the clinic, at home, or elsewhere. Finally, in-clinic techniques which work, in part, because they provide the patient with a focus of attention may fail altogether when he is alone and thus thrown back upon his own resources (as in self-hypnosis).

Nowadays no one disputes the psychological importance of an enhanced sense of control over important events (Abramson, Seligman, & Teasdale, 1978). Surely, then, learning to regulate one of the most important cognitive systems and acquiring attentional control need no special justification. Hence, meditation should occupy a central place in the management of anxiety, whether it is to be used as an adjunct to hypnosis training or as a therapy in its own right.

There is still another benefit that can be derived from meditation apart from its role as an attentional control in heterohypnosis and self-hypnosis and the physiological and psychological changes just reviewed. This was mentioned by William James in his *Principles of Psychology* (1890). James felt that it was impossible to overrate the importance of attention in our lives. What we do and experience, he said, is a function of what it is that we attend to. Our psychological reactions are the results of "the selection which the habitual direction of . . . attention . . . each of us literally *chooses,* by his ways of attending to things what sort of a universe he shall appear to himself to inhabit" (p. 424).

Meditation, then, teaches the person how to discipline his mind through the control of attention. In a very real sense, we are where our attention is. In the clinical sphere, we often communicate this concept to the patient with examples like the following: the person who has ten or more vivid anticipations of the visit he must pay to the dentist in 100 days' time can at the end of that period be said to have had at least 101 episodes of dental distress. His friend who has to face the same ordeal yet who has the ability to stay in the here-and-now has but one visit to the dentist. (Cf. the old saying "A lot of terrible things have occurred to me in my life and most of them never happened." And the one which reads, "The coward dies a thousand deaths and the brave man but one" should be rewritten as "The man with poor attentional control who is unable to acquire and hold a present-centered orientation dies a thousand deaths. . . ." Put this way, it would be too cumbersome to be pithy, but it would be nearer to the psychological truth.)

The person who leaves the present also makes poor contact with the *rewarding* events of his life—which is only to say that our attentional resources are finite (Broadbent, 1958). When we "take up residence" in some anticipated or remembered situation, our *psychological* contact with rewards or reinforcers is attenuated by the same amount. Though he might be firm on his determination to enjoy a pleasant meal or movie, the person who quickly becomes prey to all stray thoughts gives up at least some of the pleasurable potential which could be derived from the stimuli of the present.

Preparation for Meditation

Once the patient understands the rationale for meditative practice, the next step is the correct arrangement of the environment so that the technique can be used to best advantage.

The first matter is to ensure that there is a quiet environment as free as possible of noises and intrusions. The room need not be completely dark, but the lighting should be dimmed and the patient should sit facing away from the light source. More important, because less obvious, is the need for some free time immediately *after* the meditation period. If the person can allot just the 20 minutes of the meditation period before having to rush back into a busy schedule of activities, the anticipation of these will interfere with his efforts at attention centering. We suggest that the person select times for meditation which come before a stress-free, activity-free period. These recommendations do not require an elaborate justification, but there is an important point at issue here which calls for some comment. If the patient, who is tense and distracted most of the time, learns to break free of this debilitating pattern for only a couple of short intervals every day (i.e., during the practice of meditation or self-hypnosis or relaxation), has he learned anything more than how to get a brief respite from his distress? It seems clear to us that for the patient to get any substantial and sustained benefit, the advantages of meditation will have to generalize to the everyday situation. How then is this important aim to be realized if the techniques require near perfect conditions of quiet and calm? The answer is that it cannot be if the skills are not put to use outside of the special quiet times in the home and clinic. Later on we will outline a meditation technique that should be used in addition to the twice-a-day home practice periods. But before the person can learn to keep himself relaxed and maintain a present-centered attention in the presence of the "noise," stress, and demands of the outside world, he must arrange the most propitious conditions for the acquisition of these skills. That is why such care must be paid to engineering the greatest possible degree of control and, hence, the greatest possible chance of success.

The Time of Meditation

We have found that for most people it is desirable to do the first meditation (or self-hypnosis) exercise just after arising and before breakfast, and the second meditation in the evening. If possible, it is advisable to do it before eating or at least an hour afterward. Attempts at meditation (or self-hypnosis or relaxation) seem to be less fruitful and more difficult just after eating, although we do not know why this should be so. Putting off the evening meditation until after getting into bed is also to be avoided. The effects of the meditation-centering exercises when combined with a resting position on a comfortable bed are decidedly soporific (we have given the same warning in the chapter on the application of self-hypnosis techniques). Patients may even report with some pride and satisfaction that, within a minute or two of beginning the meditation exercise, they fell quickly asleep. If this happens they should be asked to do their meditation while sitting in a chair. These patients should also be reminded of the purposes of the meditation exercises: to (gently) discipline the unruly attentional processes; to practice detachment from the stream of thoughts and related motivational surges; to establish the inner conditions which are the prerequisite for self-hypnosis and self-suggestion; and, last (in our view), to enjoy these brief periods as times of unstressing and re-laxation. None of these purposes can be served unless the person is awake and doing the exercises. However, if *in addition* to the twice daily practice period—and the "mini-meditations" done throughout the day—the meditation is used as an aid to sleep, that is fine. Mental, meditation-like, and physical relaxation exercises have been used to good effect in combating insomnia (see Yates, 1980), but it should be made clear to the patient that while it is an excellent idea to use meditation as a self-control technique for sleep, or other problems, these "innovative" applications are not substitutes for regular, daily practice routines.

Posture for Meditation

Most teachers suggest that the person adopt a comfortable posture for meditation. A few insist that the cross-legged lotus posture of the yogi is ideal and others may advise the use of even more difficult positions. As far as we know there are no data to which disputants can appeal to decide the question of "the posture" for meditation. From our experience we suggest merely that if the patient is com-fortable and at ease, then that is sufficient. Some prefer a straight-backed chair and others find that they get the most out of medita-tion when they do the exercises flat on their backs. As long as the patient can manage to be at ease and avoid the two extremes of physical discomfort and sleep, he should be encouraged to experi-ment until he finds his favorite posture.

As a rule he will discover this more quickly and meditation will be easier if the shoes are removed, constricting clothes loosened, and wrist watches and spectacles removed. It is also preferable if the patient can refrain from folding his arms, intertwining his fingers, or crossing his legs. But note: some patients take advice about pos-ture to be a command to begin and stay with one position, in the belief that in meditation (as in hypnosis) the slightest twitch or move-ment will "break the spell." We make it a point to tell all patients about this misconception and point out that whenever they feel like adjusting their posture, they should do so and not worry further about it.

Summing up, there is no prescribed posture for meditation, but there are two points which can be distilled from the writings of professionals in the area: first, a feeling of physical comfort is essen-tial, for beginners at least; and, second, any posture selected must not ease the person into sleep before the end of the practice period.

Breathing in Meditation

In the literature on meditation, breathing is treated in two quite different ways. Breathing may be discussed in terms of its physical parameters and, related to this, the ideal rate, depth, pattern, and so on. Second, the person may be advised to think in a certain way about his breathing as he meditates—having the meditator attend to or think certain thoughts while he is breathing and about the process of breathing (as a certain rate, depth, etc.). As such, this is really a matter of thinking or cognition and, therefore, will be considered along with the other cognitive activities in meditation to be covered in the following section.

We can start our comments on the ideal style of breathing by recognizing two different but relevant facts about the relationship between breathing and psychophysiological functioning: very rapid breathing (hyperventilation) can produce a variety of stress symptoms—up to and including panic attacks (Collison, 1980; Wolpe, 1969); and slow breathing is associated with reports of relaxation and a sense of self-control in meditators and suggestions of calm in hypnosis (Benson, 1975). From this it can be deduced that patients should be instructed to breathe slowly while meditating. As reasonable a conclusion as this may appear to be, we have not found it to be helpful in application. We have found instead that if patients are counseled to breathe easily with as little effort as possible, slow breathing will soon result. By contrast, when in the past we have asked the patients to control the rate of breathing directly, they have reported that respiration seemed effortful and, often, they became distressed by feelings of being unable to get enough air. Here are the instructions which we have found most helpful.

"Close your eyes . . . take a *big* breath . . . let it go . . . now do that once more, this time a *really* big breath, as much as you can manage, fine, hold it . . . and now release it. I asked you to take those two strenuous breaths so that you could see how *not* to breathe in meditation. The best way to breathe is to just let yourself inhale and exhale as easily as possible . . . without effort . . . almost as though you are 'being breathed.' That might sound an odd sort of way to put it but you'll see after a while that the best breathing style is an effortless one . . . sort of an 'automatic pilot' effect. Don't worry about it; just go along with it . . . let it happen. Let me point out that you will not come to this all at once . . . just as a leaf falling softly, this way and that, finally drifts to the ground, so too will you gradually *ease* your way toward a *nice, easy*, no-worries kind of breathing. As for the depth, sometimes it will be deeper and at other times, less so. Just let it go along at its own depth and rate. Easy . . . regular . . . steady . . . over and over . . . and over again."

The form or topography of breathing has also received considerable attention from clinicians. There is a wide measure of agreement, despite the absence of experimental data, that diaphragmatic breathing is preferable to high, shallow breathing. This form of breathing is more difficult to teach to women, perhaps because they have received more admonitions than men to keep the stomach flat. If the patient is slow to grasp the idea, the practitioner can illustrate this by asking him to "imagine you are unable to move your chest in and out and the only way you can breathe is to push your stomach up, which causes the air to be *pulled* into your body and . . . then . . . let the air push its way out and your stomach will fall."

In all that we have had to say about the topography, depth, and rate of breathing, it should not be inferred that deeper or deliberately controlled forms are incompatible with meditative, hypnotic, or relaxation exercises. It is our feeling, however, that the methods discussed above are easy for most patients to understand and use. On one point all of the authorities agree: breathing techniques are an integral part of meditation.

Cognitive Activities in Meditation

The last and most important component of meditation centers on the cognitive activities in which the person is to engage. All of the well-known techniques of meditation provide the meditator with something to think about or, as we prefer to put it, a cognitive-centering device on which the attentional processes can fix. In terms of our conception, the purpose of these is to set up a "here-and-now" activity around which the person's attention and awareness can be organized. Such activities can function to help the meditator to resist the "capture" of his attention by concerns from the past and future as well as by activities going on around and within him. In short, the purpose of the cognitive activities in meditation is to set in motion the processes which are the basis for disengagement. The differences between the different schools turn on two issues: the way in which the attentional "anchor" should be used and the form it should take.

On this second issue, those meditational systems which have a strong spiritual dimension may require the student to use a special word or phrase. Teachers of Transcendental Meditation (T.M.) select one Sanskrit word from a larger number and this "special" word is to be repeated silently by the student as he does his meditation. Benson (1975) has devised a very simple "system" which requires of the meditators only that they say (mentally) the word *one* as they breathe in or out. The results (Benson, 1975) from his experiment seem to be of the same (impressive) magnitude as those reported by T.M. investigators. With respect to the aims that we have outlined, our results indicate that the word(s) used in meditation can be chosen almost at random. The only qualification to this generalization is the reasonable one that, if for idiosyncratic reasons, a patient dislikes a recommended "*mantra*," then it should not be forced upon him. As an example, some patients given the word *relax* to use with each exhalation discover that they soon start to *try* to relax. In attempting that, they only become preoccupied with their progress, or lack of it, toward the "goal" of relaxation. When confronted by this sort of a problem a more neutral word ("out," "smooth") may be less disruptive and assist the person more easily toward a *goalless* orientation.

The Unstructured Approach

There are two different positions as to the use of the *mantra* or cognitive-centering device which we will refer to as the "structured" and the "unstructured" approaches. Many teachers encourage an unstructured, or "permissive," attitude toward the use of cognitive activity and suggest that whenever the student cares to, he may (silently) say the key word. Carrington (1978), although not a T.M. advocate herself, does agree that it is best "to let the *mantra* drift in and out of awareness." We do not doubt that this can work well enough with non-anxious volunteer subjects, but our experience has convinced us that is unlikely to prove serviceable with many patients—at least not until they *acquire* the basic skills of attentional control. We have found that most patients are hyperdistractible and need constant assistance to, quietly, resist the movement of the attention away from the *mantra*. And, as so often happens in the initial stages, when they do get caught up in their anticipations and ruminations, patients need a way back out of the captivations of the future and the past. Thus, we have no hesitation in recommending a highly structured technique with anxious or restless patients.

The Structured Approach

This "structure" can be as simple as having the patient count "one" every time he inhales (Benson, 1975). Notice that the patient is not asked to let the word drift into his mind whenever he wishes. For too many patients this simply would not do, and they would spend the entire 20 minute period lost in the midst of their usual cognitive "noise." Many patients find even this an inadequate cognitive-centering device and report that they can not get past the first breath in, the first "one," before their attention is pulled away from the present by some train of thought built up around a future plan, a fear, or a past incident. They complain of having "nothing to do" when breathing out and therefore are then open to the pull of these irrelevant cognitions. For these patients there should be something onto which they can focus their attention and something to which they can return— once they have strayed from the task. We have them count "one" for the first time they inhale and say the word "out" when they exhale. The third breath in is accompanied by the number "three," and, as always, "out" when exhaling, and so on for the whole of the 20-minute period.

In teaching this meditation technique we have found that the following points must be mentioned and stressed repeatedly:

1. First, a pleasant and effortless rate and rhythm of breathing are to be established. This is the physical "platform" for the cognitive activities of meditation.

2. The cognitive cycle is not to be said aloud nor subvocally. It is to be heard, "in the head."

3. Under no circumstances is the patient to try to use the cognitive-centering activity to force out of the mind any thoughts or images. The therapist may need to spend some time on this. Meditation is *not* a technique of "thought stopping" or blocking. It is a way of training the attention to stay in the present—the "one–relax" sequence is an attentional "hook"—while at the same time learning to use the strengthened attention to come back to the present when the person has left it on an unintended excursion. What needs to be made clear is the distinction between thoughts on the one hand, and attention on the other. The attention we liken to a searchlight and the thought to what it illuminates. The attention is where—and when—we are; the thought is the (covert) activity we engage in once we are there. It is probably incorrect to say that a thought would not

arise, or at least not persist, unless it attracted some of our attentional resources. Nonconscious mental activity is an established fact which nowadays is widely acknowledged by cognitive psychologists (Shevrin & Dickman, 1980). This type of cognitive activity is, by definition, outside of our awareness. But by "fusing" our attention to a thought, or an image, we augment its intensity and life.

A simple and persuasive illustration of the difficulty, if not the futility, of thought-fighting can drive home the point.

> "Do you see this pen? [therapist holds his pen up to the patient's view]. Try not to think of my pen for the next 15 seconds. [The effect of telling the person *not* to think of the pen has but one effect: the therapist's pen, and the word *pen*, will occupy the patient's attention completely.] Well, I can see from your smile that you did not succeed. Perhaps you will fare better with my next request to fight a thought. How about your left shoe? OK? Good, for the next 15 seconds do not even once let yourself think of your left shoe. Ready? Go! [pause] Well, looks like another failure doesn't it? Let's give it one more try. Have you ever seen a picture of President Ronald Reagan? All right now give it your best: try to pass 15 seconds without hearing his name—*or* seeing his face. [Patients usually laugh out loud at the, by now, obvious futility in blocking out these motivationally unimportant thoughts and images.] More problems, I take it? Now let me point out something that you may find interesting. What happened to the thought of the pen? [By this time the pen should have been tucked quietly out of sight.] Gone, isn't it? But why?"

If the reply is "Well you made me think of my left shoe—or Reagan," the therapist should not allow the patient to persist in this misbelief. In effect this is interpreting the loss of "pen" from the mind as a capacity problem: "I cannot think of more than one thing at a time" is, in effect, what the patient is saying. In fact, as George Miller (1956) has pointed out, our capacity is somewhere around seven "bits" of information at a time.

> "Look, let me show you how easy it is for you to hold all three thoughts and images at one time: 'Ronald Reagan picked up my pen and your shoe.' You see? No, there is a far more interesting

reason why you stopped thinking about 'my pen.' And that is *because you stopped trying to stop.* It's a kind of mental jujitsu. By *not* fighting the thought, you attained 'victory.' Or, to put it another way, you withdrew your attention from it. In this case I helped you by giving you another task. When you, through regular practice, develop a powerful attention, you will not need external assistance or support. One more point. The three things I asked you not to think about (strictly speaking, not to attend to) were not vitally of interest to you today. And yet you did find it impossible 'not to think about it' when I asked you. Just think how much more difficult it is to 'rid your mind' of thoughts which are very distressing to you. So, when someone says 'just don't think about it' you are getting counterproductive advice, even if it is well intentioned. To repeat, do not try to fight off the thoughts. If you leave them alone—keep your attention on the *mantra*—the thoughts will go."*

4. Remind the patient that "failure" is a sure certainty. He will, despite his resolutions to the contrary, "wander" away from the task soon after beginning. This is to be expected. All that he needs to do, once he is aware of it, is simply and without emotional tumult pick up where he left off. Each time he returns to the *mantra* he adds another increment to his attentional controls.

5. The patient must realize that he is not being asked to "try" anything. He only has to do the meditation: by breathing easily, covertly, counting, and saying "out." The benefit derives from the execution of the technique, not its consequence of the moment. If, for instance, when he does this he experiences a feeling of deep peace and calm, fine. If he does not, also fine. To get across this notion we talk of meditation as "work," in a sense comparable to fitness training through jogging or calisthenics.

---

*In this passage we may be open to the charge of setting up an easy success for our position. By repeating and stressing the "crucial" word (pen, or whatever) we are making it almost inevitable that it will reverberate in the short term, echoic, memory. Were we to give the patient another minute he might temporarily be able to evade any thought of the to-be-avoided word. But the reader can test the validity of our contention for himself: fighting off a thought or image, even if possible, requires a great investment of effort and a high level of skill and practice. And most important, the thought-stopping or oppositional mode requires the patient to adopt the wrong attitude toward distressing cognitions. They are better handled through the "acceptance" which can lead to habituation.

The Need for a Rationale

When a patient goes to see a therapist for help with anxiety or phobias, he will expect to have the therapist explore the *content* of the problem or the specific behaviors of which the problem is constituted. He will be prepared to have the therapist point out the significance of certain thoughts or interpretations in the perpetuation of the problem (Ellis & Harper, 1975). If he is sophisticated in such matters, he will also expect to have his therapist focus upon certain maladaptive behaviors for which methods will be sought in the attempt to eliminate these and to supplant them with adaptive behaviors. Meditation, however, is directed at the structure and functioning of cognitive systems (LeShan, 1975). The aim of a meditation program is to make attentional controls stronger and more flexible and to deepen the individual's ability to make sustained, open, and undistorted contact with the activities going on within his inner and outer worlds. This is done on the reasoning that specific problems will be responded to more fully and more effectively if the coherence and organization of the cognitive control systems is strengthened. This is a much harder notion for the patient to understand and accept than the prehypnotic or relaxation functions of meditation.

Modifications and Special Techniques

The "count-out" meditation technique has the merit of simplicity. It is easy to teach and easy to learn and provides the person with a means by which he can "tame" and train his attentional processes. As with all meditation techniques, however, beginners find it difficult to do. Lawrence LeShan (1975) lists this as the first, and most surprising and upsetting, problem for the first-time meditator:

> This lack of trained discipline of our own will becomes immediately apparent as we do this exercise. In the words of one student of it, we find ourselves "itching, twitching, and bitching." We find ourselves constantly needing to change our physical position, or getting sleepy, . . . [thinking about] problems we have been concerned with for weeks, or unable to concentrate, or anything else we can dream up to avoid the discipline. (p. 55)

To learn how to keep a fixed attention—the *sine qua non* of meditation, self-hypnosis, and heterohypnosis—we practice "binding the mind staff to a place" to use the words of Patanjali, the renowned

Eastern philosopher. Before this skill is acquired, to any degree, however, the meditator will experience many difficulties. The only appropriate response to these involuntary departures from the directions to focus on the *mantra* is to "Treat yourself as if you were a much loved child that an adult was trying to keep walking on a narrow sidewalk" (LeShan, 1975, p. 54). There is no easy remedy for this "cognitive ataxia" except patient application to the rituals and routine of the meditation exercise. Nonetheless, the clinician must appreciate just how unexpected and disheartening these "failures" can be for the patient. Typically, the first demonstration goes very well. The clinician counts and says "out" (or whatever the exhalation word is) aloud so the patient does the same to himself. The novelty of the technique and the clinician's voice and presence function as powerful aids to establishing a focus of attention. This can lead the patient to expect the same satisfying results when he first does it by himself, at home. He soon discovers otherwise when he is brought face to face with his own limitations. It is then that he discovers that he has, in the colorful phrases of the meditation teachers, "an attention-span of a hummingbird" and, "the consciousness of a drunken monkey" (Ornstein, 1977).

As we see it, this distractibility is the main cause of the dropout rate from meditation programs. The clinician can take two steps that can sharply reduce this failure to persist. The first is to *predict* before the patient has his first solo meditation session that he will be unable to keep his attention fixed in the present and on the *mantra* for much of the time. Emphasize the inevitability of these lapses and make the point that each time he catches himself away from the job at hand, and returns to the *mantra,* he is, little by little, adding to his attentional capacity.

The second step is, where necessary, to modify the breath-counting technique to suit the individual's limitations, preferences, and style. In the years that we have been teaching meditation we would place the number of those who are able to persist and succeed with the breath-counting exercise somewhere around eight in ten. The remaining minority complain of one or more of the following problems:

1.   The first is an extreme sensitivity to noise when meditating. A patient of ours came up with a simple and ingenious solution to this problem. He put cotton in his ears to block out the sounds (swimmer's ear plugs will do as well). This had the added advantage of making the sound of his breathing quite audible. He reported, as

have many patients since, that the effect of this is very soothing. Some volunteer that it reminds them of the way an ocean tide sounds as it washes first up and then back down the beach. We have also experimented with a "white noise" generator. Clinical reports (Goldfried & Davison, 1976) suggest that this regular, gentle "hissing" sound is by itself a potent aid to muscle relaxation and hypnosis. Judging from the enthusiastic comments of our patients, it should find a place in meditation training: the sounds of the white noise, or breathing, are intrinsically pleasant, and they facilitate concentration on a here-and-now process. They also present the teacher of meditation with a dilemma. If his students require a completely controlled and totally encapsulated environment to establish and maintain a centered attention, such benefits as they derive from meditation will be limited to the effects produced within the daily practice sessions. Before there can be any long-term effects which generalize to all spheres of the patients' lives, they must have learned the skills of attentional control in nonoptimal situations. Otherwise the meditation will function as no more than a psychological soporific instead of a powerful cognitive self-control technique. Our willingness to use these aids at the *start of meditation training* is matched by our conviction that as soon as possible these must be phased out and the requisite controls internalized.

2. Another class of patients who have great difficulties in meditation are those who report that they cannot rid themselves of physical tension and restlessness. Unless this is reduced to manageable levels, patients find that they cannot develop the easy and regular breathing which provides the essential physical rhythm of meditation. Some patients are able to carry on effectively in the face of high levels of tension but most find it too challenging and give up meditating. The obvious solution would seem to be to program a period of deep muscle relaxation exercises just before embarking on meditation (see Appendix A). The one drawback to this is the extra time required. As it is, most patients find it quite a challenge to squeeze a 20-minute morning and evening meditation into their schedule. Asking for the addition of ten or more minutes of premeditation preparation may be asking for more than many patients will do.* The ideal solution is for the tense patient to go through the

---

*On this point, we have heard the rejoinder that will be familiar to the reader: the patient who *really* wants to help himself will rearrange his schedule to make the extra time. The basic premise of this argument is that it is pointless to try to change the behavior of the "unmotivated" patient. Our response is the obvious one. Motivation to change cannot be construed as an all-or-none thing, i.e., something that exists at full

standard relaxation procedure (Appendix A) before starting meditation. If time does not permit, or if the patient does not wish to
expend that much effort, an abbreviated form of the progressive
relaxation procedure can be used. Something along these lines will
probably have to be explored; our experience has taught us to be
skeptical of the relative utility of meditation as a way to eliminate
very high levels of muscle tension. Just which muscle groups should
be used can be ascertained by getting a self-report from the patient
as to where the tension is most noticeable. This should be supplemented by direct observation of the patient as he meditates. This can
reveal the area of greatest difficulty, which often will be in the
muscles of the hands, neck, shoulders, or face. The duration of this
practice can be as short as one or two minutes and still be enough to
bring the tension down to manageable levels.

    3. The recommended use of the cognitive-centering device
(*mantra*) is for the person to begin with the number "one" on the
first breath in and the word "out" (or "relax") on the first and every
breath out. After a few sessions the patient may come to know about
how many breaths he will take in the normal 20-minute session. This
can then become a way of timing the temporal progress of the session and thus is a possible distraction ("I'm halfway to the end";
"about two minutes to go"). When and if this becomes a concern, the
best way to combat it is to have the person count up to 20 and then
begin again at one. Recycling the count every 10 or 20 breaths
makes it impossible to gauge the length of the session by reference
to a distant target number.

    4. Other patients become adept at doing the "count-out" se-
quence without substantially disturbing their attention to the passing
parade of thoughts and images. They find that they can employ the
cognitive-centering technique in an automatic fashion and, in so doing, avoid any "cognitive-centering." If this persists, the two courses
of action open to the clinician are to alter the (auditory) *mantra* or to
switch to a "visual" technique. To accomplish the former, give the
patient an easy but non-rote computation to make on each inhalation. Two examples of these are: "begin at 100 and each time you
breathe in, reduce the number by 3–100, 97, 94, 91, 88 would be the
numbers for the first five inhalations"; or "Begin at 100 the first

---

strength or is completely absent. In fact, the desire to change will exist at some
intermediate strength between 0 and 100 percent, as will the reluctance to undertake
the arduous work which is entailed in a commitment to change. The art of clinical
practice, surely, is sensing the location of this threshold and knowing how to pace the
demands for behavior change.

time you breathe in, 97 the second time, 93 the third, 90 the fourth and 86 the fifth inhalation—in other words, what you'll be doing is to decrease the count by 3, 4, 3, 4, 3, 4 and so on, during the inhalations."

It has been our experience that when the auditory mantras do not work at all it is often because the individual has a stronger involvement with visual than sound imagery (the same can be seen in the way some attend more to the visual than to the auditory dimensions of the external world). Where this is the case, no amount of tinkering with the structure of the auditory mantras is going to accomplish very much. The "count-out" technique to them seems "thin" and lacking in substance when compared with the vivid pictures that pass across their field of awareness. For such people it makes better sense (in whichever way that word is taken) to "see" the numbers while breathing in and, similarly, to "see" the word *out* while exhaling (all of this with the eyes closed, of course). One patient we knew would "follow" the number (one, two, and so on) in through the nose and all the way down and visualize an *O-U-T* coming up from the center of the body and out of the nose. Some make the numbers and words different colors, while others prefer to visualize themselves seated in a chair and doing the meditation. With one exception, the content of these visual strategies does not appear to be an important factor; the patient's ability to center his attention onto it, is. That exception is that the inner (or outer—see below) thing at which the person looks should not be an image—or stimulus—which has the power to arouse strong emotional responses, whether positive or negative in affective tone. It is intuitively obvious that the *mantra* should not be constructed out of depressing, disgusting, or anxiety-inducing cognitions, but perhaps less apparent are the detrimental effects of some kinds of positive words and imagery. When they are not only positive but also exciting and extremely evocative, they lead to imagery, high levels of tension, and arousal. Such scenes capture the attention and control of the person instead of the other way around. These effects are incompatible with the aims of meditation whether viewed as an adjunct to hypnosis or as a technique of cognitive control.

5. All of the techniques and modifications covered up to this point begin with the first step of eye closure. The reason for eye closure is the same as that which calls for the meditation to take place in a quiet room: *physical* withdrawal from exciting, interesting,

or intense stimuli facilitates the *psychological* disengagement so basic
to the training of attention or the use of hypnosis. There is nothing
in principle which requires that eye closure must be a part of meditation, only that it is easier, especially for beginners. "Eyes-open"
hypnosis is possible, as is eyes-open meditation. Some adults, and
many young children (see chapter 5), in fact prefer to undergo
hypnosis or to meditate with their eyes open.

As a rule we do not recommend visual meditation for those just
starting meditation—the "pull" of the environment is often too
strong for those who have few attentional skills. When it is used, a
number of points should be carefully observed. The same conceptual stance applies in visual as in all other forms of meditation. The
person should let his gaze fall and stay upon some object without
getting caught up in the intellectual significance or emotional reactions associated with the object. If certain thoughts and feelings do
arise spontaneously, that is all right as long as the meditator lets
them pass and keeps or returns his attention to the object. The
object should be within easy visual access. The meditator should let
his gaze fall easily upon the object and no attempt should be made to
give it a discerning or critical scrutiny. A certain discipline must be
exercised against the urge to "jump" from thing to thing, but staring
for too long at anything is fatiguing and makes for other problems.
Individuals will differ in how long they are able to gaze at any one
thing before strain occurs. A useful guide is to switch to a new object
at the beginning of each (slow, regular) breath cycle (i.e., about once
every 10 seconds or so). It is probably advisable to do, at most, 10 of
the 20-minute meditation period in this way and to spend the rest of
the time on "inner" meditation.

6. Cognitive or visual techniques can be supplemented with
"movement *mantras*"—simple, easy movements repeated in tandem
with the main activities of meditation. Repetitive motions have long
been incorporated into many meditative practices. These have included rocking, spinning, swaying, and dancing (Ornstein, 1977)
and seem to achieve much the same sort of psychological effect as
paying sustained attention to cognitive or visual *mantras*. Many of
these movement *mantras,* however, are not practical for everyday
use, and smaller and less flamboyant actions can be used to the same
effect. The one described here involves a simple hand movement
done in concert with the person's breathing: the hands are clenched,
easily, as the breath is taken in and the tension is slowly released as
the person breathes out. This is done on each cycle for as long as the

patient wishes. For those patients who show strong evidence of "somatizing" their anxiety, movement meditation should be continued for the full meditation period.

Problems in Meditation

The most common problem, by far, is the patient's sense of failure after his first few attempts at meditation. Virtually *every* person we have seen has come back after a week of home practice with the complaint, "I tried it and I just couldn't do it." By "it" they usually mean clearing the mind completely of all stray or intrusive thoughts. This "failure" is as likely to occur with one form of meditation as with any other. "It" may also refer to their inability to reach a state of deep calm during meditation. The therapist's answer must be a restatement of the first aim of meditation: acquiring control over one's attention. It is to be expected, more than that, inevitable, that a week's practice will not be adequate. It will be nearer to eight weeks before they begin to notice any real improvement. And, it must be stressed, the improvement will be reflected in the ability to come back to the *mantra* more quickly and more easily. Therefore each loss of task orientation, in a sense, provides the meditator with a chance to acquire another increment to cognitive control. The patient must also be clear on two other points. First, the aim of meditation is not to drive out all thoughts and images from the mind by "direct attack." It is, rather, to cultivate the ability to be inattentive to and unimpressed by whatever thoughts and images that find their way into awareness. Second, relaxation is to be seen as a by-product of meditation and not something which validates the practice session. As a general rule, trying to achieve any sort of outcome is counterproductive. "Do it and forget *trying*," we tell the patient. Eugen Herrigel (1953) has written a superb book on meditation, and it is to him that we are indebted for the wonderful expressions "the artless art" and "the effortless effort" in relation to the optimal orientation to meditation. We have found reminders of this orientation to be especially useful when patients have had one, or a few, really good meditation sessions. The experiences can vary from those described as "deep, deep, calm" through to accounts which have an almost mystical flavor to the patient. The problem here is not these experiences themselves. The difficulty is using these as a standard against

which other meditation exercise periods must be measured. Then
the patients begin to "chase after" these feelings and, of course,
they are unavailable. For these people, too, the call must be to
return to the exercise—and let the effects take care of themselves.

Tension release reactions may appear in some patients. These
problems are reasonably rare but when they do emerge they can be
very troubling. After all, the last thing the patient wants or expects is
a (paradoxical) *increase* in anxiety and tension during meditation.
These reactions may be seen in patients who are very tense and
controlled. Carrington (1978) likens the reactions to what happens
when a tightly wound spring is suddenly released. As the spring
uncoils there may be jumps and tremors before it adjusts to a reduced state of tension. In a mild form, these adjustments may be
restricted to sudden and short-lived reflex movements. The magni-
tudes can range from quick, small fluttering movements of the
fingers or eyes all the way to large scale "jolts" in which the
shoulders or legs may move quite noticeably. They are often accompanied by a train of vivid but disconnected and "involuntary" images
which slip from memory almost as soon as they are succeeded by
new images. This whole pattern bears an obvious resemblance to the
hypnagogic imagery and related movements which are characteristic
of the border area between sleep and waking. As such, the existence
of this pattern may testify to a sleepy or fatigued condition in the
meditator. Since the chance of slipping from the hypnagogic condition into sleep is high, the patient should be advised to take up a
different position—less likely to promote dozing—or else to meditate
at a different time, when he is not as tired. In a more serious form,
"release" reactions may be marked by sudden spasms of anxiety
and/or disturbing images and thoughts. These may be prolonged,
especially in people who report themselves to be sexually deprived
(Carrington, 1978). We have seen depressed patients who have become extremely upset and even suicidal after meditation. When the
side-effects of meditation are serious and persistent, the first step to
take is *the immediate reduction in the length of meditation* down to ten or
even five minutes, once a day. It can be held at that level for a week
or two and then gradually increased. The concurrent use of directed
physical activity, progressive muscular relaxation, can assist the patient in the management of these episodes. The content of these
concerns can be raised and dealt with in the clinic (via the appropriate use of desensitization or flooding techniques). If none of the
above-mentioned methods works and these "abreactions" continue,

then meditation should be discontinued until the basic causes have been assessed and treated. Before leaving this topic, we would like to underscore how rare are such long-term adverse effects. Fewer than 1 percent of our seriously anxious and depressed patients exhibit them. Finally, even where they do appear, when the disinhibitory pressures are recognized and removed, the meditation may recommence with no harm to the patient.

Last, the practitioner may meet up with one or both of the two common misconceptions about meditation. In the emphasis given to the here-and-now, patients may assume that they are not to think of the past or the future and that if they do it is evidence of a cognitive deficiency. The point we make to the patient is the need to distinguish between *choosing* to review past events or future plans on the one hand, and having these intrude relentlessly and endlessly on the other. There is nothing wrong, and quite a lot right, with the former; the latter can be a sign of poor cognitive control. The second misconception is expressed as a worry that when the meditation exercises are being done and when a meditative (i.e., present-centered) attitude is held at other times, real thinking is hindered. This misconception springs from a belief that there is no cognitive or mental life outside of what happens inside of the scope of our attention or awareness. We have found that when it is pointed out to them, patients are able to appreciate that what they refer to as "thinking" is a long way from problem solving or creativity. This round-and-round repetition or skip-and-jump chattering of the "unquiet mind" is more like a succession of covert "stereotypes" and "tics" than it is to productive cognitive activity. Then we reintroduce the patient to the evidence for vital but inaccessible cognitive activities which take place outside awareness, "off stage," as it were (see Shevrin & Dickman, 1980, for a useful and topical discussion of the non-Freudian nonconscious). By keeping a focused attention and an uncluttered mind, these "silent processes" can operate more easily and successfully.

The "Outside" Use of Meditation

Patients who faithfully adhere to the daily schedule of meditation exercises should begin to reap the benefits within a few weeks. Hypnotizability scores should increase (all other things being equal), tension and anxiety should decrease, and the patient should be better able to stay in (attentional) contact with his ongoing activities. All of these changes can be reliably anticipated in the patient who has been helped to an understanding of meditation and who practices it on a regular basis. But how about the use of the meditation technique outside of the clinic or meditation room? Can it be applied at other times? And if so, when? Little has been written on this, but we have seen so many patients who spontaneously use the meditation during times of stress or periods of boredom that we have changed our ways in teaching meditation. Formerly we advised our patients to use meditation during the two specially appointed times each day. Then a patient who had occasional bouts of initial insomnia reported that he could get off to sleep faster if he did an extra meditation in bed. Others told us of coping better with frustrations and tension in their jobs if they stopped for a minute and did a little meditation. We have been so impressed with the applicability of meditation in the everyday life of our patients that we now suggest that *in addition to the two major meditation periods* a number of "mini-meditation" exercises be done each day (Carrington, 1978).

> "When you find yourself sitting behind a long line of cars in a traffic jam, or waiting in a slow-moving supermarket line, while you're taking a shower or washing the dishes, or at any of a hundred other times in the day, take a few seconds off to do a 'mini-meditation' exercise. Keep your eyes open, and carry on with whatever you happen to be doing at the time. All that you have to do is to regulate your breathing to a slow and steady rate and then count the number as you inhale and say the meditation word as you exhale. Do this for ten breaths. That is all there is to it. After you get out of bed, and before you get into it again at night, do six of these little meditations. While you do them remember that the same rules which apply to the two 20-minute meditations apply to these smaller ones: do not worry if your attention wanders, just bring it back to the mantra if it does."

Apart from helping people to cope better with the particular situations in which they do these brief meditations, such exercises confer two other benefits. The extra practice in "tougher" situations can help the person to meditate more effectively in the quiet of his special meditation place. The mini-meditations also help to establish a new and more accepting attitude toward the small upsets of our everyday existence. More generally, these exercises establish a continuity between the practice and the everyday world and thereby help to instill a meditative (i.e., here-and-now) orientation to life.

As is the case with all other techniques, the instructions and recommendations given to the patient can turn out to be the difference between a therapeutic or an iatrogenic outcome. Patients must be discouraged from using the mini-meditations only before or during times of great stress. Through associative processes, meditation might then lead to an *increase* in tension. Certainly the patients must be helped to appreciate that if he turns to meditation only when he is in difficulties, he will only have difficulty in meditation. The exercises must be done "when they are not needed"—twice each day in the peace and quiet of the meditation room—if the skills are to be available at other times. The mini-meditations are supplementary exercises and should be used in a wide variety of situations and in the presence of a range of moods or states.

Our concluding comment in this session is directed at the tasks of recording and assessment. We ask all of our patients to fill out a meditation sheet each day. On this they list the number of exercises by circling the appropriate check mark and recording the ease of meditation (see Figure 6.1).

Concluding Remarks

To some readers it might seem odd and unfortunate that we have written a whole chapter on meditation without alluding to its spiritual dimensions and purposes. In its long history, and today too, meditation has always had a close association with moral, ethical, and religious ideas. Were meditation to be defined and evaluated with respect to how well it addresses these concerns, then clearly this chapter is incorrectly labeled and should be called by another term. We would freely accept such a suggestion as would be proposed by adherents of certain schools of meditation, for example, T.M. that any departure from their regimen disqualifies the writers from the use of the term *meditation*. Indeed we have used—and continue to use—the word *meditation* with some hesitation. The word means so many different things to so many different people that, were it not for its designation as an area of study within clinical practice and experimental research, we would gladly exchange it for other less controversial terms. We prefer "attentional training" or "cognitive-

Day/Date	Morning Exercise	Evening Exercise	Rating (0 = poor, 100 = very good)	Mini Meditations
Monday	Yes/No	Yes/No		✓✓✓✓✓
Tuesday	Yes/No	Yes/No		"
Wednesday	Yes/No	Yes/No		"
Thursday	Yes/No	Yes/No		"
Friday	Yes/No	Yes/No		"
Saturday	Yes/No	Yes/No		"
Sunday	Yes/No	Yes/No		

Figure 6.1. The take-home exercise schedule for daily meditation. The morning and evening exercises are the 20-minute periods and are to be circled as soon as they are completed along with the overall rating of the patient's feelings of comfort or discomfort in the meditation period. The "mini-meditations" are brief centering exercises to be done in the midst of the patient's normal activities across the day (see text).

centering therapy." These do not have the wide currency of the word *meditation* but they are closer to the intent and operations of the training as well as the locus of change within the cognitive system. But whatever the words we choose to label these techniques, it is utterly noncontroversial that they put into the hands of the hypno-behavioral therapist—and his patients—a powerful technique of cognitive self-control.

7
The Nature
and Practice
of Self-hypnosis

All hypnosis is self-hypnosis.

—Common clinical saying

In our treatment of hypnosis up to this point we have paid almost exclusive attention to the technique, practice, and problems of heterohypnosis. Heterohypnosis is, by definition, a process which involves two, or more, people: the hypnotist and the subject(s) or patient(s). This is invariably the context in which patients make their first contact with hypnosis. Given the prevalent myths and misconceptions about hypnosis, it is probably desirable if not essential that the person should be introduced to hypnosis by a competent and well-informed practitioner.

At the same time there are certain disadvantages in any program of therapy that limits the patient's contact with hypnosis to those situations in which the therapist determines when and how it is to be employed. First, there is always the chance of excessive dependency reactions. Notwithstanding the fact that this is a problem which can develop with any form of therapy, it is a special problem where hypnosis is involved—the more so when hypnosis is presented and administered in an "authoritarian," I-am-the-expert-you-are-the-subject, manner. It may even be the case that there is something about hypnosis that threatens to trigger and perpetuate feelings of dependency in the patient. Freud believed this, and it was one of the main reasons he turned away from hypnosis despite his initial enthusiasm for it (another reason was his doubts about the reliability of the technique). There is absolutely no evidence of a possible link between the experience of heterohypnosis and the development of troublesome dependency feelings in the patient. Nonetheless, the use of *any* powerful technique, hypnosis included, which is reserved for the exclusive use of the therapist entails a serious risk for the patient that he will come to believe that his fate depends upon the therapist's skills. It is difficult to harmonize this style of therapy with current convictions, in behavior therapy at least, that the clinician's job is to teach, and the patient's job is to acquire skills of self-assessment and self-control. Traditional practices have been criticized, justly as we see it, as being hermetic and insufficiently attuned to the tasks that face the patient outside of the once-a-week 50-minute "therapeutic hour."

With the shift in attention from what transpires during this hour to the patient's active coping efforts in his day-to-day life outside the clinic, the therapist has come to be viewed as a consultant, a collaborator with the patient in devising, testing, and applying a variety of self-control strategies. The ultimate aim that guides the practitioner in these activities is to leave the patient with a strong sense of self-direction and the abilities to maintain this; in short, the aim is for the patient to become his own therapist.

In keeping with this aim, home-based programs of desensitization, rational-emotive therapy, relaxation therapy, operant behavior modification, and even aversive therapy (see Rimm & Masters, 1979) have been developed. Behavior therapists have only recently begun to consider the place of hypnosis in a broad spectrum therapy and, therefore, there is very little in the behavioral literature on the use of self-hypnosis (Salter, 1941). In fact, the published literature on self-hypnosis from all quarters is miniscule when placed against the existing work on heterohypnosis. Fromm, Lichtman, and Brown (1973) reviewed the literature on hypnosis which had been published in the major journals between the years 1958 and 1973. They found more than 1,200 articles in their search but, of these, only 24 dealt with self-hypnosis. Commenting on the dearth of clinical and experimental investigations into self-hypnosis, Johnson (1979) offered two reasons for this neglect. First, in its focus on internal direction, self-hypnosis has probably seemed less amenable to study via research designs which always call for some degree of external manipulation of the phenomenon under study. Second, the very idea of *self*-hypnosis seems to be paradoxical, implying both internal (self) and external (heterohypnosis) control. Down its long history, hypnosis has been marked by storm and controversy on all points except one: disputants have preferred to look upon hypnosis as a form of *inter*personal influence. Some insist that the laws governing this influence can be derived from social-psychological theory (for example, Barber, 1972), while others bring psychodynamic notions to bear in formulating their explanation of hypnosis (for example, Meares, 1960). Both groups, however, take the hypnotic relationship as a basic datum in their theories. A question that must be asked, therefore, is: Can hypnosis take place without the mediation of an influential or significant other? Put more boldly, is self-hypnosis possible? This must be the first question on the agenda.

The other questions—assuming an answer in the affirmative to the first—center on a variety of practical questions about the application of self-hypnosis. Before we pose these we should note the contrast between the public (i.e., experimental/published) neglect of self-hypnosis and its acceptance in clinical practice. We chose the word "acceptance" rather than "use" in clinical practice. Little is known about the ways in which self-hypnosis is integrated into therapy programs, but our informal surveys indicate that clinicians use it more as a "talking point" than as a technique of self-management. Patients will be told that "all hypnosis is self-hypnosis." This maxim is given to allay the worry in those patients who have strong fears about domination and control by the hypnotist. While in some respects this may turn out to be the case, as the evidence reviewed below suggests, the flat assertion of an identity between the two leaves the practitioner no further ahead as regards the possibility, nature, techniques, uses, and problems of self-hypnosis. The remainder of this chapter is devoted to these questions and the clinical application of self-hypnosis.

Is Self-hypnosis Possible?

The answer to this question has not been diligently sought, and until very recently the question had not even been posed. Hypnosis began with the dyad of operator and subject, and ever since, the processes of the relationship between these two have been the starting point for clinicians and researchers who have studied hypnotic phenomena. In the average person's mind no less than in the professional's, hypnosis is a form of social influence. Unquestionably this, if true, makes *self*-hypnosis a contradiction in terms and the question which forms the title of this section must be answered in the negative. There have been a few opponents of this position, the most notable of whom was Emil Coué (1922). He claimed that all hypnosis was just a variant of self-hypnosis, which was itself no more than autosuggestion.

Backers of this position (and there are few of them in clinical hypnosis) attach little significance to the nature of the hypnotic relationship while their opponents insist that without the presence of a special influence or "rapport" between the hypnotist and his patient there can be little therapeutic gain. Which is correct? More than 50 years ago P.C. Young (1927) argued convincingly that "genuine hypnosis can exist without a semblance of rapport" (p. 139). This is a fact which is well known to generations of freshman university volunteer students who have been hypnotized in hundreds of experiments by operators barely known to them. Both authors have successfully induced hypnosis easily in volunteer subjects within a minute or two after meeting them for the first time. We did not need to use any special techniques, and any competent practitioner could have done the same. The obvious and inescapable conclusion which can be extracted from all of this is that the *induction* of hypnosis does not require the existence of the heightened interpersonal sensitivity known as 'rapport." Nor does the *induction* of hypnosis require the physical presence of the operator. There are tape recorded inductions (like the Harvard Group Scale) which work well and correlate highly with the results from individually administered live induction procedures (see chapter 3). Finally, even the hypnotist's voice on tape is unnecessary. People caught up in situations of exceptional excitement or monotony can become so absorbed in these events that they slip into trance-like reactions (for example, "highway hypnosis") without the wish to become hypnotized (Spiegel & Spiegel, 1978). This is hypnosis without intent.

The *deliberate* use of self-hypnosis was first studied systematically by J. Braid, the man who coined the word *hypnosis*. He tested himself as subject using self-hypnosis as a treatment for a number of his own personal problems. His conclusion about the possibility of self-hypnosis: "inasmuch as patients can throw themselves into the nervous sleep and manifest all the usual phenomena of mesmerism through their own unaided efforts . . . there is no need for an exotic influence to produce the phenomena of hypnotism" (Braid, 1846, cited

in Tinterow, 1970). It has taken more than a century for the revival
of interest in self-hypnosis. Today it is on the threshold of immense
clinical and research popularity (Fromm, Brown, Hurt, Oberlander,
Boxer, & Pfeifer, 1981; Gardner, 1981; Johnson, 1979, 1981; Ruch,
1975) and the data coming out of the research laboratories add up
to the same conclusion as reached 140 years ago by Braid: hypnosis
does not depend upon "exotic" (external) influence nor, as Young
argued, upon rapport.

But these conclusions apply to the *induction* of hypnosis, not its
most effective utilization. Here, then, is the distinction to draw,
which can bring a resolution to the conflict. When it is drawn clearly
it can be seen that there is no incompatibility between the two views:
the *onset* of hypnosis depends largely on technique and aptitude (in
therapist and patient). Making the best use of hypnosis, on the other
hand, involves a host of factors, and a good relationship between
therapist and patient ("rapport") is a vital potentiator of these. Its
intelligent application is quite another matter from its induction.
This demands a sense of cooperation between therapist and patient
coupled with a good understanding of the patient's problems and
mutually agreed-upon goals.

The Nature of Self-hypnosis

The conceptual relationship of self-hypnosis to heterohypnosis has
been described in one of two ways. There is the already mentioned
view that "all hypnosis is self-hypnosis" and its opposite, that self-
hypnosis is just a variety of heterohypnosis (Weitzenhoffer, 1957).
Behind these diametrically opposed views is a shared assumption: in
order to understand one, whether self-hypnosis or heterohypnosis,
we only need to turn to the established body of knowledge about the
other. In particular, the prediction is that the facts of self-hypnosis
when they come to be discovered will, in all essentials, be identical
with those of heterohypnosis. The most recent research has been
directed at the validity of this assumption (Fromm et al., 1981; Johnson, 1979; Ruch, 1975) and has found it to be incorrect as stated:
self-hypnosis and heterohypnosis are not simply two names for the
same process. It follows that clinical uses of the two do not coincide
completely.

To be more precise, the similarity or the differences between
self- and heterohypnosis depends on how the particular researcher
or clinician defines self-hypnosis. The two contrasting definitions

and usages (and, thus, results) have begun with either *self-directed responses* or *self-initiated suggestions*. By self-directed responses is meant the subject's practicing tasks taught to him by the researcher or clinician. In the clinic this has been traditional usage: a patient is taught a specific routine made up of a clearly defined set of (self) suggestion and (self-directed) procedures to bring about a certain well-defined reaction (arm levitation, positive hallucination, etc.). Seen in this way, the only difference between a standard heterohypnotic induction and self-hypnosis is the presence of the hypnotist in the former and his absence in the latter (Johnson, 1981). The definition of self-hypnosis as self-initiated suggestions leaves the subject free to use whatever suggestions he wishes to use or whatever imagery and fantasies he cares to explore (Fromm et al., 1981).

The research results are not yet sufficient in number to allow for definitive statements and clear-cut conclusions about the similarity of self- and heterohypnosis nor do they allow us to say with absolute certainty which of the two definitions—and uses—of self-hypnosis holds most promise in the management of anxiety. What can be said on the basis of the recent data is that:

1. Both self-hypnosis (of either variety) and heterohypnosis are reported to involve a fading of the "generalized reality orientation" (Fromm et al., 1981; Johnson, 1981). Subjects develop an absorption (in self- and heterohypnosis) and a diminished sense of concern with and awareness of external reality and the thoughts and feelings associated with it.

2. In self-hypnosis generally, and most clearly when it involves self-initiated suggestion, there is a sense of a more expanded and less focused attention. Along with that is the tendency for self-hypnotic practices to be associated with more spontaneous and more vivid imagery than is reported in heterohypnosis. In the early stages of training there seems to be more fragmentation in self-hypnosis imagery. Johnson (1981) states that with time and practice, the self-hypnosis imagery tends to become less fragmented—a change which he attributes to the subjects' gradually increasing ability to focus the attention. Our impression—and, again, this is in accord with Johnson's work (1979, 1981)—is that at the more "permissive" end, self-hypnosis merges with the reveries of day-dreaming which can involve "poor attentional control and mind wandering with little capacity for extended thought" (Singer & Pope, 1981, p. 272).

3. Subjects in self-hypnosis say that they feel more in control and more creative than when they participate in heterohypnosis but it is still reported as a receptive state and "successful Ss do *not* seem to create their experience by active, willing, or planned decisions . . . this receptive attention is possibly one characteristic distinguishing the self-hypnosis cognitive process from active, self-directed fantasizing of the waking state" (Johnson, 1981, p. 256).

4. Subjects find that for both self- and heterohypnosis, the efficiency of entering hypnosis, its believability, and its impact increase with practice.

5. The subjects in the self-hypnosis group were inclined to doubt their ability to induce hypnosis without the presence and aid of the therapist—"Can I do it alone?" was the question the participants in the Fromm et al. (1981) study put to the experimenters.

To review the main findings, where the self-directed response paradigm has been employed, self-hypnosis and heterohypnosis show a close resemblance behaviorally and phenomenologically. There are certain differences between the two, but these have been described as "minor and specific" (Johnson, 1979, 1981). The self-initiated, unconstrained form of self-hypnosis is associated with a greater richness, fragmentation, and spontaneity of imagery.

Which form should be used in clinical practice? Our answer is: "both." It is important to give the person heterohypnotic training and the form of self-hypnosis which closely resembles this. As for the other form, Fromm et al. (1981) insist that it is "important to give the individual training in the ability to 'let go' to become more ego receptive to imagery" (p. 242). We agree with this but disagree with their final statement "that while attention is concentrative in heterohypnosis, he/she *should* attempt to use a different type of attention—free floating expansive attention—in self-hypnosis" (p. 242, emphasis added). We cannot see the justifications for limiting self-hypnosis to this "free-form" approach. It seems to us that the kind selected should depend on the clinical objective of the exercise. Moreover, we have serious doubts that very anxious and tense patients (Fromm et al. worked with carefully selected volunteer Ss) can use the radically unstructured form without slipping into the kind of self-defeating ruminations and "cognitive anarchy" which besets these sorely troubled individuals. From our experience we have learned the value in beginning with the less demanding and more structured methods rather than those which call for more self-control skills. The "graduation" from situations of greater to lesser direction and guidance must be organized with great care. As we will argue below, self-hypnosis is more readily achieved if the techniques employed are similar to those used by a therapist in induction. This is not to say that other procedures cannot be used, but in our experience patients are more able to utilize induction techniques with which they are familiar. We would go so far as to suggest to the patient that he note and employ identical induction procedures—a point which we further emphasize by suggestion in the hypnotic state. In order to reinforce this notion, the patient is directed to induce self-hypnosis at the termination of the hetero-hypnotic session. In this way, he leaves the consultation aware of his capacity to self-induce and experience a trance state, while at the same time being familiar with the sensations associated with self-hypnosis.

Self-hypnosis: Myths and Misconceptions

A lesson soon learned by clinical practitioners is that a proficient technique and clear appreciation of the place of hypnosis in multi-modal programs will, by themselves, come to nothing if the patient has not been relieved of his doubts, fears, and misunderstandings. In chapter 1 we listed these under the heading of "Myths and Misconceptions" (about heterohypnosis). The introduction of self-hypnosis can bring up in the patient's mind a very special collection of insecurities which are not necessarily alleviated by the reassurance appropriate to his worries about heterohypnosis, and an equally important but different kind of pre- (self-) hypnotic counseling is called for. The clinician may elect to deal with all of these, those presented in chapter 1 and the ones set out below, at the same time. We have found that this can be too much of an information load for some patients, and our practice is to go over the major myths and misconceptions about self-hypnosis only after the training sessions in heterohypnosis have got well underway.

The most common bit of misinformation is the belief that nothing can be achieved without the guiding presence of the hypnotist. If said aloud, the patient's thoughts would go along these lines: "I cannot hypnotize myself; someone else had to do it with me" (or, worse yet, "to me"). The best and safest way to counter this is to have the patient learn, demonstrate, and practice self-hypnosis in the clinic while the therapist looks on. We are aware that some researchers (see Fromm et al., 1981) have been able to leave it up to the subject to do it all on his own, alone. This may be an acceptable method for specially chosen volunteer subjects, but with anxious patients a much lower rate of success can be anticipated with a *laissez-faire* approach. Accordingly, our teaching program for self-hypnosis includes clinic practice before homework exercises are given. The aim of this approach is to carefully program the transfer of control over induction from the therapist to the patient (see below) so that the patient has success experiences with self-hypnosis before he begins home practice.

Prior to heterohypnosis some people worry about the possibility of being unable to exit from hypnosis ("Suppose I cannot come out from under?"). We have found it easier to settle patients' uncertainties about the effectiveness of termination procedures in heterohypnosis than in self-hypnosis, probably because the whole of the hypnosis ceremony occurs in the presence of the therapist. Patients may be told that heterohypnosis is self-terminating and that whenever they wish to do so, they can open their eyes and "come out of it." These words may help, but as the usual practice is for the clinician to decide on when and how termination is to be effected, the patient never gets the opportunity to put these assertions to the test. After a while the patient's fears about being "stuck" in (hetero-) hypnosis subside, but often this is only because of an increase in their confidence in the *hypnotist's* skills in "getting them out" of hypnosis. Thus, even after many successful heterohypnotic sessions, the patient's deep fears about *self*-termination in self-hypnosis may continue unabated. Here again the patient will gain more relief by attempting self-termination exercises conducted in the clinic than he will from a statement of the facts of self-hypnosis. We have found that all of this can be accomplished in one carefully supervised practice session in trance induction *and* termination (see below).

Hypnosis has never shed entirely its image as a kind of psychological "truth serum." People fear that once hypnotized there may be an eruption of powerful and abnormal impulses revelatory of their true but well-hidden characters. One of the attractions of self-hypnosis is that the only witness to these, if they occur, is the patient himself. For instance, more of Johnson's (1979) subjects had fears of doing something foolish or embarrassing in heterohypnosis than in self-hypnosis. The therapist may, however, run up against a similar problem in self-hypnosis. In this case, the patient fears that self-hypnosis may unleash strong and disturbing feelings because the clinical expert is *not* there to redirect and channel these reactions. These fears of "letting go" can be counteracted mainly by factual reassurance—such abreactive responses are rare and when they do appear are usually easy to eliminate with slight changes in procedure (see chapter 6).

The last in the list of these myths and misconceptions is the belief that the induction of (hetero- or self-) hypnosis constitutes, in and of itself, a powerful form of therapy. This misconception is not entirely unfounded and is therefore quite difficult to dislodge. "Neutral" self-hypnosis (self-induction without self-suggestion) in terms of its operation, results, and process shows a close resemblance to some forms of meditation which have a record of proven success in promoting the "relaxation response" (Benson, Arns, & Hoffman, 1981). However, it is not to be expected that, over and above this, the act of self-hypnosis (or heterohypnosis) will by itself add cognitive or behavioral coping skills to the person's repertoire or eliminate specific phobias. To reword slightly an axiomatic remark presented in the earlier chapters on heterohypnosis: people get treated in and not by self-hypnosis. The therapist's task in correcting this misconception is not an easy one. The positive placebo value of any technique must be fostered—good expectations are known to count for an important part of any therapy (for example, Kazdin & Wilcoxin 1976; Lazarus, 1973), especially in the early stages of application.

Structured and Unstructured Self-hypnosis: Assessment Issues and Clinical Applications

Progress in the clinical application of heterohypnosis has followed the development of instruments which give reliable and valid measures of hypnotic performance. The study of self-hypnosis is only in its infancy, a situation reflected in the meager store of information on its nature and measurement. The early studies in the literature (Johnson & Weight, 1976; Shor & Easton, 1973) were guided by a definition of self-hypnosis in terms of self-directed responses. Shor and Easton (1973) used the Inventory of Self-Hypnosis (ISH), which was first developed by Shor (1970). The ISH is adapted from the Stanford Hypnotic Susceptibility Scale, Form A (SHSS:A) of Weitzenhoffer and Hilgard (1959). In these studies the subjects were instructed to *read* the suggestions instead of listening to the hypnotist delivering them. A second and slightly different means of assessment was used by Ruch in his 1975 study. Ruch (1975) also turned to a standard hypnotic scale for the content of his suggestions. He based these on ones taken from the Harvard Group Scale of Hypnotic Susceptibility, Form A (HGSHS:A) of Shor and Orne (1962) and the Stanford Hypnotic Susceptibility Scale, Form C (SHSS:C) of Weitzenhoffer and Hilgard (1962). These investigators worked along the same lines as Shor's group in giving the subjects the suggestions to use for themselves (reworded in the first person). As noted, the findings from these reports on the whole confirmed the basic similarity of heterohypnosis and self-hypnosis.

The opposing position is set out in Fromm et al. (1981). Their unstructured style of self-hypnosis calls for a more open-ended assessment program than is necessary with self-hypnosis procedures derived from or designed to resemble heterohypnosis. The Fromm et al. (1981) paper presents a collection of results rich in implications for our understanding of the use of self-exploration and fantasy under free-form conditions. It is not clear just what clinical value they have in any cognitive-behavioral therapy program where the importance of *specificity* in the shaping of clinical objectives and in the use of therapeutic techniques assessment procedures has always been highlighted. Doubts about its use in the clinic (as contrasted with its obvious relevance as a means of studying the structure of cognition) are further sharpened when we are dealing with maladaptive anxiety. For the majority of our patients, giving only minimal assistance in self-hypnosis, or any other cognitive technique (". . . you may wish to think up suggestions . . . and experiment with them . . . [or] you may also wish at times just to remain in trance but not do anything specific" [p. 194]) would result in no more than a continuation of their habitual, high-arousing collection of apprehensions and ruminations; there are no grounds for expecting any other outcome with anxious patients. If the cognitive skills, which, collectively, produce disengagement (which Fromm and most others acknowledge to be crucial in heterohypnosis and self-hypnosis) are absent, then the therapist must devise methods to help patients acquire them. It is true that Fromm et al. (1981) did not report any such difficulties in their subjects. Their subjects, however, had been given prior training in heterohypnosis through which they may have learned some of the basic skills of hypnosis. More significantly, they had their volunteers screened and any with obvious psychological difficulties were not allowed to participate in the study.

Whichever path into self-hypnosis the practitioner selects (below we present the clinical uses to which both forms can be put), the assessment plan must connect up with every phase of the training. In our present state of knowledge about self-hypnosis, it is unfortunately the case that this assessment must rest more on clincial judgment than on quantitative measurement. In the next section we present in some detail the program we follow in teaching and assessing self-hypnotic skills.

We begin the teaching of self-hypnosis with a heterohypnotic induction. Some (for example, Ruch, 1975) claim that preliminary training in heterohypnosis may interfere with progress in self-hypnosis. Most researchers, however, have found no differences in the levels of self-hypnosis achieved by naive subjects when compared with those found in subjects first trained in heterohypnosis (Johnson & Weight, 1975). Our clinical impressions are that in patient populations, heterohypnosis, if anything, *facilitates* later performance on self-hypnotic tasks. There are other important reasons for beginning with heterohypnosis. While it is true that a person's heterohypnosis score may differ from his self-hypnosis score (although usually not by a great amount), the former is likely to be the higher of the two. Patients report that hypnotic phenomena are experienced more readily and more deeply in heterohypnosis (until they become proficient at self-hypnosis). This does not allow the clinician to administer a test of heterohypnosis and from that make a direct inference to levels of self-hypnotizability, since the heterhypnosis score will, in a large percentage of cases, be the higher of the two. The clinician can use this to get an indication of the upper range of self-hypnotic potential for that patient (assuming that no remedial training is offered). Heterohypnotic assessment can also help to pinpoint particular problems (attentional difficulties, excessive tension, etc.). Given the well-documented similarity of self- and heterohypnosis, the clinician can get an idea of just where the patient may run into problems in self-hypnosis. Another, and no less important, reason for beginning a program of self-hypnosis with heterohypnosis is to give the patient careful guidance in the experiences of hypnosis (such as the fading of the generalized reality orientation).

The last and most important reason for the inclusion of heterohypnosis is to set up the most propitious conditions for the transfer of control over the process of hypnosis from the therapist to the patient. Once the patient has been shown and experienced heterohypnosis, the therapist can take the patient through a smaller or larger number of intermediate steps in which the patient gradually assumes the role of (self-) hypnotist. The assessment task here requires the therapist to monitor very closely the rate at which the patient is able to switch roles and, hence, the rate at which he (the therapist) can "fade" himself out of the role of the director of proceedings (see below). Once this is achieved, the patient can *then,* and not before, commence home use of self-hypnosis. The therapist must then turn over the primary assessment tasks to the patient (see below). To conclude this section we will note a reminder that we often give to ourselves. The most important assessment of all is that which has to be conducted jointly by patient and therapist. Its purpose is to judge the utility of self-hypnosis in bringing about a change for the better in the patient's presenting problem(s). Any technique that fails this test of accountability cannot justify its place in the therapy program. This is only a truism, but one that practitioners in hypnosis should always keep before them. It is too easy to get so absorbed in the techniques and processes of hypnosis that success in induction can too easily be mistaken for a success in therapy.

Teaching Self-hypnosis

Step 1 is the presentation of a rationale for the operation and uses of self-hypnosis:

> "You have seen that basically hypnosis comes down to two things: disengagement and suggestion. The word *disengagement* refers to everything from first shutting your eyes, then getting quiet and relaxed, and finally focusing your attention fully and completely on my voice and suggestions. All of this was done without making any effort—actually it was done better because you didn't make any big effort. Then I gave various suggestions beginning with the induction of arm levitation to the final one to open your eyes at the end of the hypnosis. Believe it or not you can learn to do all of this at home—the disengagement and suggestions—by yourself without getting any assistance from me. And all of the objectives of hypnosis which I discussed before with you (relaxation, desensitization, and so on) can be accomplished with self-hypnosis, too.
>
> "Let's start with the first part, the one I referred to as the disengagement. As you know, this is important because suggestions work best when we are 'detached' or 'disengaged' from our usual alertness and our usual concerns. Well, you can create the same quiet surroundings, free of interruptions, at home, just as we did here in the clinic. You can take up the same relaxed

posture and adopt the same easygoing attitude. I helped you to do this here by giving you something to pay attention to which helped you to avoid getting your mind trapped in the usual collection of thoughts, worries, and calculations. I asked you to listen to my voice [or stare at that spot on the wall, or whatever focusing technique the therapist used] and to let everything else slip away. When you do the whole self-hypnosis procedure at home you may not find *this* part of the disengagement process quite as easy to do as the other steps which I just mentioned. Almost everybody comes away from the first few attempts with the feeling that self-hypnosis is not as rich and compelling an experience as therapist-directed hypnosis. These feelings of failure are almost entirely due to difficulties in keeping a steady, focused attention; getting lost in the usual tangle of thoughts is not especially pleasant, nor useful. It certainly is not self-hypnosis. If you find yourself besieged by this mental restlessness you can be sure that, eyes closed or not, you have not gone into the disengagement phase. Self-suggestions will thus be less effective because in your preoccupation with the 'passing parade' of irrelevant mental activities, you are less receptive to suggestions [the same holds true in heterohypnosis].

"The answer to this problem is to replace the externally supplied aid to a focused attention (my voice and my words) with an 'internal' one which you can supply for yourself, the meditation *mantra* [see chapter 6]. A few minutes of meditation, together with the other disengagement methods (eyes closed, comfortable posture, physical relaxation, and so forth) should set the stage for the suggestions which you will then give to yourself and allow them to work to best effect.

"OK, we've covered the first, disengagement part of (self-) hypnosis. Now, what about the second, 'self-suggestion,' part of it?"

The practitioner is now at the most important part of the rationale for self-hypnosis, getting the patient to accept the functional equivalence of self- and other-delivered suggestions. We have not yet come up with the sentences which will instill an immediate, unqualified acceptance of this proposition. People are empiricists at heart and full conviction will come only with a demonstration of self-hypnosis. Nonetheless, the right words of preparation can help to establish the belief that if the right steps are taken beforehand (to facilitate disengagement) then "it doesn't seem to matter whether the suggestions are given by someone you trust or you give them to yourself." To repeat, patients will harbor doubts that self-delivered suggestions can function in the same way and as well as those transmitted by the therapist. (If the patient has been to an untrained hypnotist or has tried to learn self-hypnosis out of one of the journalistic do-it-your-self books which extol the "power of self-hypnosis," then he may have a history of trying self-hypnosis to no avail. The therapist then has the added task of explaining why it may have failed to work. The answer can usually be found in one or more of the following: the omission of all advice for and training in disengagement, thereby confusing in the patient's mind autosuggestion with self-hypnosis; the wrong timing; and the wrong structure of the self-suggestions.)

Andrew Salter (1941) is one of the few writers on the topic to present an account of his methods for attacking these doubts. Patients find his account to be convincing and easy to comprehend. About self-hypnosis (Salter used the then current term, *autohypnosis*) he says to the patient:

> It might be clearer if we called it "auto-concentration" for in a sense that's what autohypnosis is. Your entire mind and body are concentrated upon whatever effect you wish to produce, and when your entire organism is focused upon one thing, the results may seem remarkable. We have utter concentration and *no divergence of attention,* and that's very important." (p. 434, emphasis added)*

As regards the source of the suggestions once this focusing has occurred, he says:

> It doesn't make any difference *who* gives you the suggestions. . . . The source of the suggestions doesn't matter. They may come from within or without. As long as you cooperate, with me or with yourself, the suggestions work. . . . There is no such thing as A hypnotizing B. All that A does is to tell B which roads to follow to get to his destination—hypnosis. It doesn't matter who tells you what roads to follow—whether I tell you these roads (or directions) or whether you tell yourself those roads. In any case, if you *follow* those roads, you will hypnotize yourself. (pp. 425, 431, emphases in the original)

*Salter adds this note: "I grant that this language is the worst tradition of the inspirational psychologists but it is nevertheless clearer to subjects than would be an explanation in terms of 'sensory focalization' "and 'mental set.' " We can understand and sympathize with Salter's uneasiness over the use of "inspirational" language. Salter was then, and is still today, a leading Pavlovian behavior therapist and there is no place in these schemes for the "psychology of hope and confidence." The fact that we have not been able to pin down these processes in operational terms and quantitative formulas, however, should not blind us to their "vital importance in clinical practice (Frank, 1976).

After this the practitioner can take the quick option of listing the steps in self-hypnosis, adding some guidance on the structure, timing, and specific applications of self-suggestions, and consider that the training phase of self-hypnosis has been concluded. If the practitioner has cause to believe that his patient has exceptional talent in hypnosis or prior and positive experiences with self-hypnosis, then in-clinic demonstrations and practice may be superfluous and time wasting. We have come across so few patients who fit this description that we offer the blanket recommendation of therapist-assisted practice at self-hypnosis. An easy and brief demonstration should start this practice. We have found the body-sway technique (cf. Salter, 1941) to be quite effective. The patient is asked to stand up and stare at the point where the two walls and ceiling meet. After a minute of centering ("listen to my voice, keep staring at that spot . . ."), suggestions for body sway or falling backward are given. This is one of the "easiest" of the ideomotor suggestions and within a minute or so most people will show some movement. After this the therapist asks the patient to return his gaze to the spot on the wall and to give the suggestions (swaying or falling backward) to himself. The therapist stays silent or, at most, gives a prompt or two. As soon as the swaying (or falling) is evident, the therapist stops and reinforces his earlier remarks: "There, just as I said, it's the suggestion and not where it comes from that counts. And that's the way it can work at home." In fact this is closer to autosuggestion than self-hypnosis, and while it serves as a demonstration of self-suggestion it is not exactly the same as self-hypnosis. So once these important preliminaries have been completed, training can begin in self-hypnosis proper. The main objective of this training is to transfer, very gradually, control over the hypnotic process from the therapist to the patient.

Self-hypnosis and Overt Behavior

When teaching self-hypnosis we always use an overt response in induction as an index of hypnosis. Obviously, the cognitive changes that constitute hypnosis can be evoked without the involvement of a specific motor behavior. There is no evidence, either, that if an overt response is to be used as an index of hypnosis, one behavior must be chosen in preference to another. As far as we are aware, the same assertions hold for self-hypnosis. All the same, we deem it essential to use some overt response during induction and termination (all of the examples given below refer to arm levitation because that is the one we use most often). Why are we so forceful in our insistence upon a *behavioral* index of self-hypnosis? We would not go so far as to say that without some overt behavior, self-hypnosis is impossible. That statement would be at variance with our general position and the facts of hypnosis. But the patient will not have the clinician's experience and expertise and in the early stages of home practice may be at a loss to know whether the processes of hypnosis are sufficiently far advanced for him to enter the self-suggestion phase. It is an easier task to judge whether or not the arm is coming up "unaided" than to assess the correlated cognitive changes. In training, too, there is much to be said for targeting the induction suggestions on overt behavior. The experience of "involuntary" arm levitation can allay doubts ("Was I hypnotized?") and stimulate a sense of wonderment and, along with it, powerful and positive expectations.

Self-hypnosis: Transfer of Training

The basic principle behind the transfer of training is the fractionation of the acquisition process into a number of substages so that the gap between the subject's present performance capability and the target outcome is never too great. Thus, the first step toward self-hypnosis begins with responses already in the person's *repertoire* of hypnotic skills. We start off with arm levitation in heterohypnosis as the vehicle. The first induction is carried out in the standard way (see chapter 4). Immediately after termination this is repeated, this time with the patient "shadowing" the suggestions and comments of the practitioner, word for word. The most efficient way to arrange this is for the therapist to use short utterances. For instance when the words "soon you'll notice a lightness in your arm" are spoken aloud the patient then says these very same words to himself. There are two questions of technique which arise at this point: should the words be spoken aloud by the patient and, second, should they be put in the first or second person? Donald Meichenbaum (1976) and his associates have devised a very successful strategy of teaching behavior change through the use of self-verbalizations. At first the patient's self-directions are expressed aloud, then they are whispered, and finally they are used covertly. For the vast majority of our patients this "outer-to-inner" strategy has not been necessary. Some do find it helpful, but most report that overt speech interferes with the disengagement process. Turning to the second question, some patients are more at ease if they change the therapist's "*You* are getting relaxed . . . *your* arm is getting lighter" to "*I* am . . . *my* arm is . . ." while others prefer to use the practitioner's exact words and act as hypnotist to their own subject. By and large the preference seems to be for the former, and they also report that it seems "odd" to talk to themselves in the second person.

After one or two (arm levitation) inductions in which the responses associated with hypnosis follow the delivery of two sets of suggestions—the therapist's first (aloud), and the patient's second (covert)—the therapist can change from a louder to a very much softer voice while the patient shadows these words but without reducing the (inner) "loudness" of his own delivery. After one induction the next stage is begun where the patient continues to use the same instructions and suggestions but now without the lead of or assistance from the therapist. The therapist limits his utterances to the occasional prompt and reinforcing comment. The process is brought to a conclusion by the therapist having the patient take over the whole procedure from eye closure and centering to arm levitation and termination.

The clinical training in self-hypnosis from the opening discussion about the rationale and myths and misconceptions to the final, patient-controlled, induction can be completed in one session. Although this process is brief, the practitioner may nevertheless object to using precious clinical time in this way. Such impatience is understandable but it is better not to yield to it; we have found that the continued and effective home use of self-hypnosis depends on this proper clinical training.

The Home Use of Self-hypnosis

The purposes to which self-hypnosis can be put are the same as those which can be served by heterohypnosis. That is to say, it can be used as an adjunct to all the techniques which are potentiated by heterohypnosis. These include relaxation ("neutral" self-hypnosis), graded imaginal exposure to threat situations (as in systematic desensitization and flooding) as well as with the more "cognitive" techniques (covert behavioral rehearsal in assertion therapy and rational-emotive therapy), self-delivered posthypnotic suggestion (all of these techniques are discussed in chapters 9 and 10) and, not least of all, self-exploration. Until recently we shared the bias of most behaviorally oriented therapists against that which could not be clearly specified and carefully measured. And although "inner" events were to be admitted into the clinical picture, it was always made clear that the utility of these constructs was to be judged in terms of their linkage to overt or directly observable behavioral or physiological changes. Without discounting the need to continue with this emphasis on observable behavior, it is possible to admit into our thinking the uses of "nondirective" techniques, hypnotic and otherwise. These techniques may help to give access to realms of cognition which used to be described—and disparaged—as "primary process," "daydreaming" or "reverie," or, most damning of all, "irrational." A corollary to these attitudes was that their study could not be of any possible interest to "scientific" practice. As Singer and Pope (1981) put it so well, "Professional writing about consciousness not only downplays the prevalence of thought processes which are not rational, verbal, sequential, and secondary process; but such processes are also characterized as somehow second-rate, regressive, more primitive, and often maladaptive" (p. 274). Nonprofessionals, too, have been trained to devalue these modes of cognition and share the same attitudes. "Most of us as we grew up probably were taught, perhaps directly, not to waste too much time daydreaming, not to spend our time 'off in another world.' And this devaluation of 'internal events' is reflected in much of our professional writing. We are poorer for it" (Singer & Pope, 1981, p. 276).

Erika Fromm and her co-workers at the University of Chicago have developed a method of self-hypnosis (discussed earlier in this chapter) to investigate the sorts of phenomena to which Singer and Pope (1981) refer. As interesting as it is in theory and in research, however, the specific uses to which it can be put in clinical practice remain to be determined. Fromm et al. (1981) suggest that unstructured self-hypnosis can be used to help patients become more receptive to imagery and to tolerate the feeling of "letting go." Obsessive and "uptight" patients who are constantly exhibiting behavior that surprises and upsets them may find out more about the early and, typically, poorly recognized covert precursors to these "behavioral explosions" through the use of open-ended self-hypnosis. Others, in practicing this form of self-hypnosis, may come across material that can then be explored with the clinician on a more systematic basis. The distinction we are drawing here is akin to the one experimental methodologists make between "hypothesis finding" and "hypothesis testing" (Sidman, 1960). The value and validity of the discoveries made in self-exploration can then be given more rigorous scrutiny and tested systematically with the available methods of behavior assessment and change.

There is little in the way of specific preparation required of the patient on these voyages of self-exploration apart from a willingness to go along with and accept whatever emerges. Immediately afterward it may be useful for the patient to jot down the most salient thoughts and feelings that came to him in the self-hypnosis episodes. The immediacy is important because, like night dreams, these thoughts and feelings fade very quickly. The more common use of self-hypnosis, of the structured variety, requires that careful thought be given beforehand to the development, structure, and timing of self-suggestion.

When the patient has mastered the techniques of induction and termination, he can begin to use task-relevant self-suggestions. The content of the suggestions will depend upon the problem (flying fears, public speaking anxiety, etc.) and the technique (systematic desensitization, behavior rehearsal); these are covered in chapters 9 and 10. As much planning has to go into the covert (i.e., self-hypnotic) use of these techniques as is applied in the "live" use of them. The patient and therapist together should talk over what specific suggestions are to be given in self-hypnosis. These should be written down and memorized by the patient so that in self-hypnosis he will not flounder or have to figure out what his particular objectives are (such "figuring out" in hypnosis would be expected to stimulate the processes of "dehypnosis"). In the construction of the self-suggestion monologue, the therapist should take care to see that the patient does not put in too much in the way of elaborate or abstractly stated content. The suggestions should be few in number and couched in simple language and concrete imagery (Spanos & Barber, 1976). The patient may expect that one instance of self-presented verbalizations or imagery should be sufficient. Our experience is that repetition is necessary before self-suggestions begin to work. When to give up the repetition of one suggestion before moving on to another (the next day or the next week) will depend on the patient's progress in the area covered by the content of the suggestions.

The timing of the suggestions is another important issue for which there are absolutely no good research data. On an *a priori* basis, it would seem that self-suggestion should await the completion of the disengagement phase. But how is the patient to know when this is? If there is no overt response used (such as arm levitation), then the decision must be an entirely subjective one. With an overt

response technique, we suggest to our patients that they withhold
self-suggestions until just after arm levitation (but only if they have
the sense that the arm raising was "involuntary").

   We should not leave the topic of self-hypnosis without mentioning two recurring problems (apart from those which can arise with
all disengagement techniques, the ones noted in chapters 4 and 6).
First, some patients may not know if they fell asleep during the
home practice session or were in a very "deep" hypnosis. As with
meditation, which it so closely resembles (Benson et al., 1981), sleep
is always a risk. A simple and elegant solution to this problem has
been proposed by Neil Phillips, a Sydney, Australia, psychiatrist
(1981, personal communication). After induction, the patient leaves
his arm in the raised position (standing straight up from the elbow)
and does not lower it until the termination. If he wakes to find that
his arm has returned to his lap, then he can reasonably infer that he
did fall asleep. He should then take steps to reschedule self-hypnosis
periods at other times when he is less sleepy.

Technical Aids to Self-Hypnosis:
The Role of Audiotapes

Clinical behavior therapy has been moving steadily away from the
traditional conception of the functions of the therapist. Once considered the main agent of change, he is now seen as the consultant
whose tasks are best described by the words "teacher" and "facilitator." The facilitation of specific behavioral changes if done with the
maximal involvement of the patient can promote equally important
but more general alterations in the individual's sense of self-control,
self-efficacy, and independence (Bandura, 1977; Lazarus, 1976;
White, 1959). One sign of the transference of the activities formerly
under the therapist's direction but now carried out under the patient's direction is the immense popularity of self-help tapes. There
are two questions to examine here. First, can hypnosis be carried out
via audiotapes and, second, what are the advantages and disadvantages of the home use of audiotapes?

   Large-scale research into these questions has not yet begun, but
it is widely accepted that audiotapes may fulfill a number of therapeutic roles. First, they may be used by the therapist to induce hypnosis in the clinical situation. Illovsky and Fredman (1976) describe
taped group inductions carried out on young children in a clinical
setting, and Schafer (1975) utilizes hypnotic tape recordings to aid

pain relief when changing burn dressings. The second and more commonly accepted role is their use by the patient when he is on his own. Here, the tape is used to provide hypnotic induction techniques and therapeutic suggestions, and these may be considered an extension of the heterohypnotic treatment. The hope is that through frequent usage, the taped therapy will act to reinforce the mechanisms for the production of ongoing changes in behavior. This may be of some importance when practical considerations such as the therapist's busy work schedule or the geographical isolation of the patient prevent the patient attending as often as is desired.

Tape recorded induction procedures and suggestions should not be considered as being confined to the clinical domain, for they are also extensively used in the experimental setting. Their use in this area allows the experimenter to present a standardized hypnotic induction, free from observer bias (Barber & Calverley, 1964a; Jackson, Gass, & Camp, 1979; Sheehan & Perry, 1980). The one limitation of the tape induction technique is that it does not allow the experimenter/clinician to modify his presentation in light of the moment-to-moment changes in the subject/patient responses.

The use of audiotapes for therapeutic purposes is also not without disadvantages. We have observed, for example, that some individuals quickly become bored and habituated to the tapes. Admittedly this effect can be offset by the therapist changing the nature of the induction and therapeutic suggestions at frequent intervals. We prefer another approach, namely that of stressing to the patient the importance of achieving self-control and self-mastery over his difficulties *through his own efforts* by means of self-hypnosis, and to use the tape only occasionally as a way of reinforcing the aims of therapy. Another potential problem arising from overuse of an audiotape is the danger of tape dependency. This aspect may not be as serious as therapist dependency but, nevertheless, should be actively discouraged. It is necessary that all patients be made aware of the need to avoid reliance on taped therapy even if the therapist does not supply them himself. Cassette tapes for every manner of problem and all kinds of techniques are readily available through commercial outlets. If the patient uses these (on his own) with the idea of "being changed," as many do, and not as a chance to perfect self-monitoring and self-control strategies, then the net effect will be a negative one.

Notwithstanding the potential shortcomings of tape recordings in hypnosis, we have found them to be of value in those patients whose attentional focus is so impaired that they require a taped procedure to reinforce their self-therapy; in patients who are geographically isolated and are therefore not able to attend for regular therapy; and in sportsmen for use before major competition (Willis, 1979). To round off this section, we also suggest that a tape recording be made of an actual therapeutic session, for in this way the patient is able to follow techniques and therapeutic suggestions which are familiar to him from the clinical context.

Finally, there is the question of the gadgets and gimmicks that are so closely associated with the induction of self-hypnosis (for example, rotating discs with concentric circles painted on the outer surface). If self-hypnosis is viewed as a *self*-control technique, then such external aids only serve to substitute one form of dependency (therapist) for another and even less effective one (the gadget).

8

The Anxieties: Their Nature, Origin, and Treatment Implications

There is no single problem of anxiety.
—George Mandler, *Mind and Emotion*

Any book on the clinical uses of hypnosis must pay due attention to the reader's needs to gain a measure of technical proficiency in hypnosis and an understanding of its measurement and mechanisms. All of this is important and is not to be slighted, but if the book ends with that, it has nothing to tell us about the uses to which hypnosis can be put in the treatment environment. The clinical problems that will occupy our attention all involve anxiety. The question then is: How can hypnosis be employed in the management of anxiety? Or, as our students so often ask: "What do you do once the patient is hypnotized (or once he hypnotizes himself)?"

Our intent in the remaining chapters is to explore this in some detail. In the present chapter, however, we will have little to say about specific hypnobehavioral techniques and particular points of clinical procedure. Our aim is, rather, to look past the minutiae of clinical tactics to the larger theoretical questions, for the answers to these constitute the assumptive bases of our clinical work.

In particular we wish to examine critically the popular cognitive and conditioning theories of anxiety, and to look at the evidence which is building toward a more valid account of the factors at work in the origins and maintenance of the varieties of anxiety seen in the clinic. The specific suggestions for the conduct of hypnobehavioral therapy which take up the remainder of the book will be shaped by the theoretical framework developed in this chapter.

The spur to this effort comes from the growing disenchantment with the existing behavior therapy literature on the treatment of anxiety. The great majority of the studies found there have used student conscripts and volunteer subjects. A study of the characteristics of these volunteers reveals that, as a group, they are intelligent, sociable, well-educated people who show a strong desire to be cooperative—to be "good subjects." In short, they have "the attributes that are found in those who benefit most from any form of psychotherapy" (Allen, 1980, p. 115). Too little exists in the way of experimental behavior therapy research with clinical populations. In these populations, the amount of change that can be characterized as placebo reaction is small. In contrast, the student populations are easily "cured" by almost any plausible "treatment" (Emmelkamp, 1979). In the clinical studies, improvements are more difficult to demonstrate. If a further corrective is needed against theoretical complacency and unwarranted optimism, it is readily available in the relapse rates that plague clinicians (Lazarus, 1976).

The solutions to these clinical problems require a more adequate understanding of the clinical disorders. We agree with Allen's (1980) call to give up "the myth of patient uniformity" (to use a phrase coined by Kiesler, 1966). It is also time, and this is the main thesis of this chapter, to give up another myth—that of "problem uniformity." To foreshadow our conclusions, we see the need for moving away from the conception of anxiety as *a* problem to a tripartite classification system. The three categories which we identify are phobic, cognitive, and panic-perseverative anxiety. Our aims in drawing these distinctions are clinical as well as theoretical: the treatment techniques which we use and, in particular, the uses to which hypnosis can be put usefully, will vary considerably according to which of the three forms of anxiety we are treating.

The Problem of Anxiety

Speaking of anxiety, Mandler (1975) wrote in his book *Mind and Emotion:*

> No other single topic within the domain of emotion has received as much attention or argument during the past century . . . anxiety has not only been considered as the negative emotion *par excellence* in the theoretical writings of psychological theorists but, even apart from its prototypical status as a negative emotion, it became generally the central emotional concept of many theoretical treatments in psychology. (pp. 175, 176)

On the clinical level Millon (1969) gave it the same importance: "anxiety is the primary psychological 'defect' resulting in maladaptive reactions" (p. 50). Writing from a more behavioral stance, Paul (1969) deplored the reification of anxiety and the too casual and overly flexible use of the word in clinical circles. With these reservations in mind, he was still prepared to claim: "Nevertheless, few would question the experimental and clinical importance of the phenomena asociated with anxiety or the large numbers of individuals seeking psychotherapeutic help on the basis of such phenomena" (p. 63).

For the moment and without going into any detail, it can be seen that there is a wide measure of agreement on the theoretical and clinical status of anxiety.* This consensus extends to the measurement of anxiety. Anxiety and fear,† can be expressed and measured in three response systems or channels: self-report, behavioral, and physiological. The anxious or fearful individual will report apprehension about his well-being, exhibit a variety of behavioral signs ranging from tension and tremor to full-blown attempts to escape from or avoid the threat locale, and display a collection of reactions in the cardiovascular, visceral, and other physiological systems, such as tachycardia, increased respiration rate, dry mouth, and palmar "sweating."

---

*Skinnerian behavior therapists eschew terms like "anxiety" and "depression" but they bring them back into their formulations in their discussions of negative reinforcers and negative reinforcement.

†The definitions given to fear and anxiety in this chapter are tied to our theory and consequently a complete account of the definitions we adopt must await the full presentation of our position. For now we will use the word *anxiety* to cover the many effects which flow from adverse and threatening experiences. The word *fear* will be used to denote the effects generated by unlearned ("innate") threats, as well as in connection with phobias (where phobic fear and phobic anxiety will be used interchangeably).

The anxious individual typically exhibits changes in all three response channels but the size of inter- and intra-channel correlations may only be modest and indicates a "loose coupling" across the various measures. A number of factors may operate to cause "desynchrony" between the reactions in one channel and those in the other two (Hodgson & Rachman, 1974; Rachman & Hodgson, 1974) and the clinician cannot use the activities within one channel only to judge the presence or absence of excessive anxiety. Under conditions of intense anxiety, however, more often found in the clinic than in the experimental laboratory, there are higher levels of congruence among the three channels (Grey, Sartory, & Rachman, 1979; Sallis, Lichstein, & McGlynn, 1980; Sartory, Rachman, & Grey, 1977).

Once past the general agreement on the relevance, description, and (direct) measurement of anxiety, we come to the contentious issues of its origins, nature, maintenance, and treatment. The last mentioned is the first concern of the clinical practitioner. Neither he, nor the patient, however, can act in a theoretical vacuum. It is impossible to operate entirely free of our (tacit) theories about the determinant factors operative in problem behavior, and it is better to make our hypotheses explicit than to leave them unexamined. The remainder of this chapter is devoted to a critical analysis of the speculations about anxiety contained with the most influential conditioning and cognitive theories of contemporary practice.

Anxiety: The Conditioning Theory

The year 1920 saw the publication of a landmark paper in behavior therapy. John Watson, and his graduate student, Rosalie Raynor, reported their success in establishing a conditioned anxiety reaction in the eleven-month-old boy Albert.

Albert was brought into the laboratory, put down on the floor, and shown a tame white rat. He noticed the rat and began to crawl toward it. As he approached the rat, a loud, sudden, and unpleasant noise was made to occur. The noise elicited a number of adverse emotional reactions in Albert (loss of postural equilibrium, crying). When he had recovered from his fright and tears, the rat-noise pairing was repeated, with the same results. These pairings were continued until the hoped-for change occurred and the sight of the rat alone caused the boy to recoil in distress. Tests carried out later showed that these anxiety reactions generalized to other white furry objects (for example, a Santa Claus mask) which had never been paired with the aversive noise.

Watson used the details and findings of the little Albert study and the framework of Pavlovian, or classical, conditioning to construct an account of anxiety (and of all behavior, for that matter) which is a model of conceptual simplicity. It begins by assuming that all of the stimuli, objects, and events of the world can be sorted out into two categories—neutral stimuli (for example, buzzers, tones, white rats) and unconditioned stimuli (for example, food, water, aversive noises, painful electric shock). The difference between the two is that the reactions to the unconditioned stimulus (UCS) do not need to be learned; hungry dogs, for example, do not have to undergo special training before they salivate to a food-in-the-mouth unconditioned stimulus. A neutral stimulus can only acquire significance and become capable of eliciting salivation if it is repeatedly paired with the food. Likewise, the white rat was at first a neutral stimulus, or in experimental terminology, a conditioned stimulus (CS), for Albert. By virtue of its association with the aversive frightening noise, it took on anxiety-provoking qualities.

From his study, Watson made an inductive leap from the particulars of this study to general conclusions about the genesis of all psychological problems, and beyond that to all human and animal behavior. What Watson and Raynor (1920) *did* show was how one phobia was developed. They certainly did not prove that *all* anxiety reactions arise in this way. Neither did they establish that all anxiety reactions are identical—in process, of course, and not content. Unfortunately, Watson set his mark on behavior therapy and for 50 years and more, behavior therapists have held to the belief that one set of laws would explain the origins *and* modification of anxiety. Note clearly that the second is implied by the first. The reasoning behind this conclusion goes like this. Extinction techniques—presenting the CS in the absence of the UCS—cause conditioned (learned) reactions to wane and finally to vanish. Therefore, since all maladaptive anxiety is acquired through Pavlovian conditioning, effective treatment will always involve a process of extinction. Translated into the the clinical context, therapy for maladaptive anxiety would take place in two stages. First would come the identification of the anxiety CS's, and second would be the presentation of these in the absence of aversive unconditioned stimuli. Had little Albert been treated (he was not), this would have amounted to bringing the boy into the presence of the rat (CS) without, at the same time, ever again striking the iron bar (noise, UCS).

Before we begin on the critique of Watsonian conditioning theory and its modern derivatives, the reader may wonder if it would not be appropriate to list the shortcomings of the Freudian position which it hoped to supplant. Actually, an evaluation of the psychoanalytic explanation(s) of anxiety is no easy task. The theories are constructed in such a manner as to defy all efforts at empirical falsification. It may be the case, as its defenders write, that "the chief problem . . . has been to translate [psychoanalytic concepts] into behavioral data— something experienced analysts do automatically but rarely patiently and publicly" (Redlich & Freedman, 1966, p. 59). Possibly, but the point is that psychoanalysts have not in fact done this "patiently and publicly." In the many decades since its introduction, they have not provided a single well-controlled study of the validity of the theory or the clinical efficacy of its technique. That fact alone constitutes a serious indictment of the area. One indirect test of the theory is that treatment of the surface problem instead of the "deeper" unconcious conflict of which it is a "symptom" should lead to symptom substitution. In fact the common finding is not for "substitute symptoms" to develop but the opposite. Typically, improvements of some magnitude show up in untreated areas as well (Paul, 1969). We will have little more to say about psychoanalytic theories, assumptions, and treatments except to note one *similarity* between them and the conditioning explanations. Both fail to accord any significance to the "phobic" stimulus. Both, in a sense, are "associative" theories which see the phobic stimulus as a symbol of or cue for an important "something else"—a serious deficiency in our view.

The Elements and Limitations of the Conditioning Theory of Anxiety

The biggest impediment to an analysis of the conditioning account is the easy accommodation of the conditioning theory of anxiety to a commonsense explanation of the same phenomena: it says that we owe our feelings to our experiences, and our experiences are, after all, a kind of conditioning. In this way, purveyors of the conditioning theory of anxiety may come to mistake their hypothesis for fact. There is no question that J.B. Watson did so. What is so surprising is how little change the conditioning theory of anxiety has undergone since its first exposition by Watson. A few years ago, and almost 60 years after Watson introduced the conditioning theory of anxiety, Levis and Hare (1977) reaffirmed this view:

The sequence of events required for fear acquisition is well established in the experimental literature. Its development *simply* results from the pairing of initially nonfearful stimuli with an inherent aversive event producing pain. . . . Following sufficient repetition of a neutral stimulus with a UCS, the nonfearful stimulus will acquire the capability of eliciting a fear response. At this point the nonfearful stimulus is appropriately labelled a conditioned stimulus (CS) and is capable of eliciting fear even when not followed by the inherent aversive event. (p. 303, emphasis added; see Wolpe 1966, p. 182, and Wolpe & Rachman, 1960, p. 179, for nearly identical statements)

From this overview we can glean the *assumptions* contained within this long-lived account of the genesis, nature, and modification of anxiety:

1. Any stimulus can be rendered anxiety-provoking if it is paired with a UCS or a CS already functioning as a conditioned aversive stimulus (higher-order conditioning).
2. Any stimulus that elicits anxiety has acquired its ability to do so as a result of conditioning.
3. The corollary to 1 and 2: one set of mechanisms underlies all maladaptive anxiety.
4. A treatment that is effective in eliminating any one anxiety-related problem can be used for all other problems where anxiety is the complaint.

Evaluation

Assumption 1, which states that *any* stimulus can be transformed into a conditioned aversive stimulus, has been labeled the "equipotentiality premise" (Seligman & Hager, 1972). It may come as a surprise to learn that this premise has not a shred of clinical evidence in its support. Watson, it should be recalled, used *one* stimulus—a white rat. The equipotentiality premise has its source in "general-process conditioning theory" (Seligman, 1971), identified with the names of Pavlov, Hull, Guthrie, Miller, and Skinner. These men and their disciples in behavior therapy had implicit faith in the eventual discovery of the general laws of conditioning. These laws would apply to all sets of stimuli, responses, and organisms. There was to be no place in their theory for a concern with genetic influences or evolutionary speculations about the subject's functioning in his "ecological niche." This is captured beautifully in Skinner's famous quote:

Pigeon, rat, monkey, which is which? It doesn't matter. Of course, these species have behavioral repertoires which are as different as their anatomies. But once you have allowed for differences in the ways in which they make contact with the environment [what Skinner is saying here is no more than that pigs cannot fly], . . . what remains of their behavior shows astonishingly similar properties. (Skinner, 1959)

Conditioning and Evolution: The Work of Garcia

Until the 1960s few took issue with Skinner, and the "experimental evidence" to which Levis and Hare (1977) appealed gave no one cause to disagree with the equipotentiality premise. In hundreds of experimental studies, events (for example, bright lights) shown to be good CSs for one UCS (say, food) would also work well with other UCSs (like electric shock). Watson's strong environmentalism was upheld—until the work of John Garcia, at the State University of New York and, today, at the University of California, became known. It may seem a long way from the study of taste aversions in rats (Garcia's work) to the modification of maladaptive anxiety (our concern), but the trail from one to the other is worth following because the imprint of Garcia's work and theory will be felt in this and every other area of clinical practice.

In his classic experiment (see Garcia, Clarke, & Hankins, 1974), two groups of rats were given a complex CS made up of simultaneously presented taste (saccharin), auditory (buzzer), and visual (light) cues. One group got the "bright-noisy-tasty" fluid before a shock UCS; the other had the CS complex followed by an illness-inducing UCS. All of the animals were then allowed to recover. Next, one-third of each group was tested, without the aversive UCSs, with *one* of the components of the CS complex. The animals who had the cues paired with shock showed avoidance to the auditory and visual CSs, but not to the taste. Exactly the opposite results came from the rats in the illness group: there, taste was a good CS but there was no conditioned aversion to the light or buzzer. In later work Garcia demonstrated that the temporal course of taste-aversion conditioning was very different from that which was characteristic of exteroceptive CSs and shock. For these (tones, lights, etc.), a gap of more than a minute or two could prevent conditioning, even where the "good" UCS for those cues (painful electric shock) was used. Taste-illness learning, on the other hand, can survive a CS–UCS interval of minutes and, in a recent study, 12 hours with but *one* pairing of the taste with toxicosis (Westbrook, Clarke, & Provost, 1980).

The first reaction of mainstream, general process conditioning theory was disbelief. Garcia then gave a genetic-evolutionary interpretation to his data and disbelief hardened into rejection. But the data would not go away, the replications mounted, and finally Garcia made his influence felt in conditioning theory and beyond. His thoughts on the preferential associability of taste with illness and long-delay conditioning in the taste-illness system reveal a strong concern with the biological constraints on conditioning and the evolutionary background to behavior change. With it there is a challenge to the extreme environmental position tacitly held in modern conditioning theories and most views of behavior therapy. Animals, and humans, do not begin with a *tabula rasa* enabling them to associate all events equally well. In the case of the regulation of feeding, if an animal consumes a palatable but physiologically noxious substance, he may—if he is lucky and does not die of poisoning—get ill. But the illness may not occur until many minutes or perhaps hours following consumption. Consider the problem which confronts the animal at that point in time. The eating bout is well behind him and he will probably be in a different locale. If he links up any salient stimulus present at the time of illness-onset, then one thing will happen which should not occur—he will develop an aversion to an accidental, but safe, stimulus and he will fail to learn an aversion to a truly dangerous stimulus. What he must do, to ensure the greatest chance of survival, is to link up the *taste* of the substance with the illness, for that is the most reliable cue to toxicosis. The matter of audio or visual CSs and pain UCSs were also explained in terms of adaptive predispositions. In the natural environment of most mammals, tastes do not forecast pain, but sights, sounds, and smells may be the only warning we get of the proximity of a predator. Predators, however, if *they* are to survive, will not give us a ten to fifteen minute warning of their presence before pouncing and causing pain to the surface of the body. At best they will attack within seconds of our seeing/hearing/smelling them. It stands to reason that exteroceptive cues, like noises, should associate well with painful footshock but only with a delay of seconds between the CS and the UCS.

Evolution and Phobias: "Preparedness"

When Martin Seligman heard of Garcia's work, he saw the relevance of it for phobic anxiety. Seligman proposed the dimension of "preparedness" (Seligman, 1970, 1971) as a conceptual tool for the analysis of the psychological properties of the differences between conditioning arrangements that tap into these biologically based, species-wide predispositions and those that do not. He referred to the former as examples of prepared learning (for example, taste—illness conditioning) and those at the other extreme as "contraprepared" (for example, taste—shock or tone—illness conditioning). Prepared learning is said to be acquired easily, in very few trials, and to extinguish slowly. The reverse describes contraprepared learning; in between are those associations which are intermediate in terms of speed of acquisition and ease of modification. Seligman described phobic fears as instances of *highly* prepared learning. Phobic stimuli comprise a relatively small, nonarbitrary collection of situations, all of which have signaled the heightened probability of danger in the evolutionary history of the species. As examples of the operation of more "primitive" mechanisms keyed to adaptive functioning and survival, it would be expected that they would be largely nonrational or noncognitive in nature.

As it happens, this provides a good fit to the clinical definition of phobic anxiety as a "*special* form of fear which: (1) is out of proportion to the demands of the situation, (2) cannot be explained or reasoned away, (3) is beyond voluntary control, and (4) leads to avoidance of the feared situation" (Marks, 1969, p. 3). The "irrational" or "noncognitive" quality is striking, as, for example, when the snake-phobic person shows anxiety on seeing a *photograph* of a snake he *knows to be harmless*.

Our explanation begins with a statement of these observations into a concise form: Phobic stimuli are a special class of events. There is no agreement on the exact number, but the list seldom exceeds 100 or so stimuli, and if instead of listing "spider phobia" and "cockroach phobia" we grouped them together under the category of insect phobia, the list could be shortened appreciably. Taking them individually may seem to lead to an impressively large collection, but when measured against the number of potential stimuli, the number is quite small. The reader can see this for himself by constructing what we call the "phobic fraction." To do this, put the number of *phobic* stimuli in the numerator (100 to 200 or whatever) and these plus all other stimuli encountered in the denominator. The resulting fraction is infinitely small and very informative. This is Seligman's point.

The human evidence for the special status of phobic stimuli—and the special nature of phobic anxiety—comes from recent laboratory studies (for example, Ohman, 1979) and older experimental and observational reports (English, 1929; Thorndike, 1935; Valentine, 1930, 1946). English subjected a 14-month-old girl to 50 trials of CS–UCS pairings in which the presentation of a wooden duck was followed by a loud noise caused by a hammer striking a metal bar. The child did not develop conditioned anxiety to the duck. A more systematic and ambitious attempt to replicate the findings of the Watson and Raynor (1920) study was made by Bregman study-ing under E.L. Thorndike at Columbia University. She used 15 sub-jects who were all of about the same age as Albert. Bregman used six novel objects as CSs (instead of a white rat), and a loud bell as the UCS. The bell caused startle and distress, but no anxiety was condi-tioned to the items paired with it. Bregman's failure led her supervi-sor, Thorndike (the eminent learning theorist of his day), to the conclusion that the little Albert report: "was a special case and was definitely misleading concerning the probability of leaving on the infant's plastic nature a reaction pattern . . . by any such quick and easy process of 'conditioning.' On the contrary [the effects were] so slight that they cannot demonstrate even its existence" (1935, p. 195). Thorndike (1935) finished with a humerous coda. Bregman's results, he said, "are like what parents usually get who try to shift attitudes [of children] toward a fear of matches, knives, bottles, dan-gerous spots, and the like, or toward tolerance or affection for uncles, aunts, physicians, cod-liver oil, green vegetables, keeping on mittens and the like. Progress is slow" (p. 196). Working with adult subjects, Ohman (1979) and his colleagues (Ohman, Eriksson, & Olofsson, 1975) at the University of Uppsala in Sweden have arrived at much the same conclusion. Slides depicting snakes or everyday objects were paired with a highly aversive UCS. Conditioning was faster, and extinction slower, to the snake slides.

Phobias and Modeling

All of the arguments for and against the traditional account of anxi-ety we have cited refer to direct attempts to condition the subject. Bandura (1969) has opened up the study of learning to include modeling. Behavior change can come about through direct contact with the contingencies and, equally, through the observations of others in a particular set of circumstances. More than that, hearing about the experiences of others (symbolic modeling) can have a pow-erful influence on our actions. Can (phobic) anxiety be acquired in this way? Good experimental data on this interesting question do not exist, so we must turn to clinical reports and the findings from behavior of children in their natural environments. C.W. Valentine (1946) has done extensive work in this area and he, too, puts considerable emphasis on modeling and suggestion in the genesis of anxiety. As this following quotation indicates, however, the influence of the *quality* of the stimulus is all important: "suggestion works much more easily when it is working *with a natural tendency than against one*" (p. 138, emphasis added).

Phobic Anxiety: The Ethological Position

We have seen that the data on conditioning animals and people, the self-reports from phobically anxious patients, and observational reports taken from a wide range of situations add up to serious trouble for defenders of the long-standing conditioning theory of anxiety. It is no longer reasonable to insist, in the face of these findings, that any stimulus which happens to come just before an aversive UCS will become a conditioned anxiety stimulus. The ideal candidate for such conditioning is one drawn from the small set of prepotent stimuli that are said to share one feature in common: they all (for example, confinement, snakes, heights, the dark, insects, loss of support, to name a few) appear in situations where the threat to well-being or survival is greater and has always been so in the history of the species. The implications of this work are worth considering. Although Seligman (1971) did not differentiate phobic from nonphobic anxiety, it follows from his argument that it is appropriate to do so. Human beings report feelings of anxiety in situations as diverse as taking examinations and the prospect of performing badly in a ball game. These are not likely to be "threats which have an evolutionary background" and yet the anxiety experienced in them is real enough. These more numerous situations function as cues for the operation of cognitive acts which include inappropriate self-statements and negative self-evaluation. We shall return to the origin and modification of nonphobic anxiety in the next two sections. For now we wish to point out that, according to the newer position, therapies for phobias should not be as effective for "cognitive" anxieties as are strategies directed at changing the individual's self-statements and sets. It follows, too, that with phobic anxiety some form of nontraumatic exposure to the phobic stimulus should be preferable to the modification of interior verbalizations. Both propositions have been given support (for example, Emmelkamp, 1979; Glogower, Fremouw, & McCrosky, 1978).

The data presented in this discussion strongly support the special status position on phobic stimuli and make way for the distinction between phobic and cognitive anxiety. They do not force us to rule out any chance of arbitrary events becoming phobic stimuli. There are on record instances of individuals having acquired strong conditioned anxiety reactions to tones, lights, geometric shapes, or other "incidental" stimuli. Yet these reports are few in number and usually involve the use of a supertraumatic UCS (Campbell, Sanderson, & Laverty, 1964). A large literature does exist on the outcomes from more conventional aversive procedures. Subjects given nonphobic stimuli (such as the usual laboratory buzzer) in conjunction with painful shock *do* show physiological changes in response to the pre-aversive stimulus, although when questioned post-experimentally they are unanimous in denying any felt anxiety to the CS. Hallam and Rachman (1976) gave their volunteers many tone–shock pairings and yet failed to make the subjects afraid *of the tone* (we have questioned participants in such studies and they say things like: "No it wasn't the tone that bothered me—it was the shock that I was afraid of"). Moreover, such (physiological and behavioral) responses as are established to the arbitrary CS can be eliminated by telling, and showing, the subjects that there will be no more shocks. This instructional control (see Bandura, 1969) is extremely difficult to demonstrate with phobic anxiety. As any clinician can testify, information about the true (i.e., nonaversive) state of affairs counts for less than exposure to that phobic situation.

The crux of the argument is this: phobic and nonphobic anxieties are, to some degree, mediated through different systems. It is this and not the severity of the anxiety which is our concern here. One individual's phobic anxiety may be more or less disturbing than another's nonphobic anxiety, but the selection of the key modification procedures should be determined by the kind of anxiety and not its severity.

Phobias and "Instincts": Other Etiologies

We began with an evaluation of the conditioning theory of anxiety and have concluded with a multi-anxiety theory. This calls for a new direction to the inquiry. Trying to decide between the conditioning or the cognitive explanations of anxiety implies that there is one kind of anxiety for us to understand and treat. Now we must recognize the existence of two or more forms of anxiety and ask about the determinants of each. To return to the analysis of phobic anxiety, does it come about only when the subject has the direct experience of, or modeling to, one of these special stimuli in conjunction with a trauma? From Seligman's (1971) theory we would have to answer in the affirmative. His theory admits genetic influences ("preparedness") but requires conditioning *procedures* for the transformation from predisposition to the overt expression of phobic anxiety.

One very direct way to test this is to ask people with phobias how their disorders began. On this point, Marks (1969) remarked that contrary to any of the varieties of conditioning theory, for "many phobias . . . there was no apparent trauma" (p. 92). As far back as 1950, Friedman reported traumatic episodes to have been at work in only 10 percent of his cases. In an unselected series the present authors found traumatic origins in less than 5 percent of the people questioned (not counting the special problem of agoraphobia—see chapter 11). A similarly low figure (about 13 percent) for modeling, or vicarious conditioning, was reported by Rimm, Janda, Lancaster, Nahl, and Dittman (1977). Results along the same lines have been noted in a large number of experimental and clinical reports (for example, Fazio, 1972; Goorney & O'Connor, 1971; Lazarus, 1971). These are retrospective data and thus some caution must be exercised in deciding on their validity. It is conceivable, too, that some of the respondents may simply have forgotten the crucial traumatic episode. Even allowing for these reservations, there is no question that these data are an embarrassment to *any* conditioning theory of phobic anxiety. The safest conclusion permitted by the above-mentioned findings is that conditioning, suggestions, warnings, and modeling *may* precipitate a phobic reaction. It is also the case that many phobias do not owe their origins to these processes.

More evidence for this contention comes from investigations of phobic reactions in children. Two of the earliest to emerge (fear of falling and separation fears) are universal and can be seen before the end of the first year of life. Painful or frightening stimuli imposed when the child is falling or left alone may exacerbate these fears, but they are not necessary for their appearance in the first place. Young children, especially those between the age of one and two years, when left alone in novel environments for the first time, show strong anxiety reactions and display strenuous efforts to reestablish contact with the caretaker and/or to return to a familiar environment. *A prior history of directly experienced or observed trauma is not necessary* (Bowlby, 1975). These fears can be aroused in situations that are not dangerous in the least and "can be readily allayed by actions, such as clutching a teddy bear or sucking a pipe, that do nothing effective to increase safety" (Bowlby, 1975, p. 168).

What makes this all so convincing is the massive amount of confirmatory evidence from nonhuman primates. Infant monkeys and apes are more likely to give distress cries when brought alone into strange situations (Bowlby, 1975). They also recoil from (harmless) snakes—another phobic reaction which does not seem to need an associated trauma for its onset or maintenance (Hebb, 1946). Fear of heights is still another widespread fear that makes its appearance at an early age up and down the phylogenetic scale (Gibson & Walk, 1960).

The weight of this evidence counts heavily against a single process theory of phobic anxiety and blurs the distinction between the terms phobic *anxiety* and phobic *fear*. It has been traditional to describe reactions as "anxious" if they occur in situations known to be safe and to invoke the label "fear" when objective indices of danger are present. As such, many phobias appear "silly," but only when the selective advantage of being cautious and anxious in these situations is left out of the picture:

> In the past there have been theorists who have postulated that . . . all stimuli derive their fear-arousing properties from becoming associated with pain. Not only is the theory false, but a moment's thought shows it to be hardly plausible. As a natural clue to potential danger, the experience of physical pain is in a special category. The clues to which attention has so far been directed are distal clues perceived by the distance receptors. . . . By giving warnings while potential danger is still more or less remote, these clues enable an animal or man to take precautions in good time. By contrast . . . to await events until pain is experienced may well be to wait too long . . . physical pain has the status of last ditch. (Bowlby, 1975, p. 171)

Bowlby (1975) is saying, with Lorenz (1969) and Tinbergin (1951), and this is a notion that we support, that to the eyes of the intellectual city dweller (and the psychotherapist), phobic reactions "may seem irrational and childish, and may even be attributed to pathological fancy [but] to the eye of a biologist, a deeper wisdom is apparent. Examination shows, indeed, that, so far from being irrational or foolhardy, to rely initially on the naturally occurring clues to danger and safety is to rely on a system that has been both sensible and efficient over millions of years" (p. 168).

The reader who accepts the argument up to this point would,

understandably, wonder why we are all not phobic to all of these "natural clues to threat"? If phobias are a form of "survival instinct," why don't they emerge at birth and remain in force for evermore? Some phobias are apparent at birth but most do not make their appearance until months or years later. It is no answer to cite "maturational processes," but in our ignorance about the specific mechanisms, all that can be said is that given the time required for the acquisition of the normal background experiences, most members of the species will show these reactions on *first* encounter (Hebb, 1946, p. 263). Regarding the elimination or alleviation of phobic anxieties, this poses no problem so long as we are careful not to accept the invalid dichotomy of "innate" and "learned" reactions. Environmental manipulations can potentiate or subdue phobic reactions. The latter, of course, is the clinical goal, and the term to describe the change is habituation: the waning of an "unlearned" response with repeated, nontraumatic exposure. In the previous sentence we chose the word *subdue* instead of *extinguish* or *extirpate* or any other word implying the total and final elimination following habituation. This reservation is in line with the core notions in Seligman's conditioning theory as well as the "instinct" position of Bowlby and the European ethologists. Phobic anxiety is the reaction we make to phobic stimuli which are "most clearly apparent during childhood and old age, sometimes disguised or discounted during adult life [*but*] *these biases nevertheless remain with us. From the cradle to the grave they are an intrinsic part of human nature*" (Bowlby, 1975, p. 168, emphases added).

Phobias: Habituation and Dishabituation

There are, apart from conditioning, two reasons why people remain phobically anxious, and both of these have to do with failures to habituate. Some children may have parents who are also phobic for the stimuli which frighten their children. These parents do not take their youngsters into the presence of these stimuli which they themselves fear (Windheuser, 1977). Therefore, these children do not get the opportunity to have safe exposure (and inadvertent modeling by their caretakers may add still more aversive power to the phobic stimulus). Still others may be poor habituaters and the ordinary run of nonthreatening contacts sufficient to eliminate a phobic reaction in most does not do so in these individuals (Marks, 1969; Watts, 1979).

Finally we have to address the problem of the sudden reappearance of phobic anxiety after successful habituation earlier in life—or the reemergence of reactions originally induced through traumatic conditioning and successfully "extinguished." In some rare cases there is clear proof of reconditioning involving another pairing of the previously habituated phobic stimuli with some aversive stimulus. More usually, the reappearance cannot be tied directly to experiences of extremely difficult conditions in the person's life which act to raise levels of arousal and lower the threshold for the *dishabituation* of previously mastered reactions. A patient seen by the first author had always been especially sensitive to confinement when she was a young girl. This was intensified when she saw a seaman trapped in a naval accident. Slowly, over the next few years, she managed to get over this claustrophobic anxiety. More than 15 years later the phobia reappeared, in her words, "from out of nowhere." Strictly speaking, that was not entirely correct. She was, at the time, in the midst of severe marital strife and on the day of the phobic outburst, she discovered what she had suspected—that her husband had been unfaithful to her. The evening of that disclosure she attended, with her husband, a shipboard farewell party for her aunt. She recalled being surprised at how cramped she felt in the ship. The party lasted for more than an hour, and although she felt tense and anxious pretending to be at ease with her husband, she did not leave. Then, as she stated, "it all exploded." She suffered a panic attack, shouted at her husband, burst into tears, and ran off the ship. The next day her claustrophobic fears were back at full strength and stayed at that level until she sought therapeutic assistance. Bowlby (1975) records many instances of explosive dishabituation like that seen in the claustrophobic woman. We know little about the proximal causes involved, but the following factors can play a part: *severe* interpersonal conflict; being overwhelmed by severe and realistic threats from the natural environment (hurricanes, natural disasters); and certain physiological disorders (for example, thyrotoxicosis). The impact of these stressors can be accentuated by suffering these cataclysmic conditions in isolation and are attenuated by the presence of trusted companions (Bowlby, 1975). The superstressing conditions may, as in the case just mentioned, be related to the phobia (confinement featured in both episodes) or be quite unrelated. What is also not clear is which, of all preexisting phobic tendencies, a panic will sensitize or dishabituate. Our researches indicate that separation (phobic) anxieties are the most likely "targets" for dishabituation following panic anxiety, although we do not know why this should be so (we argue in chapter 11 that many of the most prominent fears in adult agoraphobia bear a marked resemblance to the ordinary, nonpathological separation anxieties that are nearly universal in infants and young children).

Let us see where we have come in the chapter thus far. First, the conditioning theory of anxiety is workable if it is recast as the conditioning theory of prephobic stimuli (although nonevolutionary stimuli may acquire phobic properties when juxtaposed with an *overpowering* aversive condition). For these etiologies, behavior therapy techniques which facilitate safe exposure must form the centerpiece of therapy. While information and reassurance are not unimportant, phobias must be understood as "stupid" reactions which are not particularly amenable to rational analysis. Hypnosis is a technique that can function in many ways as an important adjunct to imaginal exposure techniques.

There are two routes other than conditioning that lead to phobic anxiety. Both are tied into the concept of habituation. As noted, people may *retain* their phobic anxieties due to a lack of opportunity to arrange frequent nonaversive contacts with the phobic stimulus; or the individual may not be capable of achieving habituation without special assistance (Lader & Mathews, 1968; Watts, 1979). In this case any improvement through exposure techniques, if they are used in isolation from treatments directed concurrently at the underlying arousal problems, would be short-lived. The presence of an external dishabituator would need to be detected and dealt with in order for exposure techniques to make a lasting contribution to the alleviation of phobic anxiety.

Much still remains to be done before we fully understand the origin and treatment of phobic distress. We know enough at the descriptive level to deny the claim that all phobias are the same. They differ in terms of sex distribution as well as mode and age of onset, but the source of these differences remains obscure. Indeed, we may not even be justified in thinking of all phobias as kinds of *anxiety*. For instance, observations of individuals who have phobias for scenes of mutilation or contact with cockroaches reveal an emotion reaction nearer to "revulsion" or "disgust." They are properly called phobic because of their nonrational quality. Whether or not they are accompanied by the emotion of *anxiety* is problematic. The question that must arise in the minds of clinical practitioners is: Are they modifiable by the same means, and to the same degree, as those techniques that have proven value in the treatment of anxiety? Our response is: "Yes," but obviously since this is an empirical question, it is something that can be decided only through research.

Cognitive Anxiety

In the previous section we brought together the evidence that bears critically on the conditioning theory of anxiety. The main conclusion to which we were brought was that phobic anxiety could owe its existence to a number of different antecedents. From that, it was only a short step to the clinical relevance of this conclusion: making the correct decisions about the selection of treatment procedures is tantamount to arriving at a determination about the etiology or origins of the phobic anxiety (direct conditioning, modeling, dishabituation, etc.). Phobic anxiety can be thought of as a final common path for a number of distinct antecedents (Bowlby, 1975; Seligman, 1971). Phobic stimuli and conditioned anxieties (it would be wrong to let the pendulum swing too far in the other direction and deny the *possibility* of Watsonian conditioned anxieties to arbitrary stimuli) bypass the systems of rational analysis based upon a sensible estimation of likely *present* consequence. The treatment techniques that work best are those which are built around safe exposure to the phobic, conditioned phobic, or conditioned nonphobic anxiety (relatively rare).

   Now it is time to state another implication of the theories which accord a special, evolutionary, significance to phobic stimuli. Either all anxiety is phobic anxiety or else we must admit into our theorizing—and practice—the existence of nonphobic anxieties. People can become intensely disturbed over personal criticisms—real or imaginal—such as loss of prestige, taking an examination, or speaking in public, to mention but a few of the myriad situations in which anxiety can arise and persist. Where is the "biological significance" in these situations? Any of these may contain phobic elements (for example, eye contact with strangers in public-speaking anxiety), but the major problem in them all is the apprehension of adverse consequences—during or after the person's performance—especially those which the person believes will affect important interpersonal relations. The words to note here are: "consequences" and "interpersonal." Nonphobic anxiety has a strong anticipatory tone and can involve concerns centering upon loss (for example, of the esteem of self or others, of professional status, and so on). The neutral bystander may correctly judge that even the worst possible consequences in these situations are not sufficient reason for the anxiety about them and therefore liken this anxiety to phobic anxiety (where the distress is also seriously out of proportion to the objectively assessed risks). This objection to the distinction between phobic and nonphobic anxiety is reasonable on the surface, but it fails totally to capture the most important difference between the two. Phobically anxious individuals can be given the true facts ("there's no need to worry; the snake is harmless"; "you realize, don't you, that you are in more danger in your own kitchen than you are in a modern jet airliner?"), *believe* these, and nevertheless experience little relief and show little change in their behavior. Typically the therapist will have few facts to impart about the safety of the phobic situation that this patient will not already know and accept. Once the patient understands that there is no danger at all (the harmless snake) or that the probability of a bad consequence is so low that the anxiety is excessive and unadaptive (the jet airliner), the theory which attributes phobic anxiety to anticipated danger must predict a decline in phobic anxiety. The fact is that this *does not happen.* As the patients so often say, "Isn't this ridiculous? It's all quite safe and still I go on with this stupid fear of mine." Hence it is said of phobias that "the head knows but the heart doesn't." Unquestionably the person who stays anxious for hours after social rejection is behaving no more appropriately than is the phobic individual, but the point is that he *believes* that rejection *is* a dreadful thing. In one sense, *given the beliefs or premises from which he begins* ("I must be admired and liked by all of the people in my life"), his anxiety or depression is an "appropriate" and logical outcome of them. We have taken the trouble to labor this point because of the implications for therapy which follow in its wake as regards cognitive anxiety. Mere (re)exposure to hierarchy scenes of public speaking or criticism would accomplish very little if they did not help the person to identify and alter these axioms or beliefs. It would not be very helpful either to ask a person to change his beliefs or the self-statements in phobic anxiety, when these are known to be absent or of secondary importance (Wolpe, 1981).

Cognitive Anxiety: Further Distinctions and Pseudo Battles

The foregoing may help to establish the validity of the phobic–cognitive distinction and shed some light on the key differences between them. It does not tell us whether there are different kinds of cognitive anxiety, nor what we can take from them in charting the course of therapy. The trouble is that people have got so tied down with the acceptability of cognition in behavior therapy that the debates are taken up with polemics instead of analysis. For too long, cognitive factors were neglected in behavior therapy and in all of academic psychology. In the middle 1960s critics began to relax their objections, and by 1968 there were enough people at the national convention of the American Psychological Association interested in cognitive processes in clinical problems to make up a symposium ("Cognitive Processes in Behavior Modification"). The abstract for this symposium read, in part: "The predominant conceptualization of 'Behavior Therapies' as conditioning techniques involving little or no cognitive influence on behavior change is questioned. It is suggested that current procedures should be modified and new procedures developed to capitalize upon the human organism's unique capacity for cognitive control" (cited in Kendall & Hollon, 1979). This recommendation was taken up by so many that ten years later Erwin (1978) could say that, "It is now difficult to find many behavior therapists who are not cognitivist in some sense" (p. xv). There is no question that Erwin is right. Behavior therapists are increasingly willing to bring cognitive techniques into their clinical practice. It is pointless to continue arguments that ask the onlooker to vote in an election between cognitive and behavior therapies (for example, Ledwidge, 1978). There is no sense in pitting them one against the other as though we could find a winner in the contest. It is surely past the time now when it is necessary to argue that "central" or cognitive processes are important in clinical assessment and therapy. Instead, we need to ask ourselves what the word *cognitive* denotes. If it is a word which is to be a synonym for "the mind" or "the brain"— and all of the activities therein—then we gain absolutely nothing with the introduction of that term into behavior therapy. In that sense of the word even John B. Watson would qualify as a cognitivist. Defined that broadly, it is difficult to imagine anyone who would not. To quote Erwin (1978) once more, we need to sharpen our conceptions about "the nature and grounds of the cognitivism" (p. xv). In the following section we list three different kinds of cognitive activities, and later in the chapter, the therapeutic steps appropriate to the treatment of each.

Cognitive Anxiety: Self-statements

People are able to talk to themselves as well as to others. What they say to themselves can influence their emotions and behavior (Meichenbaum, 1976). More to the point, negative self-statements can, according to their content, elicit anxious or dysphoric reactions (Russell & Brandsma, 1974; Veltens, 1968). The mere (covert) utterance of any negative self-statement is not sufficient to bring on adverse emotional reactions. But if the person believes these to be true (see Zettle & Hayes, 1980), then they can lead to trouble. The very popular rational emotive therapy (RET) originated by Albert Ellis is based on these notions. It states that psychological problems are caused by faulty patterns of thinking which occur in the form of maladaptive self-verbalizations. The person believes that, for example, "if something seems dangerous or fearsome you must be terribly occupied with and upset about it" (Ellis, 1977, p. 10). The evidence that such self-verbalization can be identified and eliminated comes from a large body of clinical case studies (although as Zettle and Hayes, 1980, point out, good experimental data for the efficacy of RET are still lacking). In the next chapter, on the use of hypnosis with exposure and cognitive techniques, we will give an overview of RET and the uses to which hypnosis can be put in this regard. The basic idea of this therapy is not difficult to grasp: the elimination of maladaptive self-statements and, with them, the anxieties they arouse.

Cognitive Anxiety: Set

Early psychologists like Wundt and Titchener defined psychology as the study of the contents of consciousness. They believed that all of the significant activities of the mind occurred in the form of images which were available to the trained observer using the method of introspection. At the end of the last century, the Structuralists (the name of that school) suffered a serious blow at the hands of a collection of people who worked at the University of Wurzburg. The people in the "Wurzburg School" (Boring, 1950) challenged the basic premise of the Structuralists—that mental activities were always registered, however subtly, in awareness. Where, the Wurzburgers asked, is the mental image which accompanies multiplication? The request to give an answer to the problem 20×10 brings forth the reply 200, but is not even *accompanied* by images. All of the examples these critics gave in support of the existence of "imageless thought" were forgotten with the demise of Structuralism (which was in its time *the* leading school). Freud built his system upon the premise of the unconscious (and Watson his with the dismissal of all "mental life"). In the rise to prominence of the behavioral schools, people lost sight of the role of nonconscious activities. Such speculation has usually been identified with Freudian theory and, as such, has been rejected. That is unfortunate because with the readmission of cognition into behavior therapy, we may be in danger of repeating one of the errors of Structuralism. The new structuralism emphasizes verbalizations instead of images but seems to assume, like the earlier Structuralists, that we are or can become aware of negative self-statements.

Undetected premises or assumptions may make up the person's model or theory of the situation. If they operate "out of sight," as it were, the therapist's task is to bring them back to awareness if possible or, if not, to set up the conditions for their modification.

Cognitive Anxiety: Misinformation

In a surprising *volte-face* Joseph Wolpe (1981), the most vigorous exponent of the conditioning theory of anxiety, recently modified his position to allow for cognitive anxiety based on misinformation:

> This information can bring about fears that are as powerful and endur-
> ing as those due to true information. Many a young man has feared
> masturbation because he has been led to believe that it will injure his
> health, and many a young woman has been afraid of sexual arousal
> because her mother has told her it was disgusting and dirty. (Wolpe,
> 1981, p. 37)

We take Wolpe's point about the misinformation which can arouse anxious reactions, but we would not hold with the strict dichotomy his presentation suggests. We have not yet seen an agoraphobic problem in which "emotional conditioning" or "dishabituation" was at the genesis of this disorder where, at the same time, this was not worsened by what Wolpe calls misinformation. The therapist must expect to encounter cases of complex phobias where misinformation is a factor, but in our experience it has never been the central problem. That criticism to one side, what is so encouraging about Wolpe's paper is the acknowledgment, by a major behavior therapist, that there are different *kinds* of anxiety and that the treatment to be used must be chosen with this in mind: "Consider the example of systematic desensitization. Since this method contains little corrective information it cannot be expected to have much effect on phobic cases that call for cognitive solutions" (Wolpe, 1981, p. 40).

We are happy to see a stimulus–response behavior therapist (which is how Wolpe labels himself) opting for a broad(er) spectrum behavior therapy. We disagree in his restriction of the "cognitive" variety to anxieties that derive from misinformation. We also take issue with others (for example, Ellis, 1977) who write as though "cognitive" referred only to self-statements. Both misinformation and self-statements can operate in psychological disorders and so, too, can nonconscious "sets." Thus, we must dismiss any idea that there is *a* cognitive therapy. Which of the cognitive *therapies* we select will be an answer to the question: What *sort* of cognitive anxiety are we dealing with?

Panic and Perseverative Anxiety

Now that the last days of uniprocess theories of anxiety can be anticipated, interest will turn to the final number of anxieties in a multiprocess model. We wish to add one more to the list which now contains phobic and cognitive anxiety, and the subvarieties of each. The one that will concern us now is "panic anxiety." The prefix "panic" may seem to suggest that the most salient feature of this anxiety is the great intensity of the disturbance. Panic anxiety is most often seen in cases of "complex agoraphobia" (see chapter 11), and typically it is characterized by extremely high levels of arousal. As unpleasant as these arousal reactions can be, it is the *unpredictability* and not the intensity per se which is the most disagreeable feature of panic anxiety. We have seen patients going through the same physiological arousal in situations of cognitive or phobic anxiety without showing the same amount of psychological upheaval, mainly because with either of these anxieties, the patient feels that he can point to the cause of his anxiety. This allows the patient to anticipate the onset of his distress. It matters not at all that the perceived causes are spurious so long as there is an *apparent* instigator. In nonclinical investigations, researchers have studied closely the effects of surprise and predictability with noxious stimuli and come up with clear-cut findings. Animals (Weiss, 1968, 1971) and humans (Lefcourt, 1973) exhibit significantly more disturbance and disruption to unsignaled than to signaled stressors of the same *physical* intensity and duration. There is no literature on panic anxiety comparable to that which exists on the phobic and cognitive varieties and thus we are in ignorance of its situational and constitutional precipitants. Clinical reports shed no light on these but they do strongly suggest, in line with the experimental literature noted above, that it is the suddenness and unpredictability of panic anxiety which render it so devastating to the patient (Goldstein & Chambless, 1978; Marks, 1969). When a person reports that, "I feel 'panicky' " (when I had to stand up and speak, or enter the elevator), he is not telling us the same thing as the patient who says "I had a panic attack." The first person "knows" *why* he was anxious; the second feels that he has been struck with a "bolt-from-the-blue."

This lack of perceived causality is not an assertion that panic attacks are without adequate cause. The locale of these causes is not known, but it is likely that they will be found in the malfunctioning of biochemical or physiological activities in the systems regulating arousal. One candidate may be the temporal lobe arousal system (Roth, 1959), or possibly the disorder may be found in the structures governing the interactions between muscular activity and arousal (Malmo, 1975). The hundreds of cases of panic anxiety we have come across in our clinical work leaves us in no doubt that some physical disturbance is involved.

The companion problem to panic anxiety is perseverative anxiety. This refers to anxiety which is triggered by situational or cognitive inputs and which then outlasts the offset of these by a considerable duration. The case of a speech-anxious man seen by us can be used to illustrate our use of the term *perseverative anxiety*. This patient never suffered panic anxiety (although he often "felt in a panic" when about to speak in public), but the extreme anxiety he experienced during public speaking occasions would "reverberate" within him for hours after the brief talk. Sometimes this was caused by excessive ruminative activity, when he would go over some detail of the speech. At other times, however, the tension and anxiety would continue through many different situations. In cases like these (the Freudian term *free floating* is often applied to "explain" perseverative anxiety), the defect seems to be in the physiological systems that are supposed to bring arousal back to prestress levels.

Here, as with panic attacks, the therapist who looks for a currently acting cognitive, conditioned, or phobic stimulus to explain the anxiety may be searching in vain. And where the patient produces a thought or points to an external cause of the anxiety, these could be the *result* of the perseverative arousal and not its cause. In cognitive theories of anxiety, the direction of influence is always central–peripheral (i.e., rational-to-emotive). The anxiety-provoking effect of negative verbalizations and images has been demonstrated, as have peripheral–central interactions where the arousal sensitizes the person and then shows up in a bias toward aversive cognitions (Bower,

1981). Where strong perseverative anxiety is in the clinical picture, we have to put into the patient's hands the psychological techniques for loosening these "sticky" control systems (Malmo, 1975) through relaxation, meditation, and self-hypnosis.

Cognitions and Phobic Anxiety: Elaboration and Inhibition

One clinical fact about phobic anxiety which proved so refractory to traditional conditioning explanations is the relatively few varieties of phobias as compared with the number that should be possible given the predictions from these conditioning theories (Bowlby, 1975; Seligman, 1971). This fact accommodates no more easily to a cognitive theory which stipulates that self-statements ("think bad") are always antecedent to unpleasant emotions ("feel bad"). We are not enlightened by this theory as to why people "think bad" about, say, harmless snakes or confinement and not as often, for example, about guns and electric outlets which (1) are far more dangerous (but, we would point out, which are new on the evolutionary scene), and (2) are likely to have been associated, in us or others, with traumas. Yet cognitions do play a role in phobic anxiety, in two very different ways. First, although the origin of phobic anxiety does not lie in the cognitions we have about phobic stimuli, the *elaboration* of phobic anxiety must depend upon verbal-cognitive processes (the snake-phobic patient reacts anxiously to the *word* snake as well as to the visual presentation of a snake). More important, cognitive factors can play a part in the control of phobic anxiety. The patient afraid of confinement will suffer more in situations where he *believes* escape is not possible (whether or not that belief is accurate) and the agoraphobic individual may feel relief if he *thinks* his wife will be home in 15 minutes instead of the hour he feared.

The therapist working with phobic patients must enter these facts into his reckoning when devising strategies for the modification of phobic anxiety. Proponents of exposure therapies (Levis & Hare, 1977; Marks, 1975; Wolpe, 1969) are correct in putting the major emphasis on getting the patient into contact with the phobic stimulus. They are wrong if they believe that what the patient is thinking plays no part whatsoever (see chapter 10).

Summary

Anxiety has long occupied the center of clinical attention, and many therapies have been devised for the treatment of anxiety-related disorders. By and large, theorists from the time of Watson and Freud have held uniprocess explanations and, accordingly, have advocated one favorite treatment for anxiety. A minority of writers who favor a technique-oriented position have argued for an atheoretical approach to treatment. This amounts to "try it and see if it works." In this chapter we have looked at the evidence which favors a third approach. This begins with problem analysis and then asks questions about how the technique proposed for a given problem makes contact with processes of the maladaptive anxiety. This analysis favored a multiprocess model of anxiety. Specifically, it postulated (at least) three different forms or varieties of anxiety: phobic anxiety, cognitive anxiety, and panic anxiety. In the next chapter, our goal is to take up in specific detail the hypnobehavioral treatments for each of these three.

9

Phobic Anxiety: Management and Procedures

We would rather be ruined than changed,
We would rather die in our dread,
Than to climb the cross of the moment,
And let our illusions die.

—W.H. Auden, "The Age of Anxiety"

The organization of the next two chapters, which deal with the clinical procedures and techniques of anxiety management, follows the lines laid down in the previous chapter on the origins and nature of anxiety. To recapitulate the conclusions we reached there, anxiety is a generic term for a collection of aversive reactions which can be grouped together under three headings: phobic anxiety, cognitive anxiety, and panic/perseverative anxiety. The layout of the present chapter is designed in accordance with the tripartite classification system we have adopted. The value of this system derives from the evidence that brought it into being and, most of all, from the *problem-focused* orientation to treatment that it fosters. It does not state, though, that a person will display only one of the three forms at a given time. It is not unusual to find cognitive and panic anxiety coexisting with phobic anxiety where all three may require clinical attention. Instead of the use-it-all "blunderbuss" strategy of an eclectic approach, however, the present system can guide the practitioner in selecting and tailoring the right modes for each problem (Wolpe, 1981).

First, we will take up the therapies for the phobic anxieties and, after that, the treatment for the cognitive forms of anxiety. Panic and perseverative anxieties are discussed in this chapter and more fully in chapter 11.

Treatment Considerations

The first step in the therapy for maladaptive phobic anxiety is for the therapist to lay down a challenge to the patient's self-devised avoidance strategies which invariably dominate the clinical picture. By the time the case comes to the attention of the clinician, the patient will have established a network of cognitive and behavioral defensive maneuvers which, in reality, perpetuate the anxiety they are designed to allay. The patient must be told at the outset that there will be no more concessions to the phobia. As for the treatment proper, insight, information about the phobia, and cognitive changes by themselves will not suffice. There is probably no other writer more committed to cognitive therapy than Albert Ellis, but he too has expressed reservations about cognitive therapies for phobias: "Pure cognitive restructuring works relatively poorly for any kind of phobia" (1979, p. 162). This awareness is, perhaps, to be expected of cognitive and behavior therapists, but it is not widely known that Freud shared the very same opinions: "The phobias have made it necessary for us to go beyond our former limits. *One can hardly ever master a phobia if one waits till the patient lets analysis influence it to give it up*" (Freud, 1959, p. 399, emphasis added). In light of these comments, it would seem appropriate to consider what techniques are best employed. Once again on broad principles of *practice* (if not theory), there is something approaching unanimity that exposure is the crucial ingredient in therapy. The basic idea is that "phobias must be faced under safe conditions of exposure" (Wolpe, 1969, p. 91; and see Levis & Hare, 1977), and "The exposure is repeated until the [phobic] stimulus loses completely its ability to evoke anxiety" (p. 91). What we have here is more than a convergence of views; there is an abundance of experimental evidence that gives massive support to these conclusions. The findings from the many hundreds of experimental investigations into the modification of phobic anxiety can be distilled to three points: (1) get the patient to reenter the phobic situation; (2) *under the right conditions;* and (3) to remain there until there is a noticeable decline in anxiety (Levis & Hare, 1977; Marshall et al., 1979; Paul, 1969).

Flooding and Systematic Desensitization

The case for exposure as the indispensable element in the treatment of phobic anxiety is difficult to resist. We are pressing this point for two reasons. First, because the evidential basis for exposure is so impressive and, second, because many clinicians turn away from the evidence and become enmeshed in "deep" analyses of the phobia. Probes into the "true meaning" of the phobia or what the patient gains by "manufacturing" the phobia (as it were), ignore all that should be recalled from the epidemiological, experimental, observational, and clinical data on the origin, nature, and treatment of phobic anxiety. We would go as far as to say that without exposure there can be no significant improvement in phobic disorders. The evidence for the value of nonexposure "placebo" therapies noted by Kazdin and Wilcoxin (1976), among others, is derived from students and other volunteers with very mild phobias. Even in these cases, however, we believe that the placebo therapies "work" by getting the volunteer subject to agree to expose himself to the phobic stimulus on the behavioral avoidance test (which all of these studies contain).

Having said all of this, it is time now to strike a balance that recognizes that exposure cannot be administered in a mechanical fashion without regard to the patient's "personality," his resources and problems, and general aspects of his interpersonal functioning. Exposure techniques are not the means of producing a "quick technological fix." If used in this way, with no attempt on the therapist's part to discover and use the possibilities for mobilizing positive expectancies (for example, Fish, 1973) and deploying therapeutic "demand characteristics" (Orne, 1962; Orne & Wender, 1968), then we believe that exposure techniques will not work. When used properly they may not either. Even a writer as committed to the use of exposure techniques for phobias as Marks (1975) acknowledges that, by itself, exposure may not be enough: "Clearly exposure per se is not always sufficient and other unknown influences are sometimes needed" (p. 69). Our aim is to review the current knowledge on these "other influences" and how they fit together with a variety of exposure techniques in the treatment of phobic anxiety.

When leaving behind the broad generalities in order to look for the correct techniques for its implementation, the reader may be bewildered by the plethora of terms in the literature. There is systematic desensitization, flooding, implosion, guided imagery, and shaping to name but a few of the labels given to exposure techniques. Marks (1972) surveyed the literature on flooding and came up with 24 different terms. Does anything of substance lie behind this array of terms? In many cases the differences between one or another of these are so slight that it would take a virtuoso in nuance to detect them. Worst of all, the proliferation of "brand names" can distract us from how they are alike in application. By making too much of slight procedural differences among these techniques, the more important similarities are obscured. What we *do* have is a family of exposure techniques, all of which have descended by one path or another from "reality testing" notions of anxiety reduction. These techniques lie along a continuum defined by the rate and conditions of exposure to the phobic scene or stimulus. The continuum is bounded at one end by classical desensitization and at the other by the most extreme of the flooding techniques.

Systematic desensitization provides for the gradual introduction of the patient to the phobic material, beginning with the least provoking scenes on a hierarchy of difficulty. Transitions from the less to the more challenging scenes are under the control of the patient. Before imaginal or live exposure is begun, the patient is taught a relaxation or coping technique, which Wolpe (1969) views as an inhibitor of anxiety. The contrasting position on exposure is called flooding and, as the name suggests, the patient is exposed to the phobic stimuli at full intensity. In its most extreme form there is no relaxation training or any other attempts to teach the patient a counter-anxiety response. The control over the duration of exposure as well as the content and intensity of the scenes is lodged with the therapist. The differences between flooding and systematic desensitization center on: (1) whether exposure alone is sufficient, or whether there must be the means available to counter the anxiety which occurs during imaginal or *in vivo* contact with the phobic events; and (2) the rate and control of exposure. These points have meaning only in therapist-directed exposure. In the home practice (which all recommend), patients rarely "flood" themselves.

The important clinical discussion is not to decide between two supposedly mutually exclusive alternatives, systematic desensitization or flooding, but rather to know exactly where along the continuum of exposure techniques the selection should be made. The consequences of making the wrong decision are, first, failing to get a therapeutic outcome (a possibility when the therapist takes such great care in being so gradual about the exposure that the patient is able to avoid effective contact with the phobic situation) or, worse, an intensification of the phobia (when the exposure is too arduous).

Flooding and Systematic Desensitization: Therapeutic and Iatrogenic Outcomes

Desensitization and flooding therapies have been used successfully to treat a wide variety of phobic complaints and, on balance, there would seem to be a slight edge to flooding (see Marshall et al., 1979). At this time the current theoretical interpretations do not permit us to choose one method and reject the other. Rather than evaluate the correctness of the contrast theory (Hodgson & Rachman, 1970), the extinction theory (Levis & Hare, 1977), reciprocal inhibition theory (Wolpe, 1958), or one of the varieties of the habituation theory (Lader & Mathews, 1968; or, the one we favor, of Watts, 1979), we will take up two questions even more pressing for clinical practitioners than a clear-cut evaluation of these theories (as important as that is, the existing evidence does not obviously support one theory against all others).

The first question is: Can any harm come from these techniques? "Symptom substitution" is the fear most often voiced by orthodox clinicians. Although there have been a few reports to this effect (Hand & Lamontagne, 1976), the weight of the evidence offers little support for this hypothesis. Thus, where a decline in the target anxiety *is* achieved, improvements, and not setbacks or "new symptoms," are readily apparent in untreated areas (for example, Paul, 1966, 1969). This suggests the operation of a virtuous instead of a vicious cycle, and is nicely expressed by Spiegel and Spiegel (1978) as a "ripple effect."

What *does* concern us more than the much debated question of symptom substitution is the problem of sensitization and relapse. A decade ago, Bergin (1971) carried out an evaluation of the outcomes reported over a period of 40 years. His conclusion was that

> It now seems apparent that psychotherapy, as practiced over the past 40 years, has had an average effect that is modestly positive. It is clear, however, that the averaged group data on which this conclusion is based obscure the existence of a multiplicity of processes occurring in therapy some of which are now known to be either *unproductive or actually harmful.* (p. 263, emphasis added)

Do these same conclusions apply to the exposure therapies for phobic anxiety?

An optimistic answer on this point was given by Shipley and Boudewyns (1980). They argue that there is no controlled research on the negative side-effects of treatment with flooding and that in their review of the case study reports of the 70 private clinical practitioners they included in their postal survey, there are no reasons to worry about flooding (and, by implication less still about the "gentler" technique of systematic desensitization). We agree with them in deploring the absence of controlled research but not with their unqualified optimism about the effects in *all* patients. First of all, as far as their report is concerned, it, too, lacks any controls. We do not know whether the clinicians who answered their survey (and not all did) were more likely to recall treatment success with flooding. Second, there are enough reports in the published literature to support a somewhat more cautious defense of flooding. For instance, failure to find improvements after flooding, and in some cases a worsening, have been associated with the use of short exposure periods (Marshall et al., 1979). Moreover, even where exposure times have been of long-duration, some phobic individuals do not get relief. Marks has published a great number of studies on flooding, most of them with very good outcomes, but he felt impelled to note that: "the uncomfortable fact remains that a small minority of patients in the author's experience have exposed themselves to the phobic situation for many hours at a time without, as far as one could tell, rehearsing covert escape or avoidance and yet without improvement at all" (Marks, 1975, p. 69). He further adds that "under certain conditions exposure *sensitizes* the subject [i.e., leads to an *increase* in anxiety] instead of habituating him" (p. 69, emphasis added).

With desensitization, too, there are reports of no improvement or worsening with treatment. In an early study, Lang, Lazovik, and Reynolds (1965) used desensitization with student volunteers. In order to ensure that individuals had no psychiatric disorders, a clinical and psychometric screening was performed on all subjects. The summary of the results in their snake-phobic volunteers shows that:

> The systematic weakening of anxiety with repeated [imaginal] presentation of a hierarchy item was the typical result. However, subjects occasionally showed a perseveration of anxiety and apparent summation with repetition [i.e., sensitization] *that presented all of the difficulties that this situation creates when it occurs in a clinical case.* (p. 402, emphasis added)

Paul (1969) in his comprehensive review of the early systematic desensitization literature noted that poor outcomes could be expected
in some cases especially where the phobias were accompanied by
"problems described as 'panic' and 'perseverative' anxiety" (p. 146).
These dangers of incorrect exposure methods were first pointed out
by Lovibond (1966) and should be recalled today.

From this overview we are left with a large number of positive
findings and a smaller number of worrying iatrogenic outcomes.
Exposure therapies are usually of benefit but sometimes do not help
to alleviate phobic anxiety. Ardent advocates of behavior therapy
may put in the comment that all other (nonbehavioral) approaches
have nothing like the proven body of findings on which to recommend their methods. There is no contesting that point, but debates
of that sort do not supply the practitioner with the information to
predict what the appropriate exposure therapy is for a given patient
and the best way to use it.

This brings into focus the important procedural matters such
as: the duration of exposure; the use of anxiety-competing stimuli;
the effect of imaginal as opposed to *in vivo* exposure; imagery instructions; and the person's understanding of the way in which exposure can help to free him from disabling phobic anxiety. Before
considering these in detail, we can ask how hypnosis can be used in
treating phobias. Hypnosis can play a valuable role at every stage of
the process, from the retrieval of key details of the phobic experience to enhancing the impact of phobic scenes and the patient's
ability to withstand the rigors of treatment without sensitization or
relapse.

By itself, however, hypnosis will not necessarily be of help and
can even lead to setbacks depending on how the therapist uses it in
the dialectic of anxiety and its antagonists. This can be seen in the
contrasting outcome of three widely cited studies, in all of which
phobic anxiety was the problem and hypnosis was employed. In one,
hypnosis was associated with sensitization and relapse in one-third of
the subjects in one group (Horowitz, 1970); in another it was merely
ineffective (Lang et al., 1965); while in a third hypnosis was associated with a significant reduction in phobic anxiety in psychiatric
outpatients (Marks, Gelder, & Edwards, 1968). What, at first glance,
might appear to be a set of puzzling and contradictory findings can
be put into some sort of order when we inquire more closely into
how hypnosis was used in the aforementioned studies. Horowitz
(1970) used *very short* exposure times (30 seconds), which seemed to
potentiate the effect of imaginal stimuli and added to the usual

sensitization effects associated with brief exposure durations (Levis & Hare, 1977). Lang et al. (1965), on the other hand, used hypnosis only in their "pseudo therapy" group. These subjects were given a "vaguely psychoanalytic" rationale and their time with the therapist was spent in discussions of nonanxiety-evoking aspects of their lives. They were hypnotized but given no exposure to the phobic scene. As expected, the subjects in the exposure group outperformed them to a significant degree. Finally, Marks et al. (1968) used hypnosis as an aid to relaxation plus coping suggestions. Relaxation plus coping suggestions is known to be useful in combating phobic anxiety, possibly through facilitating the person's willingness to undergo exposure (Goldfried, 1979).

The discrepant results in the three studies just reviewed stand as a warning against taking a purely technique-oriented approach to therapy. It cannot be the technique, in this instance hypnosis, that is to be blamed or praised, according to which of the above-mentioned reports is being considered. We realize that the current climate in clinical practice favors a technical eclecticism and therefore we have made it something of a point in this chapter to criticize the fashion of looking at and arguing first about techniques, and only secondly speculating about the processes of the problem. We disagree strongly with those like Frank (1976) who believe that "the therapists' choices [of technique] should be guided by their personal style. . . . Training programs should expose trainees to several approaches so that they can select and master the ones most congenial to their own personality" (p. 90). As an example he notes that "Some therapists are effective hypnotists, others are not" (p. 90). Just how we can use this to unravel the results of the three studies is not clear. There is no reason to believe that Horowitz (1970) or Lang and his colleagues (1965) were deficient or unenthusiastic about hypnosis. Neither is there any reason to imagine that Marks et al. (1968) were extremely proficient hypnotists (in fact they rarely use it). The discrepancies from these studies cannot be resolved, nor can the facts from them be put into order, by pointing to "personal style" of the investigators or the techniques they employed. The facts can be explained and the discordant outcomes harmonized by examining *how* the technique (hypnosis) was used with the problem treated. In essence, where hypnosis was used to encourage exposure to the phobic scene, it was beneficial.

We can close this section with a summary remark or two. It is apparent that exposure is *the* treatment for phobic anxiety. The technique may be simple enough in its implementation but the effects are far reaching. The changes can be seen and described at every level. Physiologically we may find them in a reduction in heart rate or sympathetic arousal, and behaviorally in a willingness to approach and make contact with the phobic event. Not to be neglected, and here we borrow a phrase from Frank (1976), is the restoration of morale that comes with freedom from fear.

Exposure Therapy and Patient Expectancies

The treatment package for phobic anxiety will contain exposure and anxiety-control components in a mix determined by the therapist's assessment of the patient's psychological resources and his estimate of the risk of sensitization. While exposure and anxiety-control methods will comprise the core, however, they will not make up the complete content of therapy. The justification for this assertion comes from the literature showing the clinical value of exposure-based therapies (Levis & Hare, 1977; Paul, 1969; Wolpe, 1969). Typically, in these studies there is found a *second* set of significant findings—which tend to be ignored or viewed as a "nuisance." We are referring here to the regularly demonstrated superiority of the so-called *placebo control* groups over the *no-treatment control* groups. In the former the subjects are given a bogus treatment wrapped up in a convincing or plausible rationale. The no-treatment control subjects (sometimes called "waiting-list control") are merely given the pre and post measurements in the phobic situation that all participants receive.

Behavioral researchers have underscored the statistically significant (exposure) treatment–placebo differences but have paid scant attention to the smaller but still significant difference between the placebo and the no-treatment groups (Paul, 1969). Ullman and Krasner (1975) have criticized this disdain for placebo effects noting that "Those who make the greatest use of the placebo reaction often deny its existence. Most published works on abnormal psychology, psychiatry, and general medicine do not discuss placebo reactions, and if they do, it is likely to be in terms of control groups" (p. 100). Krasner (personal communication) is especially critical of behavior therapists who have long tended to cast the experimental subject or clinical patient in the role of passive recipient of the input delivered to him in these contexts. This is a view much in line with pioneering work of Orne and his group at the University of Pennsylvania

(Orne, 1959, 1973; Orne & Evans, 1965). In their seminal 1965 paper, Orne and Evans had to remind researchers "that the subject in an experimental investigation is not a passive entity . . . [we have] demonstrated that the subject makes an active effort in interpreting the nature of the investigation and makes implicit assumptions about [the factors] which influence his performance" (p. 189). It is apparent that the clinical patient is no more passive than the experimental subject. What the *patient* thinks about himself, the therapist, and therapy can expedite or inhibit the progress of therapy. Krasner and others (Bernstein & Nietzel, 1977; Frankel, 1976) argue convincingly for the study of and integration into clinical practice of "placebo" and "demand" variables.

Expanding the scope of therapy to include placebo as well as specific treatment effects brings no increment to clinical practice unless a more precise meaning can be given to the word *placebo*. We will use it here to refer to the expectations and hypotheses the patient holds about the nature of the problem, and the credibility of the treatment proposed.

Behavior therapists, in the main, attach very little significance to the *patient's* theory of the origin, nature, and treatment of the problem, possibly in the belief that the techniques, if applied in accordance with the experimental data, will work automatically. This may be why Levis and Hare (1977), wrote: "The client is asked to imagine various scenes presented by the therapist. *Belief or acceptance of the themes introduced in a cognitive sense is not requested*" (p. 321, emphasis added). We cannot accept this orientation and indeed we cannot imagine any alternative to the following conclusion: the *very first step* in assessment is acquiring a perspective on how the *patient* sees his problem. There is much attention now being paid to the therapeutic value of a convincing treatment rationale (Rimm & Masters, 1979; Rosen, 1976). Nevertheless, the *patient's* "rationale" is still very much overlooked.

When informing himself of the patient's beliefs about the problem and what factors maintain it, the therapist should be on the alert for patients who pride themselves on being "realistic" and "rational" while berating themselves as "weak" and "silly" for being anxious when there is no real danger. These words should cue the practitioner to the fact that the patient may hold a belief in the "willpower" theory of change. Before any steps are taken toward hypnosis or desensitization, these patients must be helped to understand that phobias are not uncommon and that they are not the product of rational calculation. Most of all, the patients must appreciate the relevance of exposure therapy and the invalidity of the willpower thesis (a surprising number of patients see the point of the Auden poem quoted at the beginning of the chapter and many are so moved by it that they ask to have it copied out for them). Bibliotherapy can be a significant aid to the therapist in these endeavors. Two very good, popular books are *Kicking the Fear Habit* (Smith, 1977) and *Phobia Free* (Sutherland, Amit, & Weiner, 1977).

Lack of agreement about the definition and interpretation of phobic anxiety is one of the two major problems that must be dealt with in the preliminary stages of therapy. The other and more frequent one is skepticism that exposure, especially of the imaginal variety, will accomplish anything useful. If the patient's doubts are not reversed, the prospects for continuation in therapy are very poor. These doubts, if expressed aloud, would go something like this: "You tell me that thinking about my worries or getting an image of the fearful scene will cure me of my phobia. And you say that I can get over my fears even faster if I combine this with outside practice. Well that's what you say. But if your theory is correct, I don't see why I haven't cured myself by now. After all, I can't even begin to count the number of times I've had the phobia on my mind. And I've been in the crowded room [or whatever] lots and lots of times and all I've got out of it was more fear. Why should doing this *one more time* be any different?" The answers which should be provided are, first, "There is a big difference between making brief imaginal or live contacts with [say] confined situations and going in and *staying* in for longer and longer periods," and, second, "You've always been very fearful and uptight when you've *had* to tolerate or couldn't avoid thinking of confinement; now you're going to learn the skills which will enable you to get in touch with phobic cues without feeling that overpowering anxiety." Then two more points can be added: "Another thing—you've exclaimed how *relieved* you felt when you could get out of the crowded room or escape from the upsetting thoughts and tight spots. Well that has been a big part of the problem. Getting all that relief upon leaving closed-up places is a way of convincing yourself that escape is the only solution. What we're going to do is to go into these situations, easy ones first, and stay until the relief comes *while you're there*. One more thing: you've never *sought out* imaginal scenes of confinement and you've never gone out of your way to *enter* small rooms, etc. When you have done this in the past you've either *had* to go into the room or elevator, or else the imaginal scenes of this sort of thing have come into your mind unbidden as intrusive worries. Now all of this is going to change and you'll see that there's a world of difference between *choosing* to go as against being 'forced' to go into these situations." In short, we tell the patient that by limiting the extent of anxiety, acquiring coping techniques, and having carefully structured reentry experiences, future encounters with the phobic environment will be made on a very different footing.

Once the therapist and patient can agree upon the problem and the remedies for it, the next consideration is the correct metaphor for treatment. We owe these ideas to Fish (1973), a pioneer in the study of "placebo therapies." Fish not only attempts to sort out the patient's misconceptions about his problem and in broad terms the relevance of the suggested technique, but he also selects the idiom which best fits the patient's personality. An engineer who came to him for help with a phobia was taught deep muscle relaxation with the explanation it would act to inhibit the machinery of the anxiety mechanism. Fish sketched out a "blueprint of the system" and the engineer was quickly convinced of the validity of the rationale and was highly motivated to continue. Another phobic patient of his presented with a very different background. This person had all of the accoutrements of the counterculture—this was in the early 1970s—and had a long history of experimenting with consciousness-altering drugs. The patient was told that the relaxation training would enable him to float through the anxiety scenes as though he were on a "high," resting on a cloud. As a further example of the use of metaphors, patients who have great concerns about control can have systematic desensitization, relaxation, meditation, or any of those techniques described as methods of "self-*control*" (see Fish's excellent 1973 book *Placebo Therapy*).

The patient's beliefs about the course of change must also come into consideration. There are three models of change that give cause for concern. They are the "no-change," "all-at-once," and "straight-line" models (represented in Figure 9.1 at points A, B, and C, respectively). The no-change model is held by the patient who does not share the therapist's view of the problem and/or the structure of therapy—or his ability to make a significant alteration in his own behavior. The therapist must then put another challenge to the patient's misconceptions and set up an easy task where some tangible sign of success is almost inevitable. One patient seen by us had multiple phobias and strong feelings of helplessness. One of her anxieties centered around closing her eyes while the therapist stared at her. We began with graded practice on this problem by having her close her eyes for as long as she could. She was timed and managed

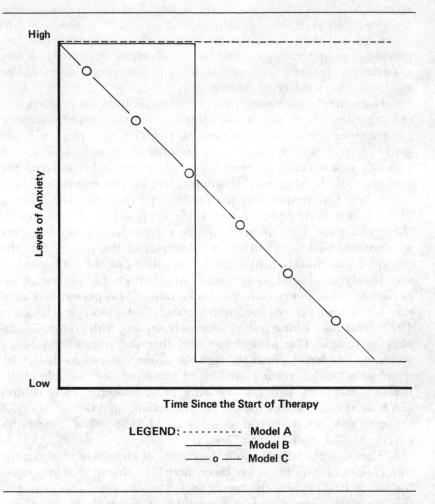

High ⌐ ‑‑‑‑‑‑‑‑‑‑‑‑‑‑‑‑‑‑‑‑‑‑‑‑‑‑‑‑‑‑‑‑

Levels of Anxiety

Low

Time Since the Start of Therapy

LEGEND: - - - - - - - - - - Model A
—————— Model B
—— o —— Model C

Figure 9.1   Pictured above are the three models of change held by patients:
the no-change model of those who feel hopeless (A); the "sud-
den-cure" model of those who expect improvement once begun
to be complete and immediate (B); and the somewhat more
realistic set of expectancies of model C. The problem with the
seemingly reasonable outlook embodied in C is that it makes no
allowances for plateaus and setbacks (see text and Figure 9.2).

this for 12 seconds. After a brief rest she was asked to try again. This time she kept them closed for 20 seconds. On the third trial she went to 25 seconds. This process was continued until she could tolerate up to 120 seconds of eye closure without tense discomfort. Improvement was graphed so that she could see the record of change clearly set out before her. She had her "no-change model" disconfirmed. The therapist seized upon this to establish an optimistic attitude toward her other, and more disabling, phobias. "Just as 120 seconds of eye closure would have been extremely difficult at first, but isn't now, so too will you find anxiety about confinement easier and easier to manage with time and practice."

The rapid-change models must also be challenged. Some patients expect a sudden and complete disappearance of their phobic anxiety (model B, Figure 9.1) while others, only slightly more realistically, believe that the graph describing improvement will show a steady fall without reverses, relapses, or plateaus (model C, Figure 9.1). Where we suspect the existence of models B or C, we draw out the function in Figure 9.2 and state, quite categorically, that the patient can expect temporary setbacks (arrows 1 and 2) and periods of little or no change (arrow 3) and that these are times when people lose hope. They may even, at times like these, feel that all of their work has been for nothing. If they can think back to how fearful they were before they began, however, the overall downward trend (hatched lines, Figure 9.2) will be apparent. We have the patient commit this to memory and give him the graph sheets so that he can consult them, and avoid loss of hope during times when upheavals in his life can provoke temporary setbacks.

Uncovering the Dimensions of Phobic Anxiety

A silent assumption contained within all theories of exposure therapy is the belief that if desensitization is to work, the patient has to make contact (imaginal or *in vivo*) with the actual threat situation, or ones that closely resemble it. Another way of putting that assumption is in the form of a statement that relevant exposure is to be preferred to irrelevant exposure. The person who is phobic about heights or confinement would benefit little in these areas from exposure to scenes of mutilation even if they elicited anxiety which he learned to master. That, at least, is the assumption. Most of the evidence supports it but there are published studies (for example,

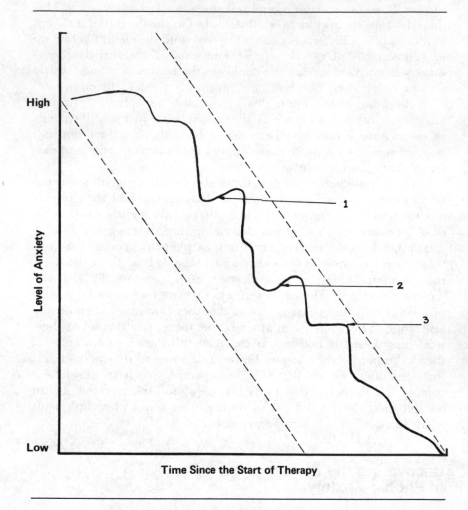

Figure 9.2   Pictured is the overall pattern of improvement (hatched lines), the local or temporary setbacks (arrows 1 and 2), and the plateau effect (arrow 3) which can undermine the patient's morale and motivation to continue unless he is forewarned of their likelihood.

Watson & Marks, 1971) where patients exposed to irrelevant scenes did as well as those treated with a more orthodox flooding routine with symptom-relevant material. It is probably best not to be unduly restrictive on this point and insist that only relevant, and preferably, real-life exposure will do. But by the same token, it is likely that, overall, the use of relevant material will lead to better results.

Oftentimes, the dimensions of the problem will be apparent to both patient and therapist. The patient may be quite aware that this problem is a fear of flying, to give an example, and in particular, heights (fear of flying is not a unitary phenomenon; for some the confinement or loss of support sensations in flying may be the most aversive). The patient may not be aware of the name of the phobia but it will often be easy enough for the therapist to pinpoint the trouble with a question or two. On occasion, however, the therapist can be misled, especially by pliant, "cooperative," and quiet patients. One such case was that of a man who complained of extreme anxiety when riding in the subway. On first analysis it seemed a clear instance of claustrophobia. The fewer people on the subway, the better he managed it, and the more crowded it was the greater the anxiety and the more his desire to escape. Fortunately, before we jumped to the (incorrect) conclusion of claustrophobia and began a hierarchy of few-to-more people and less-to-more-crowded situations, we stumbled upon the fact that the patient could tolerate an all-female crowd more easily than a subway car full of male passengers. Further questioning revealed that the real fears were of eye contact with males, especially those to whom he felt inferior, and an intense fear of homosexual content. Obviously, we would have been seriously mistaken had we assumed a "simple" fear of crowds and confinement and proceeded with a hierarchy of claustrophobic scenes.

To safeguard against selecting the wrong theme or dimension, there are two important questions that must be put to the patient:

1. After sketching out a scene based *closely* on the patient's description of an anxiety-provoking situation ask: "What would make this even more anxiety provoking?" and,
2. "If you could *not* get away from this situation [place, time, etc.] what could you do to make things better?"

Stress this point: "You can do *anything* to make matters better or worse." Many patients can enter into this more completely when hypnotized. Once hypnosis has been induced, we introduce them to the "magic wand technique." They are told: "With this 'magic wand' you can do or change whatever you want. Anything. Let your imagination take over. You can ask for rain, wave it, and, presto, it will start to rain within the room. Of course I realize that that is probably not something you'd want to do, but I mentioned it just to give you the idea of the control you have with your magic wand. As another example, you could make everybody in the room deliriously happy or, if you so wish, temporarily deaf." The therapist then gives the scene in some detail and notes the changes the patient makes. This technique can give valuable clues as to the critical and not just the apparent dimension of anxiety (phobic or cognitive) and what anxiety-control reactions the patient may have been using or the therapist could use in imaginal presentations.

The rationale, procedures, and the techniques of dimensional analyses proposed for phobic anxieties work just as well where the anxiety is the outcome of earlier traumatic conditioning or where a patient feels anxious and confused about a situation without at the same time being able to give or recall any details of the traumatic environment. Stampfl and Levis (1967) mention many cases of "repression," which they interpret within the context of the two-factor theory of avoidance. Just as experimental subjects can be taught to avoid externally presented stimuli associatively linked to conditions of great trauma, people can also learn habits of cognitive avoidance. This can be assumed without invoking Freudian notions of repression stemming from intrapsychic conflict.

We gave only tentative acceptance of the arguments of Stampfl and Levis (1967) until we had direct evidence of "repressed" (or avoided) traumatic memories. The case concerned a New Zealander, then living in Australia, who sought help for a variety of debilitating performance anxieties. One session, while hypnotized and going through some very stressful hierarchy scenes which related to his fears of failure, he suddenly began to breathe rapidly and deeply. Within a few seconds his right arm began to rise slowly from the chair, although no suggestions to that effect had been given (20 minutes earlier hypnosis had been induced through the levitation and lowering of that arm). By the time the arm again came slowly to the vertical position—this time without suggestions from the therapist—the patient was showing signs of being under great stress (pallor, sweating, rigid trembling of the arm). These lasted for a minute or two and then with a sigh his right arm fell back heavily to its original resting position on the chair. During this short period, the hierarchy scene was discontinued in favor of simple reassuring comments and instructions to breathe easily. Hypnosis was terminated gradually and the patient was asked what happened. In his words: "In the middle of the public speaking I started to get very, very anxious about everyone staring at me . . . I froze . . . and then all of a sudden I recalled an incident which happened in New Zealand 25 years ago . . . it was just rugby practice and I was in the dressing room . . . there was a big game scheduled in a few days time . . . I had been very anxious about the game and worrying that being too anxious would make me a liability to the team . . . I wanted to play, but for the good of the team I decided to tell the coach about my anxiety and let him make the decision . . . I waited until he was away from the others and caught him in a corner of the dressing room and told him . . . he looked at me and laughed and said in a loud voice, 'Hell I'd never even thought of playing you for more than a few minutes at the most, you're not that good!' . . . It was so humiliating . . . the funny thing is this is the first time I have thought of it in years. . . ." He walked out of the dressing room without mentioning it to anyone, and did not even think about it on the day of the big game.

The pattern of extreme, sudden trauma and a subsequent (cognitive) avoidance of the cues associated with dreaded situations conforms to the scheme presented by Stampfl and Levis (1967). After a few more exposures to the football scene, this time done deliberately, the patient showed a marked improvement in his current anxieties even on difficult hierarchy scenes with which he had been struggling for a number of sessions, suggesting that they could have been second (or higher-order) conditioned aversive stimuli based on the earlier trauma. Levis and Hare (1977) hypothesize that these can acquire aversive potency through their association with first-order anxiety cues.

Hypnosis and the Guessing Technique

What struck us as particularly interesting about this case was that the imagination of the (conventional) hierarchy scenes without hypnosis did not precipitate any recall of the avoided (i.e., "repressed") memories. We have found again and again that anxiety-eliciting material gains extra impact in hypnosis (cf. Bower, 1981). In the case of the New Zealand man, neither the patient nor the therapist had any intimation that such highly charged matter would explode in the middle of an exposure scene centering on other well-recalled events.

Two of the indices of "repression" are an intellectual awareness that a problem dates from a traumatic event without there being clear recall of the episode or appropriate affects excited by it. The therapist can only guess at the dimension, but whether or not correct in his intuitions about these and details of the (hypnotized) hierarchy, the patient will be unable to corroborate, through recall or feeling, the accuracy of the therapist's material and/or the affect associated with it.

In imaginal exposure the therapist has to help steer the patient on a careful middle course between excessive anxiety to the scenes and a too distant "cold" recall. If the patient's immersion in the scene is so great that he is submerged in anxiety, then relaxation/control techniques must be added to guard against sensitization (later in the chapter we will present a number of these anxiety-control techniques). When dealing with "uninvolved" recall, or no recall at all, as with the New Zealander, the very opposite is needed—i.e., some way to evoke a moderate, but not excessive, level of anxiety. Anxiety can be clinically useful when it assists recall and gives the patient a sense of competence in coping with stress (Meichenbaum, 1976).

Once some part of it is uncovered—retrieved might be the better word—it can be used as the basis for more detailed probes. These can serve two functions: to discover and bring the scenes into awareness so that they elicit anxiety reactions which can then be presented and re-presented until the distress and related avoidance diminish. The method we use in this "search-and-expose" operation is called the "guessing technique" (first reported by Farmer & Blows, 1973). It rests on the well verified assumption that our experiences, once coded into memory, may for whatever reason not be available to unaided recall. A number of experimental studies have indicated that guessing can be a powerful technique for increasing the probability of veridical recall (Kintsch, 1970).

The guessing technique is a simple one to apply and explain. First the patient is hypnotized and "age regression" suggestions are given; by the use of that term we are not subscribing to the popular view that hypnosis can reinstate the psychophysiological functioning of an earlier developmental stage. There is another meaning that we intend. Age regression suggestions and cues can help to reinstate the context surrounding earlier experiences. This is a memorial, or recall, account of age regression. Used in this way it can operate to lower the threshold for the retrieval of memories and their associated emotional reactions. When the patient is "at" the right age, the therapist then commences with the guessing technique. It begins with a series of questions, given one at a time, and couched in the form of a choice between two mutually exclusive options. The options are structured in such a way as to exhaust all of the logical possibilities about the particular aspect of the environment which is being probed. Since it is a "forced-choice" technique (cf. Dember, 1965), the patient does not have the option of stating "I don't know" or "I'm not sure." The introductory questions are organized around the contextual details of the target place and time. The justification for this is the evidence demonstrating that recall is facilitated by the preliminary recall of the incidental surroundings of the situation (Anderson & Bower, 1972). The recall of these "trivial" and non-threatening background cues can also serve as a kind of desensitization, preparing the person to recall and cope with yet more difficult material. In the manner of a hierarchy, the therapist begins with questions designed to elicit details of the time of day, the arrangement of the furniture, and so on leading up to questions about the cognitively avoided events.

To exemplify the operation of the guessing technique we will take some of the details from a case seen by the first author. The patient was a 40-year-old woman who complained of inability to achieve orgasm in intercourse. She was able to masturbate to orgasm but only if her partner was out of the room. On the advice of one practitioner, she tried having her partner stimulate her with the sort of vibrator technique which she had used successfully on her own. This resulted in intense anxiety and a loss of sexual arousal. Efforts to desensitize her to this proved fruitless and it was decided to investigate the possible influence on her present sexual functioning of a number of sexually traumatic experiences from her early adolescence. Behavior therapists have viewed such suppositions with skepticism, preferring to stress the value of a "present-centered" orientation to therapy. This emphasis on the current environmental and cognitive antecedents to and consequences of behavior has paid off handsomely, but at a cost. The unfortunate by-product of a resolutely ahistorical stance has been a neglect of influences from the distant past which can nevertheless make their mark on the individual's present functioning (cf. Ahsen & Lazarus, 1972). That certainly seemed to be so in this case. As a girl, she had been sexually assaulted on many occasions over a six-month period by her stepfather. The patient could remember going to court to testify against him, but nothing at all of the numerous attacks he made upon her. It was revealed that she had excellent recall of the events of her life prior to and after this time, which ruled out the existence of a generalized memory deficit. The guessing technique was outlined to the patient, at which time it was stressed that she should answer "without trying to remember or recall" (or even guess) and "to choose without thinking or debating" within herself. Some of the questions were: "When you were 13 [the time of the attacks] did the attacks occur at night or some other time?" (Answer: "At some other time.") "Was it in the morning before 8 A.M. or at some other time? (Answer: "Before 8 A.M.") The finishing questions were: "Was he naked, or did he have on any clothing?" (Answer: "Naked.") "Did you pretend to be asleep during the attacks or did you let him know you were awake?" (Answer: "Pretended to be asleep.")

As can be seen, the questions used in the guessing technique are framed as dichotomous alternatives covering all logical possibilities. The reaction of the patient as the answers come forth will depend on the distance of the probe from the central trauma and the rate of recall and the attendent emotions associated with the return of these memories to awareness. In the case described above, the recall was gradual and well within the patient's coping capacity.

We have used the guessing technique with and without hypnosis. Based on our experience we would suggest that in hypnosis the patient can retrieve more of the events more easily than is possible without it. This conclusion could also be reached on *a priori* grounds. The disengagement from irrelevant distractions and the inhibition of "rational controls" in hypnosis lend themselves to the processes of the guessing technique.

Type of Exposure: Imaginal versus In Vivo

The phobic patient has to be requested or urged (not forced) to reverse his avoidance tendencies and deliberately to place himself on the path toward the phobic stimulus. There are two modes through which this can be engineered: imaginal or live (*in vivo*) exposure. It stands to reason that the closer the conditions of treatment are to those in the phobic situation the better are the results. This reasoning finds support in the experimental data. Where imaginal and *in vivo* exposure treatments (of the same duration, etc.) have been compared, the *in vivo* variety has usually turned out to be superior (for example, Emmelkamp & Wessels, 1975). Notice, however, that this is a judgment of the relative merits of the two. There are many studies demonstrating the clinical efficacy of imaginal treatments in their own right (for example, Paul, 1969) and many, too, where no differences were found between the two types of exposure (Levis & Hare, 1977). So any conclusion that imaginal/fantasy exposure techniques are of no value can be rejected. There are still other reasons for continuing to use imaginal exposure techniques. The therapist can reproduce, in the clinic, conditions that may be impractical or impossible to arrange in real life (for example, for those who have flying phobias or a dread of being stared at by a group of strangers). Many problems can present insurmountable technical difficulties for any attempts at live presentation. Then there are the patients who are excessively fearful and unable to enter the phobic environment except under the most carefully controlled conditions which the therapist can produce with imaginal exposure. We should not overlook the possibility that imaginal exposure may have one *advantage* over *in vivo* exposure. If applied correctly, patients given imaginal exposure (in hypnosis preferably) may show improvements in untreated as well as treated phobias (results similar to this were reported by Crow, Marks, Agras, & Leitenberg, 1972). That possibility to one side, the fairest conclusion is that, on balance, live exposure is preferable. Hypnosis has a role to play in assisting the patient to make the most complete contact with the phobic scene so that he can immerse himself in it. With the focusing that comes with hypnosis, interfering cognitive activity is reduced and hypnotic imaginal contact is thus more nearly like real-life exposure.

Building the Hierarchy

Hierarchy construction is a necessary part of the treatment for phobias regardless of where on the continuum the exposure is concentrated. The items will vary from the easier to the more difficult. Having items that give a range of difficulty allows the practitioner the option of going more slowly with patients who might be "sensitizers."

In earlier days much care was taken in the application of time-consuming methods of hierarchy construction in the belief that the distances between one item and the next had to be psychologically equal. There is no evidence supporting the need for elaborate efforts at quantitative exactitude. The "scaling" of items on an ordinal hierarchy of easy-to-moderate-to-difficult should suffice. The number of items overall can vary from 7 to 15 depending on the needs of the patient. Where difficulties emerge, the therapist can expand an item by introducing coping techniques (see below) or by introducing more detailed elaboration (see Appendix B).

The process of hierarchy construction and therapist–patient communication can be facilitated with the use of the "fear thermometer" (FT) technique or the SUDS scale (subjective units of discomfort). The patient is told that anxiety, like anything, can be measured. Words ("bad," "very anxious") can give a general idea of how much anxiety is associated with a phobic stimulus, but numbers can do this with less chance of semantic ambiguity. The use of numbers (0 = no anxiety and 100 = the most anxiety) also conveys an attitude to the problem which in itself is therapeutic: it says that "your problem is that you are more anxious than you need to be; the difference between a phobic disorder and 'normality' is one of degree and not one of kind."

The process begins at the zero end of the FT with the therapist eliciting the details of a calm, relaxing scene *from the patient* and not from a "handbook of relaxing scenes." When the dimensions of the problem have been revealed, the therapist should then put together a scene which ranks in the upper reaches of the FT. Care must be taken not to *tell* the patient: "OK, now that we have a zero scene, here is one at the 100 level." It is better to say to the patient: "Well, how would you rank *this* item?," and if it is below 100, "what could you add, or take away from the scene to get it up to 100 (on the FT)?" Once the two end points are established the ones in between can be filled in. If the patient is unsure of what details are most upsetting, or which scenes rate where on the FT, he can be given homework assignments to go as far as possible into the aversive environment and rate the elements on the SUDS scale.

Hierarchies can be organized around the distance of the patient from the phobic stimulus ("spatial hierarchies") or the amount of time the patient spends in or near the phobic environment ("temporal hierarchies"), or they can be focused on a common mediational feature ("thematic hierarchies" as, for example, in fears of "going crazy" or being criticized). Which of these three the therapist uses will rely upon his judgment about the essential, as opposed to the peripheral, sources of the phobic anxiety (Paul, 1969, p. 68).

We have found that most hierarchies will involve all three themes (see Appendix B). All may be relevant, but the most important is the temporal theme. When the duration of contact with the phobic scene is too short, the patient may not habituate to the scene and some will show *increments* to their levels of anxiety.

Imagery in Exposure Techniques: Content, Structure, and Problems

A sufficient amount of evidence exists in favor of the supposition that there is a degree of functional equivalence between imaginal and *in vivo* stimuli. In light of this evidence, "behavior therapists have . . . found it clinically useful to substitute imaginal events for virtually every term in various learning paradigms: eliciting stimuli (Wolpe, 1958, 1969), complex responses (Suinn & Richardson, 1971), positive as well as aversive consequences . . . and so on" (Wade, Malloy, & Proctor, 1977, p. 17).

The argument is no longer "do imaginal events have a place in behavior therapy?" That matter has been settled. For that polemical question we can substitute the more functional one: "What factors influence the effectiveness of 'cognitive stimuli' in fear reduction techniques?"

Imagery is "a complex and poorly understood cognitive process" (Wade et al., 1977, p. 17) and after decades of use in the clinic it is only now beginning to receive systematic study. We do know that the brain mechanisms underlying verbal and nonverbal activities are functionally and anatomically distinct (Gazzaniga, personal communication; Paivio, 1971; Sperry, 1969). Language stimuli can get access to either system, but the arousal and functional value of the words in scene description vary directly with their concreteness (Paivio, 1971, p. 266). Therefore, the first rule of exposure imagery is that the hierarchy and relaxing scenes should be given in specific detail. "You're on the beach and feeling relaxed" will be less evocative than the more detailed and pictorial ("concrete"), "You are walking along the hard flat wet sand just down by the water; from time to time the tide washes over your toes and sometimes up to your ankles . . . the sun warms your shoulders and back . . . your hair is just a little damp." Similarly, when describing the phobic environment, the depiction should be tied to a detailed map of the environment (table, chairs, windows, the color of carpets and furniture, etc.) with all of the modalities used. There is no rule that all of the inputs must be verbal. Wherever possible the sounds, touches, and smells of the imagined scene should be incorporated to lend a touch of realism (for example, recordings of planes taking off, sounds of thunder and storm, etc.). The purpose of all this is to get the most relevant *content* into the hierarchy scenes, for it is this and *not the clarity of the images*, as such, which will make the difference between easy and difficult scenes.

Most but not all patients are able to produce clinically useful levels of imagery. Some, though, claim they get no images at all. If patients are in fact unable to generate *believable* images, then they must be considered bad candidates for imaginal exposure (interestingly, our figures reveal that roughly the same percentage, about 10 percent, of poor imagers are also unskilled at hypnosis). The practitioner must withold a quick judgment on this until he determines that the deficit is a general one and not simply specific to a particular image. The way the patient deals with a neutral image will tell the differences between the two possibilities. If he can get a clear image of his living room or automobile but not the hierarchy scene, then the trouble may lie in a "cognitive avoidance" (not necessarily under the deliberate control of the patient). The remedy in that case will be downward extension of the hierarchy to include much easier items. Our practice is to give all patients a brief (two to three minute), neutral, standard scene before moving on to the first (i.e., easiest) phobic item. The one we have found most serviceable is the following: "It is just getting on to early evening and the sun is setting on a mild day. There is a hushed feeling . . . the few clouds in the sky hang motionless, lit from below by the soft light of sunset . . . the colors are breathtaking . . . flamingo pink, mauve, lovely pastel colors . . . the whole horizon is bathed in a golden tawny light . . . higher up, the first stars are golden against the backdrop of the royal blue sky. . . ." Afterward we ask the person to describe the things *he* saw (it is not safe to assume a one-to-one correspondence between the suggested scene and the one actually visualized and experienced by the patient, so after the first standard and the first phobic scenes the patient should be debriefed and questioned about his reactions).

Hierarchy Scene Presentation: General Guidelines

Once hypnosis has been induced, the therapist should quietly but firmly instruct the patient on the right attitude to the suggested images. First, the therapist should be sure that the patient understands the importance of accepting the images as they arrive without striving to make them conform in every single detail to the therapist's narrative: "In a while I'm going to sketch out some scenes for you to picture. You may get all or possibly only some of what I have suggested. And the scenes may come and go, fade and return. That's OK. Don't worry about it. Just be sure that you don't try to bring the scene to mind. It'll come and go of its own accord."

Second, the patient will be asked, before the onset of the phobic scenes, to give the preselected signal (for example, raising the right index finger) when the FT rating climbs above, say, 50: "When we get to the hierarchy scenes involving the airplane flight, the anxiety at times may climb above 50. When it does I'd like you to indicate this to me by raising your right index finger. Do that now . . . good, fine—that's just what you'll do if the FT rating goes over 50, or thereabouts." In connection with anxiety signaling, the therapist *must take the greatest care not to imply that by signaling anxiety the patient will displease the therapist or that by doing so the patient is confessing failure or weakness.* We also go to some lengths to disabuse the patient of the belief that therapy will go faster if he does not signal. Men may need more reminders of this (reminders and instructions are given before and reinforced during hypnosis), perhaps because they see it as less masculine to admit fear (see Marks, 1969, p. 78). The correct behavior for the therapist once anxiety is signaled is a matter of some disagreement. Should the therapist immediately terminate the scene and have the patient engage in relaxation or other anxiety-inhibiting activities? This is the orthodox practice. At times it may be counterproductive if the patient interprets it as: "I see that you are experiencing some difficulties with the scene and I'll terminate it right this instant because you are too fragile, psychologically speaking, to cope with it. It is too dangerous for you to be very anxious." This is tantamount to reinforcing an avoidance strategy and may inculcate an excessively cautious and vigilant orientation in the patient. Of course, we have to be aware of the dangers of sensitization at higher levels of anxiety. Our practice is to keep the patient "in the scene" when he signals anxiety, but to "dilute" it or add anxiety buffers (see below) and then to remove these gradually *without* terminating the scene.

The above-mentioned considerations point to the need for watchful and flexible behavior in the therapist. This may help to explain why flooding (or other exposure therapies) *are not as effective when the phobic scenes are presented by tape recording* (Levis & Hare, 1977, emphasis added).

Duration of Exposure

Once finished with dimensional analysis and item construction, the next job is to make a decision as to the duration of exposure. Without question, this is one of the most critical factors influencing the effectiveness of exposure therapy (Levis & Hare, 1977; Marks, 1972). By and large, long duration exposures are preferable to short ones. It is at this point that specific guidance becomes difficult to obtain. Some researchers have called exposure times in the vicinity of ten minutes "long," while these same durations have been called "short" by other workers (for example, Miller & Levis, 1971). Information about the optimal exposure time is of great practical as well as theoretical interest. Where exposure to the scenes is not of a sufficiently long duration, anxiety *increments* may occur (for example, McCutcheon & Adams, 1975). One solution would be to choose an exposure duration value already shown to be effective in a well-controlled study or to exceed the duration of the longest effective exposure time reported in the literature. This is similar to the strategy proposed by Levis and Hare (1977). As conservative as this is, it still suffers from serious flaws. It fails—and this is the most serious limitation—to distinguish between "nominal" and "functional" exposure. Nominal exposure refers to the length of exposure as measured by an external clock, and functional exposure refers to the real (i.e., psychological) exposure time. The nominal (set by the therapist) and the functional (achieved by the patient) exposures may not be equal. Patients may engage in a variety of avoidance tactics ("thinking of something else") which reduce the functional exposure while, naturally, having no effect on the nominal exposure. The first author once worked with a patient who would go to sleep once the imaginal exposure to the hierarchy scene began. He received—until this was discovered—zero functional exposure and 20 minutes' worth of nominal "exposure" (where there is a chance the patient is asleep or inattentive, a request to "take one deep breath" is preferable to asking the patient if he is "awake").

Individual differences in coping processes are also left out of any recommendations of specific exposure durations. A given exposure duration may "work" for one patient and not for another—or for a particular patient one day but not the next. The wisest and safest strategy is to continue with a particular scene until the clinician is satisfied, first, that the patient has made "true" contact with the imaginal scene and, second, that there has been a reduction in anxiety *as reported by the patient*. As a rule this is unlikely to occur until at least five minutes have elapsed. Anxiety can be expressed in three ways: self-report, behavioral, and physiological. These three are loosely coupled (Lang, 1969) and are capable of independent change (Hodgson & Rachman, 1974). Therefore the clinician has to decide on the criteria for scene termination. Some (for example, Marshall et al., 1979) favor physiological criteria, but most clinicans will not have the time, the expertise, or the equipment to gather the necessary data. We are not urging that every therapist rush out to purchase a polygraph or an EMG device, although the experienced therapist could obviously put these to good use in deciding when to terminate a hierarchy scene. More important, there are published reports of scene durations of sufficient length to bring about a marked reduction in physiological anxiety reactions without having anything like the comparable effect in the domain of self-reported anxiety (for example, McCutcheon & Adams, 1975). Since it is the patient's perception and interpretation of his physiological arousal and overt behavior which is the main criterion, the final judgment should be based on the patient's self-report (behavioral tests, though important, may tell us more about the strength of the "demand characteristics" than the feelings of fear).

Now we come to another question of judgment. What degree of change should be counted as a therapeutic "reduction"? How low in absolute terms should the anxiety be? There is no published research on either of these two questions. A rule of thumb that we have found useful is to continue with a given scene until the anxiety rating drops below the 50 and preferably below the 30 level on the fear thermometer. Marshall et al. (1979) take a different stance. They believe that "exposure should be continued for some time past the point of return to baseline [i.e., no anxiety] responding" (p. 245). This seems a too conservative recommendation. The job of exposure therapy—of all therapies in fact—is to help the patient to *cope* with anxiety, and the total elimination is not necessary and may not even be desirable (some level of anxiety may be useful as a cue to the use of self-assessment and self-control strategies).

All of this relates to the question of the in-clinic assessment of anxiety. A complete program of anxiety management demands, whenever practicable, that the patient also be involved in outside practice. In it each contact with the phobic situation should be noted in the three channels of assessment. We cannot say which physiological response to monitor. Any physiological change (pulse rate, dryness in the mouth) to which the patient is sensitive can be used, if relevant, but we have found that patients are capable of making global ratings of general as well as specific physiological arousal and of keeping these independent of self-report and behavioral data ("When I tried it, my heart was pounding at about the level of 90 on the scale and I had very anxious feelings, let's say about 90 there, too. Then I remembered that if I just 'let it wash over me' it'd pass. Right away I felt better—down to about 50 on the FT, although my heart kept racing for a few more minutes. Even though I was able to calm myself mentally, my body anxiety stayed above 70 for some while. And all the while after that, I kept myself in the room and didn't shake at all any more"). By having the patient take readings in all three channels, the therapist can get an idea of where extra remedial work might be required.

We have identified the duration of exposures to the phobic environment as the essential (but not the only) ingredient for the alleviation of phobic anxiety. We must also make it clear that exposure is no guarantee of good results. There are some patients who do all that is asked of them, who have the highest expectancies, who are steadfast in the face of long-duration imaginal contacts in the clinic and scrupulous in their adherence to *in vivo* practice schedules in the phobic environment, but nevertheless get little in the way of measurable relief. For these patients exposure to the phobic stimuli is a necessary but not sufficient condition of change, and the therapist must build into the therapy program some anxiety-coping strategies.

Before we get to these, we would like to offer one last remark on the duration variable. There is no clinical dictionary or code book to which the therapist can turn to find a predetermined assignment of just how long to sustain a scene, or live contact, or when this should be terminated. We endorse the words of Marshall et al. (1979) on this question: "The need [is] to make exposure dependent upon individual subject characteristics" and "it would . . . be unwise clinically to terminate exposure if the subject still reports feeling anxious" (p. 245). This is a complex judgment and will have to do with the patient's perception of his efficacy or control. Thus, by still another path, we arrive at the question of the control of anxiety.

Control of Arousal and Anxiety: Reduction and Elimination

Systematic desensitization was the first, most widely publicized and analyzed, of the exposure therapies for anxiety. Given that fact, it is surprising that its originator, Joseph Wolpe, was so seriously misunderstood in his explanation and use of the technique. Many believe, erroneously, that Wolpe insisted on the inclusion of progressive relaxation as a means of inhibiting any anxiety during phobic imagery. What Wolpe (1969) did call for was the use of some method of anxiety inhibition. He named progressive relaxation, feeding, pleasant imagery, among others as candidates, but his commitment was to the principle and not to any one technique. He was, therefore, advancing a *conceptual* argument about the necessary conditions for anxiety reduction, and not endorsing a specific procedure (such as progressive relaxation) as being essential. Wolpe's fears about excessive anxiety and avoidance have received ample confirmation. There are the reports of sensitization mentioned earlier in this chapter, and the many findings that deliberately inducing high levels of anxiety does not add to the outcome of exposure (Hafner & Marks, 1976). Nor must we forget the repeated mentions in the literature documenting the phenomenon of panic-induced clinical relapse occurring during exposure or during great stress after the successful conclusion of therapy. The ever-present danger of relapse highlights the importance of teaching all patients stress-management techniques. One of the first of the reports of post-cure sensitization was made by Watson himself. Some time after the little boy Peter was "desensitized" to his fear of rabbits (Jones, 1924b), he was hospitalized for two months with scarlet fever. A few days after he was released from hospital he was taken back to be retested—recall that his fears had been eliminated with the "retraining" Jones (1924a) provided. On the way to be seen by Jones, he was badly frightened by a barking dog and *all* of his fears returned (Watson, 1930, p. 174).

As for the evidence that exposure by itself ("sheer exposure") has worked successfully, we take the point of those who note that these claims, about clinical phobias, usually agoraphobia, ignore the existence of a very potent anxiety inhibitor—the presence of the therapist in the clinic or nearby (Marshall et al., 1979). In our view there is no profit in the endless debates as to whether or not an anxiety-inhibiting stimulus was or was not present during the patient's contact with the phobic stimulus. It is enough to note that the evocation of high levels of anxiety in therapy is not essential and not helpful and may sensitize the patient. Moreover, high-stress therapies are aversive to the patient, a state of affairs which can threaten his continuation in therapy (for example, Horne & Matson, 1977, obtained good results with flooding yet the subjects said that it was so unpleasant that they would not recommend it to their friends).

Decisions about the inclusion of anxiety-inhibiting techniques during exposure depend on such factors as the patient's response during exposure, a history of sensitization reactions or panic attacks, his ability to tolerate, comfortably, higher levels of anxiety, and the intensity of the fear. Where any or all of these are in the picture, there is evidence to suggest that relaxation or its *functional equivalent* should be included *and taught properly** (Moore, 1965; Morganstern, 1973, 1974; Schubot, 1966).

Anxiety Control Methods

The methods of anxiety control fall into two categories. There are those which alter the anxiety-eliciting properties of the scene content (or the actual environment in real-life exposure) by adding or subtracting key elements. The other, indirect, path is through the use of procedures designed to lower the patient's level of physiological arousal. Meditation and progressive relaxation techniques have been used most extensively and effectively. We have given a detailed account of their application in chapter 6 and Appendix A, respectively. Drug-assisted relaxation is used much less often, but it does have a place in certain selected cases (Hussain, 1971). These techniques can make a significant contribution in their own right. Consequently, their use need not be limited to the role of adjuncts to exposure. There are a number of intra-scene techniques which are also useful.

Modeling

Watching another person approach and make contact with an anxiety-provoking stimulus has therapeutic effects and increases the willingness of the fearful observer to do the same. Live demonstrations accomplish this (for example, Bandura, Jeffrey, & Wright, 1974) and more recent reports suggest the same for covert (imaginal) or symbolic modeling (Rosenthal & Reese, 1976). Another variety we use is "participant" covert modeling, which begins when the patient is hypnotized and told that a trusted figure is at his side as he goes into the feared situation. This is in contrast to "observational" modeling, which has the patient "look on" as the model approaches the phobic simulus.

*We are aware that relaxation and other coping techniques have been tried and found to be unnecessary *as taught*. Closer investigation reveals that often the "teaching" program is given no more than a few minutes (for example, Riddick & Meyer, 1973) and it is unlikely that *any* complex skill can be acquired in so brief a time. In the studies in which live, and not taped, coping skills are taught for *at least* two sessions, significantly better results are obtained (Borkovec & Sides, 1979). Moreover, coping techniques, even if unnecessary in getting the patient through the hierarchy, may help him to fight off relapses, which occur all too often post-therapy.

Although the published research data does not indicate a difference between coping and mastery behavior of the models (for example, Kornhaber & Schroeder, 1975), our feeling is that having the (imaginal) model first exhibit and then overcome his fears is preferable to seeing a model stride confidently into range of the phobic situation displaying obvious lack of concern at every step of the way. "You are standing well away from the cliff. A person who seems to be quite frightened of heights walks very slowly toward the edge . . . he stops, looks back . . . takes a deep breath and seems about to turn back . . . pauses, seems to collect himself, and then moves even closer to the edge. As he gets to a place which is still a safe distance from the edge, he freezes once he sees how far the drop is . . . but he decides to stay there and stick it out . . . the seconds and minutes go by [see chapter 10 for the time-expansion imagery] and he walks back toward you with a big smile on his face, delighted at having overcome his fears. He then decides to test out his newly won skills and has another try. This time he shows some anxiety and hesitancy but much less then before." The use of either covert modeling procedure should not be continued indefinitely; eventually the patient must enter the phobic environment "unaided" (Reiss, 1980), both in the scene and *in vivo*.

Distancing

Extremely anxious patients can get exposure to the phobic stimulus and protection from it at the same time with "embedding techniques." These too begin in hypnosis with suggestions that the patient is in a pleasant scene. The idea is for the patient to have a "daydream" about the phobic stimulus within the relaxing scene: "As you lie there resting comfortably on the gently sloping hill, warmed by the sun, you begin to drift into a reverie . . . you see [the phobic events] and it's so vivid . . . you can feel the closeness of the room. . . ." If the patient gets too upset at any time the therapist can remind him of where he is, on the hillside: "You can notice the azure sky and the deep emerald green of the grass and the crowded little room seems a long way off; you can still see it but you are more aware of the breeze against your face. . . ." The patient can get involved in the disturbing scenes but within the all-encompassing pleasant scene. This scene-within-a-scene technique gives added distance from the phobic stimulus and the anxiety elicited by it. A variation of the daydream method has the patient view the feared event or object on a TV screen, so that he can bring it into clear focus or not, as he wishes.

Covert Reinforcement

In his early studies for fear reduction in animals, Wolpe (1958) used feeding to speed the progress of the animal through the (live) hierarchy environments. We have seen the same sort of facilitation in patients, especially when eating or drinking something sweet. The timing of the consumatory response is a matter of some interest. We tell patients to drink the orange juice or eat the chocolate only once they have made some movement in the required direction or have remained a little longer in the disturbing place. Assuming the efficacy of covert as well as overt reinforcement (for example, Steffens, 1977), it can be suggested to the patient that he is very thirsty and the water, lemonade, or whatever it is that he prefers to drink is near or next to the phobic object. For a variation on this theme, the patient can approach the feared object while eating or drinking (on occasion, we have had the hypnotized subject drink something pleasant while imagining a hierarchy scene).

The Behavior of the Patient

Clinical research (for example, Marshall, Stoian, & Andrews, 1977) emphasizes the relevance of the patient's (imaginal) behavior in fear reduction. Specifically, patients improve more quickly if they are asked to interact with or engage in actions in the phobic situation, whereas patients given passive exposure procedures do not cope as well, and tend to experience more anxiety.

Humor

Being able to see the lighter side of the picture is something notably absent in anxious patients. As a rule, they exhibit a solemn and humorless demeanor. If they can be induced to smile or laugh as they take up the challenge of the exposure routine, they can get a more balanced perspective. We go out of our way to use humor and whimsy to take some of the "deep seriousness" out of the proceedings (a flippant attitude is, of course, uncalled for and the patient must not think a joke is taking place at his expense). A direct suggestion to smile or laugh is unlikely to work, so the therapist must look elsewhere for a stimulus to a humor response. Two possibilities are adding elements to the scene which are amusing (for example, having all of the people on the plane start telling jokes, which the therapist recounts to the patient) or by having the patient recall an amusing incident while "in" the scene.

Cognitive Avoidance:
The Use of Hypnosis to Induce Anxiety

For *all* patients the final scenes should be given with suggestions that the therapist's presence is difficult or impossible to notice: "You can hear the words but it's as though they're coming from inside your head. You're all by yourself in [the situation]." All "aids" should be removed before exposure is concluded (Bandura, 1977, p. 202) and that includes the support from the proximity of the therapist.

Where studies demonstrate the relative superiority of flooding over desensitization, it may be the case that the "gentler" techniques allow the person to avoid a full confrontation with the threatening environment. Under certain circumstances the best course of action is to "force" the patient into (vicarious) sustained contact with the things he fears, especially in those patients who report no anxiety at all during exposure to relevant scenes.

Where avoidance continues, "response prevention" may be employed. This is a method for eliminating fear reactions, and which originated in laboratory research. In brief, what this entails is confining the subject in the presence of the feared stimulus (Baum, 1970). The longer the response is prevented, the greater the reduction in avoidance behavior. These techniques have been used to good effect in the elimination of crippling obsessive-compulsive disorders where the therapist forcibly intervenes to interfere with the execution of the compulsive ritual (Rachman & Hodgson, 1980). The counterpart in imaginal exposure to response (i.e., escape) blocking can be achieved through suggestions of immobility. Suggestions of bodily heaviness and immobility start the procedure: "Your legs are so heavy . . . perhaps you could move them but it certainly wouldn't be easy . . . it's as though they're stuck to the ground with a powerful glue . . . your arms are hanging heavily at your side . . . it would be impossible to raise them . . . even your voice won't work. . . ." The patient is "locked up" inside the phobic scene without defensive resources, by himself until the effective contact is established and sustained. Needless to say, this response-prevention technique has special and limited application with patients who have serious but circumscribed phobias which they chronically avoid.

Fears and Phobias in Children

The same problems that we encountered in our analysis of the origin and treatment of adult phobias are met in the literature on children's phobias with one important addition: the treatment of phobias and anxiety in adults has been intensively researched over the past two decades, whereas there is a virtual absence of experimental data on treatment methods for these problems in children. The situation was so disheartening when Miller, Barrett, and Hampe (1974) reviewed the existing work that they chose to give their chapter the title: "Phobias of Childhood in a Prescientific Era." Five years later Ollendick (1979) voiced a similar conclusion. This state of affairs is indeed ironic when it is recalled that the dominant schools of clinical practice, psychoanalysis and behavior therapy, began their theory-building with the study of phobias in children. The names of little Hans (Freud, 1959), little Albert (Watson & Rayner, 1920), and Peter (Jones, 1924b) are known to all. What is puzzling is why these groundbreaking reports have not excited investigators to the same systematic research efforts as have been aimed at the adult varieties. For this reason this section on the treatment of children's phobias and anxieties, unavoidably, will contain fact and speculation in equal proportion.

The difficulties begin with the definition of phobias and their distinction from fears on the one hand, and anxieties on the other (Berecz, 1968). In adults, fears are distinguished from phobias in two ways. In fears, there is a concensus on the existence of a present danger, whereas in phobias there is not only the absence of danger but the realization by the individual that his phobic concerns are groundless. Children by comparison *may believe* that the phobic situation *is* dangerous. There is a risk in pressing into service with children categories which serve well in the adult case. As is known from developmental psychology, children are not miniature adults. Methods of treatment that work with adults may not be helpful for children—or may even have effects diametrically opposed to those obtained with adults (for example, Jersild & Holmes, 1935).

Frequency and Kind

Epidemiological work has revealed that mild to moderate fears are almost universal in children up to the age of 12. MacFarlane, Allen, and Honzik (1954) found mild to moderate fears in 90 percent of their sample, a result very much in line with earlier research (for example, Jersild & Holmes, 1935). Multiple fears are common, with findings indicating 2 to 5 per child (LaPouse & Monk, 1959) and in one survey of rural British school children up to 7.5 per child. Typically, girls report more fears than boys (Ollendick, 1979), but whether this is a true finding or an artifact of boys' unwillingness to report fears is still unclear.

In most children these fears are reasonably transient and of a mild to moderate intensity—facts which are not grounds for dismissing the importance of these fears. Ollendick (1979) says, and it is an entirely reasonable claim, that although

> it is common for children to exhibit a number of fears throughout development [and though] these fears dissipate through natural exposure to the feared stimuli, [they] should not be ignored since even mild to moderate fears cause psychological discomfort and may evolve into more persistent and excessive fear. (p. 163)

Estimates of the percentage that fall into the "persistent and excessive" category vary from 5 to 8 percent (Agras, Sylvester, & Oliveau, 1969).

The kinds of fears reported by children vary with age. Sudden noises and loss of support (Gray, 1971) are two of the first to emerge. Fears of separation from mother or caretaker appear in virtually all children after 6 to 9 months of age—regardless of the child's experiences or culture (Bowlby, 1975). Separation fears, in normal circumstances, continue up to age 3 and decline slowly after that. At age 3, fears of the dark, the strange (especially when in the dark or alone), and small animals begin. Social fears (of school, failure) typically have their onset with first schooling experiences. After showing a decline across the years 7 to 11, many of the common fears make a reappearance at age 11 to 12 (Miller et al., 1974).

The prognosis for untreated fears is a function of their severity. Early studies reported a complete disappearance (habituation in our terms) of mild fears within three years (Hagman, 1932; Jersild & Holmes, 1935). The term "in remission" might be more apt in view of the frequent reappearance of phobias in stressful circumstances (Whitehurst & Vasta, 1977) and their quick rates of reacquisition when paired with aversive unconditioned stimuli (Ohman, 1979; Valentine, 1930). For more excessive fears, the prognosis for untreated phobias is not as good. Agras et al. (1969) carried out a five-year follow-up on untreated phobias in adults and children. They found that 100 percent of the children's sample improved to some degree (37 percent of the adults were actually *worse* at follow-up). These figures, however, are not all they appear to be; fully 60 percent of these children still showed mild to moderate fears.

The phobia that attracted the greatest attention is school phobia. This is probably because the school-refusing child will come to the notice of legal authorities. The term *school phobia* was coined by Johnson, Falstein, Szurek, and Svendson (1941), and in most respects it is an unfortunate one. It implies the existence of a similar origin and treatment for all cases of school refusal, a position that cannot be reconciled to the facts. Some children balk at going to school because of some real or fancied threat associated with it (for example, an unsympathetic teacher; taunting classmates), and in a real sense they *are* afraid of school. With other school refusers, the problem is not so much going to school as it is of *leaving* home (Kennedy, 1965; Vaughn, 1957). A question which will separate the two is: what does the child do on Saturdays, Sundays, and holidays? Children with separation anxieties are likely to give signs of unease and fear whenever they have to leave home and guardians. Davidson (1960) suggests that these children are "mother-philes" rather than "school-phobes." This form of school phobia, called Type II by Kennedy (1965), is likely to involve very complex mechanisms and more associated disorders than are other childhood fears and phobias (Bowlby, 1975; Gelfand, 1978; Johnson, 1957). In a large number of cases, there is a history of parents fostering an overdependent style of life in the child. For a vivid description of the clinical picture, the reader should consult Waldfogel (1959). The incidence of school phobia has been put at 17 per thousand school-age children (Kennedy, 1965), and between 2 and 8 percent of the referrals in some child clinics are school phobic (Kahn & Nursten, 1962).

Not only is this type of school phobia difficult to treat once well established but it also defies simple explanation. Those, like Vaughn (1957) and Davidson (1960), who downplay the fear of school as such, are probably on the right track, as they are in highlighting the excessive attachments of these children to their mothers. We wonder, however, at the insistence on *mother* attachment. School phobic children may also exhibit considerable father and home attachment. Perhaps we can get more insight into the nature of the disorder by asking ourselves this question: when a "school" phobic child attains the age of 17, 18, or older—when school attendance is no longer mandatory—and still retains all of the features of the problem, what name would then be given to his condition? A clinician would have no hesitation in answering: agoraphobia. This is our view, and thus many of the methods known to be of value in the management of agoraphobia could be applied to these children (see chapter 11).

Treatment

The first large-scale treatment, and in many respects still a model for present-day practitioners, was conducted by Jones (1924a). She treated 70 phobic children with one or more of these five techniques: (1) elimination through disuse (by keeping the phobic stimulus away from the child); (2) punishment through social ridicule; (3) verbal persuasion; (4) direct reconditioning (by bringing the child gradually into closer contact with the phobic stimulus while giving food or reassurance); and (5) social imitation. Only two of the five were always successful: reconditioning and social imitation—by having the child observe a fearless model.

In contemporary terms "direct reconditioning" and "social imitation" would be translated into "exposure" and "modeling," respectively. These, plus operant and cognitive techniques, complete the list of therapeutic procedures which have recorded some successes in the treatment of children's fears and phobias.

Exposure Techniques

With adults' fears, the therapist can range over the whole continuum of exposure techniques from careful systematic desensitization to the extremes of flooding. Therapists concur that exposure to the feared situation is also imperative with children, but there are strong doubts, which we fully share, as to the use of techniques of the flooding variety. Ullmann and Krasner (1975) remind the therapist that the more arduous exposure techniques can lead to an association in the patient's mind between the therapist and fear, and Graziano (1975) argues that there are serious ethical/humanitarian questions raised, if only because the children do not have a choice as to whether they will remain in or leave a flooding-type exposure treatment.

The evidence for the less demanding systematic desensitization techniques is mixed, with some (Hatzenbuehler & Schroeder, 1978) claiming that its value has not been proven, while against that there are a number of uncontrolled clinical case studies that report successful outcomes (Freeman, Roy, & Hemmick, 1976; Lazarus & Abromovitz, 1962; Ollendick, 1979). In one large-scale study (Miller, Barrett, Hampe, & Noble, 1972), systematic desensitization was compared with a "psychotherapy" condition and a waiting-list control. Overall, the results indicated that both treatment groups were significantly more improved (most of the participants were "school phobic") than the no-treatment children but were not different from each other. However, since the children in the "psychotherapy" group were "encouraged to . . . formulate behavioral strategies for coping with stress and the affect accompanying these efforts" (p. 271) and parents were advised to use response cost procedures for phobic behavior (for example, denying television viewing on the day of school refusal), the *true* differences between the treatment groups may have been minimal. It is especially interesting that the younger children in the Miller et al. (1972) study improved much more than did the older children aged 11 and over. This is in line with the strong urging of experienced practitioners that no delay should be allowed in treating excessive fears in children (Kennedy, 1965).

If speed is necessary in returning the child to the feared situation, it is also true that care must be taken to equip the child with anxiety-inhibiting skills or else to arrange for secure conditions (Watson & Rayner, 1920, were unable to elicit a conditioned fear reaction to the white rat when the little boy was allowed to suck his thumb). First, the child must trust the person (parent or therapist) who asks him to give up his avoidance habits. The number of possible anxiety-inhibitory techniques is limited only by the ingenuity of the therapist. Jones (1924a) used feeding during exposure, while others were able to teach children muscle relaxation (Kondas, 1967). Lazarus and Abromovitz (1962) used imagery in an innovative fashion with a school-phobic child. They had the child attempt, in imagination, longer and longer trips away from home while accompanying a comic book hero on a "secret mission." The hero took the child into the vicinity of the school and then "had to" leave for periods of increasing length while carrying out the secret mission. Thus, the exposure was graded and the child was given progressively longer periods alone without his guardian. By way of general guidelines on "emotive" imagery, Lazarus and Abromovitz (1962) recommend images that arouse feelings of self-assertion, pride, humor, and affection.

To our knowledge no one has yet combined graduated exposure techniques with hypnosis. In view of the high hypnotizability of children, their wholehearted entry into fantasy techniques, and the cumulative evidence favoring exposure techniques for children's fears, the use of hypnosis-assisted procedures of this sort would seem long overdue. We also see the merit in taking a lead from the work of primate ethologists who have shown the value of contact comfort in fear situations (Harlow & Zimmerman, 1959; Menzel, personal communication).

Modeling Techniques

The exposure to the feared situation (direct or vicarious) can be given added value if it includes the use of another person. The fearful child may derive some comfort and security from the presence of someone else (Hill & Hansen, 1962; Wolfenstein, 1957). Modeling influences also work to reduce fear. Imagining, seeing a film of, or actually witnessing another person go into the avoided environment and *interact* with the feared stimulus has a reassuring and fear-inhibiting effect on the child observer. The behavior of the model may be a factor, although this point is still in doubt. Nevertheless, our results prompt us to suggest the use of a model who is somewhat fearful in his earlier interactions, and less so as he spends more time in contact with the feared stimulus. One other dimension of the modeling procedures which may count is the age of the model. Kornhaber and Schroeder (1975) compared adult and child models and found greater fear reduction in those children who were in the peer-modeling condition.

In the fear situation, the child patient or his model must not merely be exposed to the fear-eliciting agent. It is essential that the child be engaged in positive interactions at the same time (Holmes, 1936; Jones, 1924a, b). The child can benefit still further if he is given cognitive techniques of anxiety inhibition. Kanfer, Karoly, and Newman (1975) gave a group of five- to six-year-old children, who were mildly phobic to dark, three different kinds of sentences to say to themselves while undergoing exposure to a darkened room. Some of the children were given verbalizations of self-competence ("I'm brave, I can take care of myself"). Others were asked to use verbalizations describing the dark as pleasant ("the dark is a fun place to be"). The third group uttered nonrelevant statements ("Mary had a little lamb"). The findings of interest were: the children given exposure and competence sentences were significantly better than those given exposure plus counterattitudinal or distraction sentences. More evidence for the place of cognitive strategies in the behavior of the model (and, of course, in the child patient) is given support by the work of Jakibchuk and Smeriglio (1976). Their socially anxious child subjects benefited from vicarious modeling only when the model spoke aloud to himself, in the first person, about how he felt and what he was trying to do. These data go well together with those of Kanfer et al. (1975) in highlighting the importance of nonpassive exposure if the child is to derive significant gains from treatment.

The Role of the Parents

It is unlikely there will be lasting improvement in the child's behavior unless there is an *in vivo* practice built into the treatment program (Tasto, 1969). This is tantamount to saying that the therapist must secure the cooperation of the parents, or guardians, of the child. His success in doing this will depend, among other things, on counseling the parent against: self-blame; adherence to the willpower theory of fear reduction (some parents, especially fathers, hold to the belief that the child is just being "silly" and can be coerced into "being sensible"); and, last, the belief that if they do nothing about it the fear will go away. Parents can adversely affect matters by inadvertently modeling the fear which they are trying to eliminate in the child, so the therapist must be sure there are not stressful (dishabituating) circumstances leading to a reinstatement of fears eliminated in the clinic.

In this brief review of the origin and treatment of children's fears, we have looked at a literature—and our own practice—which has focused exclusively on children's fears once they have come into the excessive range. It is to be hoped that researchers and practitioners will take up the advice of Bandura and Menlove (1968) to investigate *preventive* strategies. Up to the present little has been done in this direction. Poser and King (1975) did find promising results from their efforts at fear reduction before children were exposed to harmless snakes and, more significantly, Melamed and Siegel (1975) successfully used symbolic modeling in preparing children who were about to undergo surgical procedures. The children in the symbolic-modeling group showed less in the way of self-reports of fear, lowered physiological reactivity, and fewer postoperative problems than the control-group children. These results are very promising and should be followed up in other areas. For example, it is common for most children to experience quite considerable distress before starting kindergarten or regular school. Perhaps it may be possible to immunize children to these and other age-related techniques employed in "stress innoculation" programs (Meichenbaum & Cameron, 1973). This ounce of prevention may be worth many pounds of cure.

Phobic Anxiety: A Last Comment

The treatment of choice in phobic anxiety is reentry into the phobic environs and exposure to the anxieties elicited therein. This is where the battle is fought, and the patient must have as much support as he needs (provided by meditation, relaxation, hypnosis, emotive therapy, or any other means of anxiety control) consistent with the ultimate goal of remaining in and no longer avoiding the phobic events. Psychoanalytic clinicians have always held that this is too simple a prescription. The facts have proven them wrong. But, while the treatment procedures may be reasonably simple in application, the psychological changes brought about in exposure are often complex, and the last word about the theory of change has yet to be spoken. Hence, strident certainty about the mechanisms of change is out of order, though there is a position on the treatment of phobias which we can endorse without reservation: "Inumerable persons whose lives are disturbed by phobias . . . could have cured themselves if at the start they forced themselves to do repeatedly what they feared. . . . In many cases, phobias are never conquered because of the inability of the patient to fight hard enough" (Alverez, 1951, pp. 556–557, cited in Berecz, 1968). The therapist's job, finally, is to help the patient to go into this battle.

10

Cognitive Anxiety: Management and Procedures

Do not let us fear things too much, for we often suffer more from the things we fear than from those which really come to pass.
—Abbé de Tourville, *Letters of Direction*, 1939

In this chapter we will take up the important but still controversial problem of cognitive anxiety. Of these words, *anxiety* is the better understood. There is no question that we are still a long way from a complete enlightenment on the operation of individual differences in the interactions among the self-report, behavioral, and physiological systems which make up the construct, and yet, in a general way, judges can agree with confidence as to whether or not they have a very anxious person before them. By comparison with the conceptual fuzziness surrounding the term *cognitive*, definitions of anxiety are a model of clarity. We shall try to sift out a working definition of cognitive from the many statements about it before looking into the systems and techniques of cognitive-behavior therapies.

In broad terms, cognitive is a word which is synonymous with the processes of the mind, or brain. The definition is sharpened in most systems by the exclusion of reflex actions (for example, sneezing, automatic postural adjustments, startle reactions). Such *reactions* are "driven" by the eliciting stimuli, show a stereotyped form, and will make their appearance under the appropriate conditions unless forcible restraint is applied. Just as most definitions exclude these "stimulus-bound" outputs, there is agreement on what activities of the organism *are* to be included in a definition of cognition. A partial list would have to include the inter- and intrapersonal use of language, the operation of long-term memory, and the systems subserving planning and choice behavior. So what differentiates the reflexive from the cognitive systems is not the involvement of the brain, nor can the difference be stated as one between the "simple" (i.e., reflexive) and the complex (i.e., "cognitive"); both kinds undoubtedly involve complex brain circuits. In this chapter, we will adhere to a definition of cognition that follows the one proposed by Hebb (1949): Cognitions are subject-directed, semi-autonomous, central ("mental") activities and operations the contents of which are based on past experiences, which form the basis of planning and expectations, and which determine the judgments and evaluations that we make of ourselves and others. Cognition is thus used as a synonym for "higher mental processes."

Applying this distinction between cognitive and noncognitive is easy enough when contrasting such reflexive behaviors as postural adjustments and such cognitive ones as planning a speech. The question of phobic reactions, however, presents some problems. Where no effort is made to inhibit them, they show the qualities of being "stimulus bound," their existence does not depend greatly on teaching, and they are intimately connected with the survival of the species (Bowlby, 1975). Nevertheless, phobic reactions are modifiable by the "downward" influence of higher mental processes through the processes of habituation. The key difference between cognitive and noncognitive reactions may be this: phobic anxiety reactions (pain would be another example) can be *influenced by* our beliefs and expectancies based on past experience, but they cannot be explained away as "all in the mind". Cognitive anxiety, on the other hand, is that anxiety which owes its very existence to the person's *beliefs and evaluations* of events—more than it does to the quality of the events themselves.

Therapy for cognitive anxiety—the anxiety caused by our interpretations of the important events of our lives—aims to modify unpleasant affect and maladaptive behavior by changing the associated pattern of thinking that is responsible for our distress. At a glance, there might seem to be little to distinguish cognitive therapies from conventional psychotherapy. For example, the mental processes of the patient are viewed by psychoanalysts as the locus of his problem and the arena of therapeutic change. On closer inspection the similarities turn out to be more apparent than real. Cognitive therapies are short-term and highly structured instead of long-term and non-directive; present-centered instead of oriented to the (patient's) past; and aim at the modification of specific difficulties rather than global "personality change." Furthermore, the cognitive therapies are grounded in a concern with empirical evaluation and, in this, they share more with behavior therapy than with any variety of psychoanalysis. Indeed with the long-standing use of techniques like (imaginal) systematic desensitization, flooding, and covert modeling, behavior therapy might seem to have been more cognitive than it realized for these many years. This closeness in outlook is increasingly noted and is the chief stimulus to the efforts to bring about an integration of cognitive and behavior therapies. The choice between and the use of either will have to do with the problem at hand. In the case of therapy for phobias, the aforementioned exposure techniques aim at the elimination of the anxiety reactions which are directly linked to environmental stimuli (or their imaginal equivalents). Since cognitive anxiety starts with the patient's view and not the external stimulus, cognitive therapies give less significance to the objective events of the patient's life than to his judgments about them. For that reason they set as their target the alteration in these judgments, which mediate between the reality of the patient's world and his feelings about and reactions to it.

The most popular and widely practiced of the cognitive therapies was devised by Albert Ellis. For his starting point Ellis quotes the maxim of the stoic philosopher Epictetus (60 A.D.): "Men are disturbed not by things, but by the view they take of them." The clinical intent of this message is obvious. When a patient reports a feeling of anxiety, the therapist's job is not to pay undue attention to the environmental stimuli which might *seem* to trigger his distress ("I failed to do well"; "they said awful things to me"). The therapist who follows Ellis' approach will, instead, spend his efforts in ferreting out the patient's cognitions about himself and others ("the view they take of them"), informing the patient of their irrationality (a word Ellis favors), and setting him on the road to challenging and changing them. For example, if a person interprets all of his behavior and that of others as indications of whether or not he is liked, he may give unqualified credence to the belief "unless I am respected/liked/loved by everybody my emotional well-being is threatened, and *that* would be intolerable". Ellis (1962) argues that all emotional misery can be traced to the existence and continued application of one or more maladaptive evaluations (for example, "It is a dire necessity for an adult human being to be loved or approved by virtually every significant other person" and "Human unhappiness is externally caused and people have little or no ability to control their sorrows and disturbances," pp. 61 and 72; see Ellis & Harper, 1975, for the rest of the irrational beliefs on the list). The following exchange between therapist and patient will give the flavor of Ellis' rational-emotive therapy (RET):

Therapist: "You say that you're so worried about the upcoming examination that you can't sleep and you're snapping at everyone at home. Well let's imagine, for the moment, that you *do* fail. What then?"

Patient: "I don't even want to *think* about that. If I failed I'd freak out; I couldn't cope. I couldn't go on."

Therapist: "But what would *happen?*"

Patient: "Well my folks would raise hell and I'd be unable to face my other relatives."

Therapist: "But *why?*"

Patient: "I just told you, everyone'd put me down or scream at me."

Therapist: "And *that* would make you feel anxious and upset?"

Patient: "Yes."

Therapist: "Let me ask you a question. If I failed an exam would you put me down? Would you say I was worthless?"

Patient: "No."

Therapist: "Even if you did, would it prove that I was 'worthless'?"

Patient: "No."

Therapist: "Suppose just before the exam you, for argument's sake, developed an overpowering interest in a business venture and lost all interest in schoolwork. Would you still consider yourself a failure?"

Patient: "No, I guess I wouldn't."

Therapist: "That's interesting. Before you told me that the *failure* would cause X amount of anxiety. But, in our hypothetical situation, you still failed, only in this

case you stopped caring and felt less anxiety as the
result of this change in attitude. Can't you see that
with all of your interest tied up in this new project,
you were telling yourself something different about
your failure. For example, 'Well, the test was on material I couldn't have cared less about; I just did it to
get it out of the way.' What I'm suggesting to you is
that the way you *perceive the failure* causes your anxiety. I'm *not* saying that it wouldn't be nice to get a
very high grade. But what's 'nice' and what is *absolutely* necessary for your happiness are two different
things."

   In this Socratic dialogue the therapist's task was to identify and
expose the fallacy of unverifiable, irrational beliefs while, at the
same time, highlighting them and not the failure per se as the real
problem. Again and again the patient is told: if you want to feel
better you're going to have to change your thinking.
   Ellis (1962) recommends the ABC teaching technique as an heu-
ristic device, analytic tool, and vehicle of change. The "A" is the
activating event from the environment (failure, criticism, etc.); the
"B" stands for the beliefs and thoughts which intervene between the
perception of and reaction to the activating—or "outside"—event;
and under "C" the therapist writes down the patient's emotional
reactions. In the example just given, the A is the failure, the B is the
patient's self-statements and beliefs ("I couldn't cope"), and C is his
anxiety, irritability, and insomnia. The *true* causal link is between B
and C, and while the patient may come into therapy also fully convinced that there is a causal relationship at work, he believes that it is
between A and C. Once the patient has been won over to the therapist's analysis, he is given clinical rehearsals and homework exercises
with the ABC*D* paradigm. The D stands for "disputation," and the
rational thoughts which can be used to attack the irrational beliefs
("So I didn't do well on the exam; that's unfortunate but I did do my
best and it *is* possible to do badly on an exam and still be happy in
life. And in any case I'll soon be started on a new life").
   Ellis and most writers on cognitive therapy (for example, Postman, 1976) assert that the medium for these irrational beliefs is the
internal self-sentence and self-instruction: "The main stuff of the
mind is sentences . . . when we are thinking, we are mostly arranging
sentences in our heads. When we are thinking stupid [the equivalent

in this quote to Ellis' "irrational"], we are arranging stupid sentences" (Postman, 1976, p. 3). Thus, RET invites the epigrammatic summary "new sentences for old" as the cure for the psychological dysfunction, which can also be stated succinctly as "think bad—feel bad."

Evaluation of RET

RET theory and therapy rests upon three assumptions. The first (the others are discussed later in the chapter) is that negative self-statements can elicit aversive emotional reactions. This contention has received support in a number of experimental studies where subjects were given self-verbalizations with depressive (Veltens, 1968) or anxiety-toned material (May, 1977; May & Johnson, 1973; Russell & Brandsma, 1974). There is one serious qualification which we wish to note here. Negative self-statements will reliably succeed only when the self-referent verbalizations are not too discrepant with the subject's beliefs about himself (Rogers & Craighead, 1977). Let us consider what this fact tells us about the best ways to reverse negative self-statements.

Implications for Therapy

The use of task-relevant statements or positive self-evaluation cannot be too far out of line with the patient's beliefs about himself at a particular point in time or they may be rejected as irrelevant and thus will be ineffective. For instance, the student who believes that it is totally and completely catastrophic to do poorly in an exam should not be given a disputatious self-verbalization in which he tells himself that "exam performance is a matter of no concern to me" and that "I will be quite at ease before, during, and after the exam." It is likely that he will derive more assistance from one that is reasonably congruent with his belief, not completely in discord with reality *and* that can help to move the negative beliefs further in the desired direction (for example, "I sure hope that I'll do well . . . I'll probably be pretty upset if I goof up . . . but I'll live through it . . . I'll probably be on edge when I get into the exam room . . . my heart will be pounding . . . that'll remind me that I should do a 'mini-mediation' exercise" (see chapter 6).

Hypnosis and the Direct Modification of Negative Self-beliefs

In some cases the application of carefully structured self-sentences plus efforts to alter the patient's beliefs through behavior change produces only modest improvement. In these instances we have had some success with the presentation of the same (moderately discrepant) statements in hypnosis, when the patient's ability to rouse oppositional self-statements/beliefs is low. In hypnosis, or when drowsy (or meditating), the person seems to be more open to counter-attitudinal statements. An intriguing instance of this was reported in a study by Barber (1957), demonstrating that people were very suggestible when in a drowsy condition or in hypnosis. One of Barber's subjects said to him, "I was just sleepy enough to believe what you were saying was true. I couldn't oppose what you wanted with anything else" (p. 59). More findings of this sort were reported by Felipe (1965). Useful overviews of similar studies can be found in Budzynski (1976) and Suedfeld (1980). It bears mentioning, once more, that even with sensory deprivation or other disengagement techniques, the practitioner must be mindful of the need to use only moderately discrepant suggestions and to gradually "shape" the individual toward the desired beliefs (for example, Myers, Murphy, & Smith, 1973).

Changing Self-statements About Arousal

The second assumption in the RET system is that not only *can* negative self-verbalizations lead to dysphoric moods but that clinical anxiety and depression *are* caused in this way. This is a much stronger claim. We seriously doubt its validity in the etiology and maintenance of *phobic* anxiety, though they may *add* to the phobic anxiety with the use of negative self-statements. For nonphobic anxiety, the RET assertion is more plausible but still a difficult one to prove. Supporters of RET cite the evidence showing that psychologically disturbed individuals endorse more irrational beliefs than better adjusted people. This fact, however, can be given an entirely different interpretation, which was well put by Goldfried and Sobocinski (1975). In some cases, aberrant thinking can provoke feelings of anxiety, but in others the converse is true. As Goldfried (1979) wrote in his review of this work: "It is possible to argue that heightened emotional arousal and unassertive behavior sensitizes an individual to certain irrational beliefs, rather than the reverse" (p. 124). Bower (1981) has recently reported research data in support of this proposition: once a mood change is produced, it functions to "search out" and select memories and evaluations that fit in with the quality of that mood. When an anxious mood is induced, irrespective of the method by which this is done (Schacter, 1966), the threshold for negative cognitions drops. Hence, the thinking-to-feeling change (rational-emotive) spells out one possible relation between thoughts and feelings. In certain circumstances, the reverse is also possible: negative self-statements may *follow* mood shifts as well as cause them.

Implications for Therapy

Patients with what we term panic-perseverative anxiety, to indicate its probable indebtedness to a malfunctioning of the arousal-regulating systems, may well report "faulty cognitions." But even the most conclusive evidence of their presence would not establish the indications for RET if such self-statements were the end-products of runaway arousal reactions. Although relabeling techniques can free the patient from catastrophic interpretations which further heighten the arousal-induced anxiety reactions, the main thrust of therapy should be toward arousal-management strategies (supplemented, perhaps, with pharmacological interventions, see Liberman & Davis, 1975). Hypnosis would certainly have a role here—as a means of dampening arousal reactions, and not, as in the previous case, to alter self-statements and beliefs.

The final assumption on which the advocacy of RET rests is that it is the treatment of choice for cognitive anxiety. The evidence here is equivocal. Smith and Glass' (1977) meta-analysis of almost 400 studies shows RET to be the second most powerful technique, after systematic desensitization. (As a balance against unqualified acceptance, see the Zettle & Hayes, 1980, review for a discussion of the conceptual and methodological problems in the RET literature.)

Overall, though, RET, with all of its limitations, has rapidly developed into one of the most popular cognitive therapies. The clinical and laboratory data, taken as a whole, justify this popularity. Our experience is that, with certain modifications (some of which have already been mentioned), RET makes a significant addition to the clinician's methods for dealing with anxiety.

Nonverbal Cognitions and
Cognitive Therapy for Anxiety

Our greatest dissatisfaction with RET is in its depiction of cognitions
as covert verbalizations. *Is* it correct to say that "The main stuff of the
mind is sentences?" (Postman, 1976, p. 3). If it is not, then the clinical
implications of broadening the definition of cognitive to include nonverbal processes are worth careful examination. One very obvious
limitation of the cognitive-verbal conceptualization is its omission of
thought that occurs in images. The cognitive psychiatrist A.T. Beck
(1970; 1971) mentions the case of a woman whose fear of going for a
walk by herself was exaggerated by images she had of herself falling
to the ground with a heart attack, and another in which a student's
fear of leaving her college dormitory was worsened by images she had
of being attacked as she did so. Less anecdotally, the extensive research with patients who have had all of the interhemispheric connections cut—the "split-brain" procedure—has established beyond a
doubt the existence of two cognitive systems, one dealing with verbal
and the other with visual (i.e., imagery) cognitions.*

We will have some suggestions to offer about combating maladaptive imagery later, but the more important matter of cognitive
"sets" deserves prior attention. A set is a predisposition to react to
environmental and cognitive stimuli in a certain way. It can be lik-
ened to a filter or template which *facilitates* the search for certain
kinds of cognitive or environmental data and *screens out* inputs that
are not compatible with it. The clinical importance of sets derives
from their (usual) operation outside of the person's consciousness.
The idea of nonconscious cognitions may sound like a contradiction
in terms to some, and to others like an attempt to revive the unhelpful idea of a Freudian "repressed unconscious." For the last-men-
tioned reason, behavior therapists have carefully avoided speculations about the existence of nonconscious processes. We use the
word "unconscious" with some trepidation because, even with the
aforementioned clarification, readers may think we are alluding to
the *psychoanalytic* unconscious.

We appreciate the need to approach warily the notion of psychological processes taking place outside of awareness. A long time
ago William James (1890) reminded us that "the unconscious is the
sovereign means for believing whatever one likes in psychology and

*There is some evidence that verbal inputs make contact with the (right hemisphere)
imagery system but only if these words are in a concrete, pictorial form (Budzynski,
1976).

turning what might become a science into a tumbling ground for whimsies" (p. 163). As we know, Behaviorism reacted by rejecting unconscious mentation and driving out consciousness along with it. The subsequent enthusiasm for theorizing about the unconscious by workers from a collection of popular schools (for example, psychoanalysis, primal-scream, and gestalt therapies), who show an indifference bordering on contempt for methodological rigor and empirical validation, must have been taken by the early stimulus–response theorists as confirmation for their righteous rejection of all types of cognition. Current thinking has shifted from this position, and the place of cognitive processes in the explanation and treatment of psychological disorders has won wider acceptance (Bandura, 1974; Lazarus, 1977).

With the return of (conscious) cognition to psychology, attention has turned to nonconscious thought. This interest was stimulated by laboratory research on attention, memory, perception, and hypnosis (Deutsch & Deutsch, 1963; Dixon, 1971; Harter, Seiple, & Musso, 1974; Hilgard, 1977; Libet, Alberto, Wright, & Feinstein, 1967; Nisbett & Wilson, 1977), where workers have found the need to make reference to cognitive processes which go on outside of awareness. We have not the space to discuss this work here, but we urge the reader to study the paper by Shervin and Dickman (1980), who conclude their review of this research with the remarks:

> The clear message [from these data] . . . appears to be that behavior cannot be understood without taking conscious experience into account and that conscious experience cannot be fully understood without taking unconscious psychological processes into account. The laboratory and the consulting room do seem to be sharing at least a common wall, which may in fact turn out to have a door in it. (p. 432)

Why should any of this be of interest to the cognitive behavior therapist? The answer lies in the fact that the patient will have great difficulty altering a process that he doesn't know exists. We will give two examples for the reader to "try on" in an effort to give an intuitive, "*verstehen*," understanding of what it is like to be trapped in a nonconscious set. Do both examples as quickly as possible.

Example 1: An empty bus leaves the depot for its day's run. On the first stop it picks up 10 people . . . next stop it picks up 20 people . . . then, on the next, it lets off 10 people . . . next it picks up 30 people . . . then it lets off 20 people . . . next it picks up 40 people . . . then it lets off 30 people . . . next it picks up

50 people . . . then it lets off *60* people. The question is: how many *stops* did the bus make?

Example 2:   A little boy is wheeled into the emergency room at the hospital. The surgeon came in to prepare the child for the operation and looked down at the boy exclaiming in suprise "Son!" Now here is the problem: the surgeon was *not* the boy's father. How could that be?

On first hearing the bus example, listeners respond with sur- prise to the request asking for the number of stops. Why? Because, *without being told to,* they find that they have assumed that the task was to keep an accurate running total of the number of customers on the bus despite the fact that no such instructions were given *explicitly.* More important still, they report being completely unaware of the bias in their information gathering. They did not know what they had directed themselves to do. Likewise, clinicians often en- counter in their patients a tendency to search the array of cues in a social encounter for the ones relevant to their anxiety or depression- related concerns. Beck (1967) calls this "selective abstraction" and indicts it as one of the principle cognitive problems shown by his patients (for example, the anxious patient who is set to perceive, note, and recall only the unhappy moments of an experience).

The second example is an instance of another, and in clinical problems, a more insidious disorder. In the first example we saw the operation of "a set to attend selectively." The set biased the informa- tion that was taken in. With help it is possible to "catch oneself" and then to "go back" and reanalyze the data (for example, "let's see, how many stops *did* it make . . . nine!"). The second is an example of "a set to interpret" which is exceptionally difficult to change without special preparation. The answer in the second example, which few people get, is that the person is the boy's *mother.* Why is this obvious answer so elusive? Because of the hidden assumption: "all surgeons are men" which channels and traps our thinking. What we respond to in sets like these is *not* the problem given to us but the (insoluble) problem which we give to ourselves, *without knowing that we do so.* To give a common clinical example, there is the patient who complains of outbursts of anger followed by self-reproach and anxiety which he attributes to what others said to him. He will be quite unaware of the hidden assumptions that he brings to bear (for example, it is *as if* he says to himself "they *should* not be so sharply critical . . . this means I have failed again . . . things will be awful now"). These hidden statements are the functional causes of his anxiety, but until the patient realizes this and takes the correct steps to break these negative sets he will remain in a cognitive trap. This is not to suggest that there is an unconsciously motivated inhibition of admitting these assumptions into awareness. In our conceptualization both kinds of sets are, to repeat, *traps* which lead the person blindly into self-defeating habits.

The clinical point we want to make in conclusion is that maladaptive cognitions can be the cause of psychological misery and behavior disorders. *Some* of these cognitions are embodied in negative self-statements which, regardless of their origin, must be pinpointed and more adaptive self-instructions instilled. In other patients, cognitive anxiety will be linked to the use of disturbing imagery (Beck, 1970, 1971). Last, the cognitive distortions lying behind evaluative (i.e., "cognitive") anxiety may operate as persistent and powerful interpretive sets. Being prey to one kind of distortion does not immunize the patient against being ensnared in any of the others, but each will respond *best* (if not only) to selected clinical techniques: positive self-statements and task-relevant self-instruction; counter-anxiety imagery; and "set-breaking" procedures, respectively.

It is a good deal easier to defend these propositions in principle than it is to convince the patient that his cognitive habits influence his sense of psychological well-being. *Some* beliefs are easily reversed because they are amenable to factual disproof. An intelligent woman we once saw for an obsessive-compulsive disorder believed that she was well along the road to insanity and would soon need to be incarcerated. With a few brief examples of psychotic speech and thinking taken from Neale and Oltmans (1980) and an explanatory overview of obsessive-compulsive problems, she was relieved of this cognitive anxiety (but not, of course, her presenting problem). Likewise, *some* sets may be undone by logical challenges and disconfirmatory data (as in the surgeon example). Typically, though, the clinical challenge of cognitive anxiety amounts to a good deal more than merely imparting facts. By the time they get to the clinic, anxious individuals will have developed well-learned avoidance habits that perpetuate the cognitive-affective-behavioral problem.

The activities in the cognitive-affective loops lead them to the defensive actions they take, thus further diminishing their ability to deal with events smoothly and efficiently, and so on into the classic vicious cycle. Thus the therapist is faced with a patient who will have become dependent on others for "assistance," estranging him still more from rewarding interactions with his environment. This picture of cognitive anxiety is best described by an interactionist model wherein behavioral disorders serve as "confirmation" of the dysfunctional cognitive schemes out of which they arise. If the patient becomes anxious, then that is taken as proof of his irrational beliefs. Conversely, if the patient can be convinced to "stand his ground," as it were, then this will weaken his allegiance to the distorted picture which makes up his "cognitive map." This is a plea for cognitive-*behavior* therapy as against "pure" cognitive therapy.

Therapy for Cognitive Anxiety

Cognitive-behavior therapy can be divided into four stages: the rationale; the defense; the application; and the evaluation.

Rationale

The first step in therapy is explanation. A therapeutic explanation is one that does three things. It lays bare the processes of the problem; it brings therapist and patient to a common point of view; and it gives an explicit statement of how the patient can make use of the recommended techniques to eliminate that problem. "Rationale therapy" begins but does not end with the delivery of information to the patient. If cognitive anxieties were due simply to the patient having the wrong information or an insufficiency of facts about his problems, then cognitive therapy could be started and finished in one session.

Once the therapist discerns the problem in broad terms, his first job is to work with the patient in developing a shared outlook on the nature of the problems and the steps that must be taken to rectify them (Meichenbaum, 1976). During this reconceptualization phase the therapist tries to get the patient to come "to view his problem from a different perspective, to fabricate a new meaning or explanation for [its] etiology and maintenance" (p. 241). If this is done properly, the clarification can waken feelings of hopefulness and faith (Strupp, 1970) that the situation is *not* past repair, that he is *not* stuck in his misery, and most important of all, that he *can* do something to take control of his own feelings and actions. There are a number of major obstacles and misconceptions that block the patient from a *re-cognition* of his problems. If he is not won away from these, only limited changes can be anticipated. Let us say this again: the promise of RET and the other cognitive techniques that appear in this chapter will not be realized if the patient does not understand *and accept* the premises contained within them.

Blaming the Event

The first variety of in-principle rejection of the cognitive thesis is seen in patients who think of their problems in stimulus–response terms. They believe without question that their emotional distress is caused by a particular someone or something around them (the "external event," [A] in Ellis' ABC paradigm). They show no awareness of the intervening sets and self-statements that they add following contact with the external event. It is their conviction, however, that "he [they or it] made me anxious," which is as big an obstacle to progress in therapy as their lack of awareness of the critical cognitive antecedents. In the language of RET, their spurious, causal analysis has only two terms: the "outside" antecedent event (A) and the emotional consequences (C).

The therapeutic strategy to counter this is simple in principle and is best exemplified in a number of vignettes which illustrate the cognitive-RET thesis. The examples given should be presented as a gentle challenge, the purpose of which is to show that even if the external event is left unchanged, by modifying his own cognitive activities the patient can eliminate the maladaptive emotional reactions.

The therapist does this by duplicating the "A" conditions while showing that they do not necessarily lead to the "C" of his problem. For instance, if the anger–anxiety complex (C) followed Mr. X's pungent criticism (A), the therapist allows that this was so, and then attempts to enlighten the patient on the difference between *correlation* and *causation*. ("Yes, it is true that after A, C followed but that does not *prove* that A caused C; that the harsh words made you anxious.") To make the lesson clear, he can ask the patient to imagine that just before the encounter, Mr. X had been given news of his daughter's death. The patient when asked to put himself back to the moment of the unpleasant exchange with Mr. X and give his affective-behavioral responses to the *very same actions and words of Mr. X,* is likely to reply that his response at C would be very different indeed (sympathy, or at least less anxiety and anger). This is the time for the therapist to introduce the "B" phase (cognitions, interpretations), for *that* is what distinguishes the first from the second A–C sequence. We have invented obviously implausible but instructive stories for patients who are slow to see that the functional sequence is B–C and not A–C. For example, "Just before he met with you that day, someone said to him "if you don't yell at Mr. P [the patient] I'll put a bullet through you.'" And then we go to the same Socratic method, using it to prod the patient to see that when he changes his thinking, this leads to a change in his affective and behavior reactions.

If the patient misinterprets the examples showing that he, incorrectly, believes that *another* external event (the news; the threat) mitigated his anxiety, then the therapist must continue to pursue the theme until the patient finally grasps the principle. (For example, have the patient imagine that someone had said to him "I'll bet you could not keep from being upset if Mr. X does such-and-such. In fact, I'll put down a $1,000 bet on it." Once again the patient is asked to say how he would react. The therapist will be looking for some awareness that he did not *have* to feel and behave that way. Once the patient accepts the point behind these more extreme examples, the therapist has his foot in the conceptual door and he can move to examples closer to the patient's own problem.)

For patients slow to grasp the point, we use a technique we refer to as "externalizing the misery." The idea behind it is this: by the use of carefully contrived examples which employ humorous exaggeration, the therapist strives to focus the patient's attention on the bodily (i.e., physiological) constituents of anxiety. The purpose of this is to prove to the patient that he, and no one else, is the one responsible for his own emotional reactions. The corollaries to this are drawn out and stated explictly by the therapist.

> "Your upsetting feelings do not help you in any way, do not change the situation in any respect. So your disagreements with Mr. X, or the point in your argument, is in no sense advanced because you are suffering greatly while you deliver your message." This can be illustrated by the following sort of dialogue: "What you wrote down under 'C'—sweaty palms, trembling, tension headache, anxiety—all refer to changes that went on *inside your body*. Ask yourself this question. How could Mr. X have caused all of these changes? Must it not have been *you* who made all of that happen? I agree, it might seem that your feelings were caused by Mr. X. But that is because his harsh words came first and your bad feelings occurred afterward. And this is just where the problem lies. Just because one thing occurs be-

fore another, it does not prove that the first caused the second. Consider this 'silly' example, which I hope will make the point. Suppose you had blinked your eyes during Mr. X's tirade, would you say that he *made* you blink them? All right, instead of speaking about a collection of responses which together made up your anxiety, we put all of the bad feelings and responses in one place and make the cause *very* obvious and clear [this is emphasized when unconscious sets are at work]. We'll imagine it works this way: each time something unfortunate happens (you do badly on an exam, or get rejected by your lover, or Mr. X criticizes you), you give yourself a punch in the right eye and keep on doing so for 5 to 10 minutes afterward—the usual length of your anxiety episode. If I were to come along and ask you why you were hitting yourself in the face, and if you were to reply 'Mr. X made me' (or 'getting the wrong answer made me hit myself'), would you expect me to think that a very sensible answer? Would you agree with it if someone said the same in reply to a question of yours? [patient answers "No"]. No, I didn't think so. Well, you see, all that I did was to collect all of the misery and put it in one place on the *outside,* instead of in many places inside of your body. And just as you could learn to stop cracking yourself in the head each time your wishes weren't met, so too can you put aside the internal knocks which you inflict upon yourself."

When the patient sees the point of this and is able to reorient himself, then the next steps in cognitive therapy can take place.

Believing in Distress Without a Cause

There are other patients who are aware of being unhappy and yet when questioned on the perceived cause, confess themselves to be unaware of any likely reason for feeling as they do. They may be able to supply particulars on their problem in very general terms ("I worry too much"), or to specify its behavioral and affective referents ("I get very tense, I can't get to sleep, and sometimes my heart starts to race"). The therapist's efforts to find situational precipitators meet with the blank response, "I don't know" (or, "I've always been this way"), suggesting a complete ignorance of any external or cognitive precursors. The incompatible theory here is a theory of "no causation." It, too, blocks the patient from recognizing the role of cognitive mediators.

In passing, a patient's complaint that "it just happens" is not to be dismissed in every case. Some patients do suffer from chronic anxiety which has much to do with poor arousal-control techniques coupled with "sticky" regulatory controls (Malmo, 1975) as it does with the use of unrealistic or irrational interpretations. For the patient who knows only that he has a problem but can supply no answer as to its likely causes, begin by having him keep a homework diary. This should include hour-by-hour mood ratings, and where the SUDS ratings climb above 50, the setting events (the who and what of the situation) and the consequences should be put down in some detail (in fact, all patients should be asked to do this homework). Systematic changes in aversive moods and associated behaviors which co-vary with the patient's activities provide the data for a challenge to the belief in a "causeless" anxiety. Although the particular words and examples may not always be the same, the underlying ideas in the following passage are invariably used and are useful in the therapeutic challenges to this theory. "Two sessions ago, when I asked you what you thought was making you anxious, you answered that it was nothing in particular; that you were always that way. Well, if that is so why is it that you are more anxious on Sunday and Monday evenings, early in your teaching week, than you are on Friday and Saturday nights?" The point of this exercise is to establish the situational cues which, together with the homework data, count as evidence against the causeless theory. The therapist, naturally, will take care to dissuade the patient from then switching to the opposite stance, "blaming the event." Once the environmental correlates of the problem have been identified, the search for negative cognitions can then get underway.

Objection: Cognitive Therapy Is Too Cerebral

The patient may misunderstand the thrust of the therapist's remarks, believing him to be saying "get rid of all emotions." The patient will ask, in so many words, "Doesn't this mean that I'll become cold, mechanical, and unfeeling?"

Reply. "Not at all. There are many emotions—laughter, surprise, love, sexual feelings, excited interest, feelings of calm and competence, exhilaration, which are a wonderful part of life. What I'm asking you to consider is this: how vital a part of your life is anxiety, anger, frustration, and depression? Do you really want to tell me that doing without them will make you 'cold and unfeeling'?"

Objection: Cognitive Therapy Is Unrealistic

Patients who are satisfied with the first defense often bring up a second challenge: "Sure, sure," sometimes said in sarcasm, "I'll just say to myself 'how wonderful it is to be yelled at, or fail an exam, or that I like being unable to sleep.' "

Reply. "No, cognitive therapy is not a denial of reality. If Mr. X is abrupt and unpleasant, then that's the way to describe him; failing a test certainly isn't passing it." The therapist should add that it is, in this imperfect world, probably unavoidable that some anxiety will occur when we fail, when we are criticized, or when things we hope for do not eventuate and stressors show up in their place. Some events, for example, the loss of a loved one or the threat to one's economic well-being, are justifiable causes of anxiety and depressed feelings. But the long-term perpetuation of such emotion *is* maladaptive and indicates the *active*, though perhaps unrealized, use of "catastrophic cognitions" (Ellis & Harper, 1975).

Objection: Cognitive Therapies Don't Work

This is the last objection raised by most patients after they have been convinced of their contribution to their own distress but, all the same, say in resignation, "Fine, I'm now convinced. But if I 'say' the right things to myself, I'll still feel the anxiety when next [such and such] happens."

Reply. The patient is now ready to start the next stage of cognitive therapy. The therapist's best tactic is to agree to the patient's point that just saying something that seems like the right thing will not work (cf. Rogers & Craighead, 1977). There are two reasons why it will not. First, the belief underlying the cognition may still be partly intact ("sure I'm responsible for my anxiety . . . but it *would* be awful if so-and-so rejected me"). Second, there is a (cognitive) habit component which dictates the need for continued practice of the competing (adaptive) habits, and, third, the adaptive cognitive habits may not generalize from the quiet and order of the clinical setting to the disruptive conditions of the problem environment.

Application: Special Techniques for
Modification of Self-statements

Some years ago, when we first used cognitive therapies with our patients, we went through the recommended steps in the accepted textbook manner. With mildly to moderately anxious patients this treatment package worked, but in too gradual a manner. Severely anxious patients derived very little benefit. Goldfried (1979) mentions that this is often the fate of traditional cognitive-behavior therapy programs with extremely anxious individuals: "highly anxious clients frequently report that they are too anxious to think straight" (p. 134). So, too, said Meichenbaum (1976): "Having clients merely cognitively rehearse the [correct] self-instructions [and] saying that they could overcome their fears did not lead to consistent behavioral and affective change" (p. 252). His research showed that in nonstress situations, patients in a group trained only in the correct self-instructions (who, of course, had been given and accepted the ABC rationale before entering into this final stage of therapy) reported minimal anxiety, "indicating that they were calm and in control" (p. 252). When the demands upon them were increased,

> their self-reports of anxiety precipitously rose with the consequence of a rearousal of their fears. The initial bravado which followed from mere self-instruction training gave way when the task demands increased. In comparison [patients] who rehearsed the self-controlling strategies *and who then had an opportunity to use them in confronting a stress* [electric shock] significantly reduced their fears following treatment. (Meichenbaum, 1976, p. 253, emphasis added)

Notice that Meichenbaum only stipulated "a" stress. This suggests that the quality, or the relevance, of the stressor used in expanded cognitive behavior therapy need not bear any close relation to the quality of the real-life stress. The results of Meichenbaum and Cameron (1973) fit in with this premise, though Meichenbaum went on to qualify this claim: "Saying the 'right' things to yourself may not be a sufficient condition for change. One may have to 'try out' these self-statements gradually *in real situations that are similar to the criterion task*" (Meichenbaum, 1976, p. 253, emphasis added). We take this to mean that nonspecific stress training known as "stress inoculation" *and* ecologically valid training are both required. We work on this assumption and have had gratifying results combining the two. The vehicle we use for this is a modified flooding-implosion treatment, which we will illustrate with the problems of nonassertive behavior. We added the word *implosion* because the therapist often has to make inferences about the underlying thought processes and, second, because often quite "unrealistic" imagery is used (see below) as the "therapeutic stressor."

Self-statements, Cognitive Anxiety, and Assertive Behavior

The absolute number of clinically relevant negative self-statements remains a matter of speculation (Zettle & Hayes, 1980). Patients seek help for social, public speaking or sexual anxieties, and as many problems as there are specific situations in which self-defeating cognitions can operate. The common factors in the preponderance of cases are: an overconcern with the negative evaluation of others; a drastic overestimation of the possibilities and consequences of failure; and a fear of losing control when provoked. These are examples of unassertive behavior. This reveals that cognitive anxiety and problems in assertiveness often go together.

It has not been the practice in the behavior therapy literature to link unassertiveness and cognitive anxiety. Cognitive therapists have expanded more of their efforts on ways to find and reverse negative self-statements than they have on pinpointing the behavioral concomitants of cognitive anxiety. Assertive trainers have done something like the opposite, centering their efforts on overt behaviors marked as assertive or unassertive. Writers of this school tend to see unassertiveness as a skills deficit calling for direct behavioral interventions. That, at least, was the position until recently. Over the last few years a contrasting position on unassertiveness has been advanced. It begins with a very different assumption, which is that what the unassertive lack is the confidence and not the skills to behave in the appropriate fashion (Linehan, 1979). Otherwise, how is it that unassertive people can surmount performance deficits when strong pressures are placed upon them for adaptive/assertive behavior? It is interesting to note that at such times they reported feeling anxious about what others would think of them (Alden & Cope, 1981; Alden & Safran, 1978; Rodriguez, Nietzel, & Berzins, 1980; Schwartz & Gottman, 1976).

Probably the wisest lesson to draw from this research is that there is a place for two models of unassertiveness. Some people, but not most, will do better with therapies derived from a skills deficit

model. For the remainder, assertiveness problems are better described by the response-inhibition model. This says that the goal in
therapy should be to reduce the anxious apprehension about the
consequences of assertive behavior.

Stress Inoculation and Cognitive-Hypnotic Techniques for Assertive Problems

The first step in this extra training, when the more conventional
measures mentioned earlier in the chapter fail to work, is the construction of a stimulus hierarchy. All of the guidelines already presented (SUDS technique; duration; scene construction) apply here
with the one important modification: "static" hierarchy scenes
should be avoided. The patient who is afraid of being mildly assertive to one person will likely be more afraid of being mildly assertive
to two people, and so on. If the scenes are rendered in this fashion,
however, with the only programmed changes occurring in the external situation (few-to-more people in the audience), two important
elements will be left out: first, what the patient fears the others will
say or do and, second, what he will say or do himself. After all, if
cognitive anxiety is produced by what the person says or how he sees
himself in a given situation, little benefit can be expected from reex-
posure alone. Another difference from phobic exposure procedures
is that when cognitive anxieties are the target, the content of the
scenes need not be realistic (anymore than the beliefs underlying
them). For example, the fear of negative evaluation may be based on
self-sentences or images of catastrophic outcomes which have never
nor are ever likely to come to pass. We get our patients to imagine
these in a way that will generate high levels of anxiety. Images may
be of scenes of the outwardly mild, nonassertive patient screaming at
the top of his voice, hurling objects around the room, lunging at his
tormentors, and generally losing the control that has always been his
chief worry. We then get the patient to visualize scenes of the most
extreme abject compliance. In short, we have them deliberately visualize and "practice" the two major behavioral problems of the nonassertive: overcompliance (Alberti & Emmons, 1974) and aggression
(see Lange & Jakubowski, 1976). Curiously, by practicing the
"wrong" responses, patients can learn to acquire control over them.

Developing the right material for our "implosive" hierarchies
(Levis & Hare, 1977) can pose problems. Unlike phobic cues, which
can be clearly delineated, aberrant cognitions and belief-related be-

haviors may be difficult for the patient to recall and/or to "feel" in the quiet and calm of the clinic. The patient may be unable to recall the material for the scenes in sufficient detail or, if they are recalled, they may have no affective impact. For recall or for the generation of strong affect, we use the technique Bower (1981) employs to facilitate the recall of, and emotional responses to, imaginal events. It will be recalled that he found reliable mood-memory relationships, so that by eliciting the desired mood (say, anger or anxiety), people were better able to retrieve the relevant memories and cognitions than when they tried to do so "cold." Bower (1981) used hypnosis to generate these moods. As he found, "the advantage of hypnosis is that almost any emotion can be produced quickly and at an intensity one can vary by instruction and . . . keep it going for many minutes" (p. 131; and see Isen, Shalker, Clark, & Karp, 1978).

After high levels of arousal and anxiety are evoked in the patient, while hypnotized, he is asked to silently repeat the appropriate and psychologically congruent adaptive self-instructions *while the anxiety is maintained* for another minute or so, and then reduced while the appropriate self-instruction is repeated. Finally, and again in hypnosis, a realistic depiction of an assertive scene is elicited and the realistic and reasonable self-verbalization is used to terminate the scene.

Throughout, the patient must be advised on *how* to view the aversive scene. In particular, it is important to instruct the patient to attend to his bodily responses as well as to the stimulus details of the scene (Bauer & Craighead, 1979; Lang, 1977). This will have the effect of increasing physiological arousal—a useful part of the stress training method of altering "irrational beliefs."

The reasons for the value of stress induction have not yet been clarified, and a number of hypotheses can be advanced. It is possible that the person becomes "inoculated" to stress, so that by practicing the right self-instructions in the face of stress, greater generalization effects are made possible; that by, paradoxically, practicing the "wrong" responses one gets an increased sense of control over them; that the patient is helped to discriminate the correct from the incorrect cognitions and behaviors; that conditioned fear reactions connected to the patient's own behavior are neutralized; or that his worst and most catastrophic cognitions come to fruition and yet he survives; or all of these. Further research will be needed to elucidate the mechanisms behind stress training in the modification of irrational beliefs. For clinical purposes we are satisfied that Meichenbaum (1976) is correct and that mere rehearsal, especially in the more difficult cases, will be insufficient. The technique should always be concluded on a realistic note—although the use of extravagent but humorous imagery may aid the patient in his recall during his encounters with out-of-clinic stressors. (For example, a patient who worried incessantly about what others thought of him when he spoke to them was given the image of the viewers feeling sleepy and very tired after having a good meal. Instead of thinking about him they were fighting to keep their increasingly tired eyes open.)

To review, negative self-statements and images *must be understood by the patient* to be a significant contribution to cognitively based anxieties. Rehearsing the correct self-verbalization and images is the basis of this therapy. In the more severe forms, stress-inoculation training (Meichenbaum, 1976) in hypnosis (Bower, 1981) is proposed. Clinic role-playing and role-reversal are additional components and, finally, homework assignments complete the package. The evaluation can be carried out, as with phobic anxiety, in three channels: self-report, behavioral, and physiological [if self-report assessment data are gathered, we recommend the Gambrill & Richey, 1975, and the Rathus, 1973, Assertiveness Scale (see Blanchard, 1979)].

Application: Special Techniques
for the Modification of Sets

The opening moves for cognitive "set" therapy are the same as those for problems arising out of negative self-statements and catastrophic images. The big difference is that sets are usually not in clear awareness and, thus, are especially difficult to detect and modify.

Negative sets can be disrupted by positive self-directions embodied in verbalizations and images, so we are not suggesting an *absolute* separation between the therapeutic techniques which can be used against self-defeating sentences and those for negative sets. Indeed, treatment procedures for the two often overlap; however, sets by their very nature are resistant to treatment.

What we have found to be essential in "set breaking" is for the patient to be clearly aware and have a detailed knowledge of the kinds of situations in which he habitually and unconsciously "slots in" his interpretations. When he is able to recognize the early signs of dysfunction, he must then slow down and use the adaptive, task-oriented reminders developed in the clinic. This will prevent the dysfunctional cognitive-behavior reactions from "firing-off" in ballistic fashion. A patient of ours, a lawyer, was subtly harassed by his (nominal) subordinate and would overreact to him and later feel awkward and worried. He began to dread his twice-weekly meetings with this person. All of the orthodox cognitive therapies and assertive training was of little avail as he would find himself reverting to his old habits of backtracking (overcompliance) and attacking (ineffective emoting and aggressive behavior). The patient complained that "before I knew it I was doing and saying all the wrong things—just as always." Effective management of this patient's problem involved an imaginal-slowing technique which gave him control, at first in the protected situation of the clinic, and then in his office environment. The technique of time expansion (Kroger & Fezler, 1976) proved to be a valuable adjunct. In this technique, the words we use emphasize the slowing of time *and* behavior. In the case of our lawyer patient it went like this: "Time is slowing down . . . slowing [therapist lengthens the pauses between his words and utterances] . . . each second seems like many . . . when you breathe in and out the whole cycle takes a little more than a second . . . time is expanding . . . and everything is slowing . . . you can see the people in your office . . . moving like in a slow-motion film . . . very graceful." The therapist can probe to check the effects before and after time expansion suggestions by having the patient make an estimate of when 30 seconds has elapsed: "I'd like you to tell me when 30 seconds is up starting now . . . don't count or try . . . just let the answer come into your head when it does. . . ." Each patient can thus be used as his own control. Most people, *before* attempting this in hypnosis, will judge 30 seconds to have passed when in fact less than 20 or even 15 seconds of clock time has elapsed. After three to five minutes of time expansion imagery the next estimate is likely to be much longer; often when 50 to 60 seconds has passed on the real clock the patient will signal that the perceived time lapse is 30 seconds.

Time-expansion imagery can be utilized to slow down the psychological clock in anxious and depressed patients, so that first it better matches the objective time and then slows still further. Once achieved, the crucial scenes can be run through in *very* slow motion and the patient can "see" the problem as it begins to unfold. It may be helpful to "freeze the frame" and stop all of the participants in mid-motion and have the patient "insert" the correct self-instructions. We sometimes supplement this set-breaking technique by linking salient environmental cues to adaptive self-statements. For instance, the lawyer was told in hypnosis to "hang" self-control cues on objects like the phone and important others. So when the "difficult" colleague next came in, the patient would "see," tied around his colleague's waist, a sign with the message "don't trap yourself this time!" Again, these reminders are designed to function as "bell ringers" and enable the patient to develop self-awareness early in the "automatic" cognitive-affective-behavioral response chain (and the earlier caught, the better).

The ideas behind set-breaking are not new to psychology, though they are to the clinical literature. The early (experimental) Gestalt psychologists discovered the two principles which apply as well in the clinic: Negative sets and "stupid" behavior can be strengthened by *increasing* drive or arousal and *speeding up* the proceedings. By contrast, flexible and "creative" solutions emerge when the subject is calm and at ease and moves carefully through the steps examining his premises and self-directions at every step of the way (see Woodworth & Schlosberg, 1954, Chapter 26). The very same conditions are propitious for breaking resistant and persistent sets. Get the patient to reduce drive or arousal, go very slowly at first, adopt a deliberate (even excessively so at first) manner, and use self-instructions and self-evaluations at all times. Finally, positive sets can become as well established as the negative ones.

The Psychological Clock: Anxiety and Depression

We have been gathering data for publication on the perceived time estimates of the anxious and depressed people we have seen in our clinics and in the experimental laboratory. One finding that has come up with impressive regularity is that very anxious and depressed individuals run a "fast clock." That is to say, when (say) 30 seconds have passed on their clock, often 15 or fewer seconds have elapsed on the real clock (in one case a woman given this task gave the signal indicating that she thought 30 seconds had passed when the stopwatch time was 6.2 seconds!—cf. Einstein's illustration of relativity: for a man sitting on a hot stove a second seems an eternity, whereas for two lovers an eternity seems to last a second).

An interesting speculation on anxiety and depression can be made from these observations. If it is the case that a drop in the rate of reward plays a factor in anxiety and depression, then when a subject's psychological clock, for whatever reason, begins to run more quickly (i.e., when arousal is increased), then his rate of reward, which is computed as the number of pleasant events achieved within a period of time, will show a decline. To give a simple illustration, if we say, arbitrarily, that five pleasant events in a half-hour period contribute to a person's well-being, then when his internal clock begins to run faster than the objective clock, and 30 minutes feels like, say, an hour, then the *functional* rate of reward has been halved. One implication from this is that meditation and neutral hypnosis will, if they function to slow the individual's clock (as is suggested by clinical evidence), also operate to increase the *functional rate* of reward. Another related issue, and one which is contrary to popular intuition about the nature of depression, is that depressed as well as anxious people show indices of being in a high arousal state (Wolpe, 1979; Lovibond personal communication). Thus, time-expansion techniques might be useful in cognitive therapies for depression.

Cognitive and Phobic Anxiety: Summary and Assessment

We have only a few remarks to add to these two chapters. Phobic anxiety and cognitive anxiety have been the subject of vigorous research and clinical analyses. Out of this work have emerged two formulas, one for the treatment of phobic and the other for the treatment of cognitive anxiety. Both sets of recommendations have an attractive simplicity to them, and positive data have been reported for each. Simply, when the phobic patient undergoes extended exposure to the phobic stimulus, his anxiety will, ultimately, be extinguished. An equally direct treatment has been proposed for cognitive anxiety: the substitution of adaptive self-statements for negative self-statements. We have deliberately used the word *simple* but we have stopped well short of the term *simple-minded*. There are too many findings in favor of the efficacy of both (for their respective problems) for us to be anything but impressed with the clinical value of these techniques. However, there are also too many refractory data to justify an attitude of theoretical or clinical complacency. Rohrbaugh, Riccio, and Arthur (1972) presented some of the first, in what is by now, a large body of evidence that exposure by itself "cannot be uncritically assumed to reduce anxiety" (p. 125) and Meichenbaum (1976) felt impelled to entitle one section of his paper on cognitive therapies "When Self-instructions Fail" (p. 251). Both kinds of techniques, for safe exposure and positive self-statements, can work, but there are enough data available to indicate that often something more is needed. And disagreeable though it may be to confess it, we are not always able to specify the particular components of that "something more." As a starting point in the search, we can think of no better words to guide us than the ones used in the title of a recent paper by Michel Hersen (1981): "Complex Problems Require Complex Solutions."

11

Agoraphobia: Theory and Management

There's no place like home.

—Dorothy, *Wizard of Oz*

The subject of this chapter is the treatment of agoraphobia. We have elected to consider agoraphobia separately because of the special problems that set it apart from all other phobic and anxiety disorders. From the clinician's perspective, it is unique because there is no other phobia that is more incapacitating or more difficult to treat (Marks, 1969; Mathews, Gelder, & Johnston, 1981). In Albert Ellis' (1979) laconic phrase, "agoraphobics are difficult customers" (p. 164).

Our aim here is to begin with a recounting of the important facts of agoraphobia, including data on incidence, prevalence, mode of onset, and clinical course. From there we will be in a better position to identify and challenge the many persistent myths and misconceptions which have become embedded in the conventional clinical wisdom about agoraphobia. We will conclude the chapter with our model of agoraphobia and the main avenues of therapy to which the model points. Most of the treatment section will be devoted to the management of panic attacks. This is the part of the syndrome that clinicians often overlook—even though it is of dramatic salience to patients, who see panic attacks as *the* problem of agoraphobia. As is well publicized, exposure techniques are the treatments of choice for the phobic components of agoraphobia. The reader looking for information on this part of therapy can refer to the guidelines presented in chapters 9 and 10 and to Appendix A for step-by-step directions for the use of relaxation therapy.

The Clinical Picture

Agoraphobics are, first of all, anxious people. A list of the situations that evoke anxiety would include traveling in buses, trains, planes, and elevators; walking unaided away from home or home surrogate (for example, the patient's automobile); having to wait for any length of time in stores, on bridges, in traffic jams, or in any place where confined, especially in the absence of a trusted companion. In specific detail the list is almost endless. To it we could add barbershops, hardware stores, visiting relatives—or worse, strangers—and many others. Some writers have treated these as separate problems (for example, Glick, 1967), but that leads to an unnecessary and unjustified proliferation of phobias (barbershop phobia, bridge phobia, shopping phobia, and so on). Questionnaire and test data (Hallam & Hafner, 1978; Marks, 1969; Shapira, Kerr, & Roth, 1970) and clinical observations (Marks, 1969) reveal that the superficially numerous and seemingly distinct stress environments can be tied to two themes: phobic anxiety associated, first, with separation from home (or other "safe" places) and, second, with separation from certain support/attachment figures.

Of these two "separation phobias," the inability of the patient to tolerate (more or less) long trips from home has attracted more attention. Indeed, it is often discussed in the behavior therapy treatment literature as though it *is* agoraphobia. To the significant others in the patient's life, it is likely to be the *constant* demands for their presence and support which is the most visible part of the syndrome, and the one which is most burdensome to them. Hence, they would nominate excessive dependency and person separation as the essential problem. To the agoraphobic, as distressing as the two separation phobias can be, they fail to compare with recurrent panic attacks as a source of psychological misery. These attacks may be predictable but more usually they have an "out-of-the-blue" quality (Goldstein & Chambless, 1978; Zitrin, 1981). These paroxysmal anxiety reactions are marked by tachycardia, hyperventilation, extreme physical tension, and behavioral and cognitive disorganization. They are accompanied by feelings of dizziness, weakness in the legs, and premonitions of being on the threshold of insanity and/or death. There is one word that agoraphobics use again and again to describe their feelings about panic attacks: "terrifying." The attacks are usually short-lived, rarely lasting for more than 10 minutes. It is not the duration so much as the *unpredictability* and *intensity* which give them their enormous impact. There are three significant consequences that flow from these attacks. First, they deepen or re-evoke separation concerns (place and person). As Emmelkamp points out "panic attacks [can] undo the effects of weeks of desensitization treatment" (1979, p. 85). Second, they instill a generalized apprehension which agoraphobics describe as a "fear of fear" (Weekes, 1977). Third, panic attacks are demoralizing as well as frightening. If they recur frequently, the patient often lapses into depression.

In mild cases, panic attacks may be rare or absent altogether (though they will have been in the clinical picture at an earlier time in virtually all sudden-onset cases—which are in the majority). The presence or absence of panic attacks is the clinical feature which distinguishes the refractory from the manageable instances of agoraphobia. From the valuable Goldstein and Chambless (1978) paper we will borrow the terms "simple" and "complex" agoraphobia to describe cases which respectively present without or with panic attacks (our use of these terms is not exactly what it is in their paper). Phobic and panic anxieties make up the core of agoraphobia. Other anxieties, cognitive in our scheme, center around apprehensions of panic attacks and worry that during an attack they may exhibit grossly inappropriate behavior in the presence of others (screaming, crying, losing control of bowels, and looking foolish, stupid, or "crazy" to strangers).

We have given an overview of the major and most disabling problems of agoraphobia. However, the list is not exhaustive. Fear during sexual intercourse may cause avoidance of all sexual activities. Depression has already been mentioned and will be of admitted concern to the patient. In cases of complex agoraphobia, depersonalization reactions and obsessive preoccupations may be harder to detect. Because these seem "crazy" to the patient, he may fail to disclose them to the clinician unless directly, but gently, questioned about their presence. The social consequences of agoraphobia are proportional to the severity of the phobic separation anxieties, the frequency of panic attacks, and the depth and duration of the depressive reactions. The more incapacitating forms of complex agoraphobia impose social disabilities that can profoundly alter the patient's life. He may be unable to travel to work, visit friends and relatives, or tolerate the absence of attachment figures. Predictably, this generates tensions and family disharmony, for the attachment figure is usually a spouse or close relative. Social isolation is inevitable, which places still more burdens upon significant others. Anger toward attachment figures is frequent, especially when they attempt to leave the agoraphobic alone. The demands that the agoraphobic makes upon significant others are frequently recognized by him as being quite unreasonable. Such insight, by itself, is not likely to lead to change. Two vicious cycles are thus established. Anger toward attachment figures will be succeeded by anxieties about loss of support. Then when the significant others prepare to leave in order to pursue their own duties, errands, or pastimes, "clinging" behavior is intensified and anger ensues, followed by more anxiety ("have I made them so fed up that they'll leave me for good or ignore my pleas in the future?"). The second vicious cycle centers around "travel" worries and chronic tension which lower the threshold for panic attacks and lead to autonomic hyperactivity ("autonomic firestorms" as one patient so colorfully put it). Thus, the patient's confidence and his willingness to attempt taxing journeys, alone or with dependency figures, is weakened still further. From this outline of the clinical picture we can see that if agoraphobics are "difficult customers" for the therapist, it is equally true that agoraphobia is a difficult business for the patient.

The Onset, Prevalence, and Clinical Course

The prevalence of agoraphobia has been estimated at six per thousand (Agras et al., 1969), which would put the number in New York City at somewhere around 45,000 people. As impressive as this figure is, it may be too low. Resolution of the diagnostic/classifactory confusions surrounding agoraphobics (see below) has yet to reach the mainstream of clinical research and practice. Another problem that may depress the estimates is the inability of seriously handicapped agoraphobics to leave the house, and their ignorance about, fears of, and reluctance to "confess" their problems to outsiders (cf. the worry about seeming crazy in the eyes of strangers). All of these factors singly or in combination could have contributed to the surprisingly low clinical "catch" rate in the agoraphobics we have seen. Of the 100 patients in our sample, over half had not had any therapeutic assistance apart from house calls from, or visits to, the family doctor for tranquilizers for "bad nerves." Fewer than 10 percent had been diagnosed or treated for agoraphobia.

The ratio of females to males has been put at three to one (Marks, 1969), but the sex distribution figures may also be different from the published estimates. These rest on the assumption that males are as ready as females to admit to panic and phobic anxieties. We believe this to be a questionable assumption. It *may* be the case that females may constitute a higher proportion of the more serious cases. The pressures upon men to get out to work each day may provide them with a form of exposure therapy and enable men to keep free of the vicious cycle pattern. Women may be more vulnerable to this because they can get others to do the travel tasks for them. Certainly, it is the case that single women are less often housebound and, thus, less agoraphobic than their married counterparts.

In the overwhelming number of cases, for males as well as females, agoraphobia has a sudden onset. The process begins with the first panic attack. The specific precipitators are not known, although it is usually possible to identify significant stressors just before the first attack. There may be sudden shocks associated with the unexpected loss of a close relative, the breakdown of an important relationship, or one of a number of very taxing physical stressors. One predominant stressor which should be noted is that associated with obstetric complications in labor. Others are drug-induced panics (for example, from LSD) or after attacks of Ménière's disease. The close connection between stress and onset prompted Roth (1959) to refer to agoraphobia as the "calamity syndrome."

The panic attacks will be followed within days or a few weeks by the emergence of the separation phobias. If the condition endures it may, as Slater and Roth (1969) point out, evolve into a "process" with the full complement of problems which together make up the syndrome. There are agoraphobic conditions that run a brief course and remit completely without treatment. If the condition persists for more than a year, the chances of "spontaneous remission" are very small (Marks, 1969; Mathews et al., 1981) and certainly well below the 66 percent figure cited by Eysenck (1952) for all "neurotic" disorders.

In the "permanent" cases, however, agoraphobia follows a dynamic and not static course. Patients will recognize this and complain about it, but usually without being able to pinpoint the causes of the fluctuations. In the present state of knowledge, the therapist is not much better off. Some of the variability can be linked to one or more internal and external events. Phobic anxiety will be increased and the threshold for panic anxiety will be lowered if the patient contracts influenza, mononucleosis, or hepatitis. Why this should occur is not known. Curiously, no such changes accompany any decline in physical well-being. For example, broken limbs, headaches, and painful stimuli appear to have no discernible effect on agoraphobia and, curiously, where there is very high fever there may be a temporary lifting of phobic anxieties.

The external correlates of variability and fluctuations have already been detailed. All that we wish to do here is to raise one more point. The more predictability we can bring into the patient's life, the better. Even if the therapist has an understanding of the causes and correlates of the easing and intensification of agoraphobia, it will be of little therapeutic benefit if the patient remains demoralized (not too strong a word) in his ignorance.

With all of the complex and unknown influences at work, it is no easy matter to arrive at the correct mix in a multimodal treatment program for agoraphobia. The job, difficult though it is, is made a little easier if the myths, misconceptions, and confusions about agoraphobia are cleared away. The most prevalent of these are listed below.

Agoraphobia and the Fear of Open Spaces

In Webster's *New World Dictionary,* "agoraphobia" is defined as fear of being in the open. This is the definition given by most general psychology (for example, Price, Glickstein, Horton, & Bailey, 1982) and abnormal psychology texts (for example, Page, 1975). Widespread though this definition is in the minds of all but a few nonspecialists, it is wrong. An agoraphobic patient of the first author offered an eloquent comment on this misconception. He said: "Before I went to university I thought agoraphobia was some species of exotic plant; when I was in medical school I was told that it was a fear of open spaces. Now that I've been an agoraphobic for 10 years I know that both definitions are wrong." What is more puzzling still about this misdefinition is that agoraphobics, if anything, are more afraid of *closed* spaces where these are perceived as barriers to the homeward journey. Whatever the reasons for its popularity and persistence, the definition of agoraphobia as a fear of open spaces is, to reiterate, incorrect.

Agoraphobia and Depression

The phobic and panic anxieties of agoraphobia seldom appear without some degree of clinical (i.e., nontrivial) depression. By itself that observation is not very enlightening. The challenge is to unravel the connection between the two. Should the dysphoric mood be understood as a *response* to the physiological stressors and psychosocial consequences of agoraphobia, or are we dealing with a depression of the *endogenous* variety, in which a biochemical disturbance is presumed to be etiologic? If the latter, then the focus in therapy would be on the depression, with the agoraphobic anxieties relegated to a secondary place in the treatment program. From a therapeutic standpoint, this is a vital consideration. When agoraphobics do get to treatment facilities, it is our experience that they are most often diagnosed and treated as depressives. The confusion between the two is not at all difficult to understand. Commonly, anxious people get depressed about their concerns and clinical depression is often associated with tension, agitation, and apprehension (Beck, 1967, p. 200; Slater & Roth, 1969, p. 97). The differences, though often hard to recognize, are predictive of the response to treatment interventions. For example, so-called endogenous depression can benefit from electroconvulsive therapy (ECT) but, in general, "ECT is probably not effective at all in [those] who lack signs and symptoms of an endogenous subtype" (Scovern & Kilmann, 1981, p. 285). When administered to agoraphobics, ECT is not only "not effective" but positively noxious. It produces a constellation of problems, some persistent and severe—the worst of which is depersonalization (Slater & Roth, 1969, p. 97). *ECT treatment should not be used in agoraphobia.* The depressive reactions seen within it, however prominent, are best construed as the "reactive" depression of perceived and *actual* helplessness (Seligman, 1975). This conclusion is strengthened by the correlation between falls and rises in depression and the improvements and setbacks the patient experiences in coping with the phobic and panic anxieties (Emmelkamp & Kuipers, 1979). The proven value of imipramine and other tricyclic drugs (Zitrin, 1981) does not detract from this assessment. The tricyclic drugs are most commonly used as "antidepressants," but that does not mean that they always act in this way. For example, tricyclics are useful in the alleviation of pain and the treatment of some forms of enuresis. Their value in agoraphobia is in reducing panic attacks and not depression (Klein, 1964, 1967; Zitrin, 1981). Thus, although agoraphobics do get depressed, the major treatment efforts must be centered on the elimination of the anxieties. When this line is taken, it is found that as personal competence improves, the depression declines. To cite but one instance, there is a recent study by Emmelkamp and Kuipers (1979). They organized their treatment program around the modification of agoraphobic anxiety. They wrote in conclusion that "the amelioration of depression as *a consequence* of behavioral treatment for phobias is particularly noteworthy when seen in the light of the frequently mentioned connection between them" (p. 354). One caveat is worth noting: agoraphobics are extremely sensitive to "failure" experiences and are easily plunged into gloom when unable to overcome the separation phobias or panic. The therapist must take care not to ask too much of the patient, especially in the early stages of therapy.

Agoraphobia: A Clinical Entity or a Collection of Different Problems?

Agoraphobic patients bring a number of problems to the clinic, the foremost of which are anxiety and depression. Why not, in that case, dispense with the word *agoraphobia* and call the condition "anxiety plus depression"? Why add another term to our clinical vocabulary which says, in effect, that there is something unique not captured by the two categories of anxiety and depression? Although we would disagree with the implied answers to these questions, they are nonetheless reasonable ones to ask. *Do* the component problems of agoraphobia make a distinct cluster or are they separate entities?

The clinical and psychometric evidence is that they do (Marks, 1969; Mathews et al., 1981). The first accounts of agoraphobia (Westphall, 1871) bear an unmistakeable resemblance to contemporary descriptions (Marks, 1969). In clinical terminology agoraphobia may be termed a syndrome*; the behaviors which index it correlate

---

*We are not unaware of the limitations of the syndrome concept (Neale & Oltmans, 1980, p. 18). Despite these, and its origins in the medical model, it can be retained with profit as a descriptive term, and not as a kind of explanation. Agoraphobia used as a syndrome can be a "bell ringer" for the clinician, reminding him not to overlook all of the major features of the disorder.

with each other and cohere across measurement occasions (Eysenck et al., 1975). What *has* made for confusion is the use of the word *agoraphobia* to designate the whole cluster (phobias, panic attacks, depression, insecurity, and the rest) at one time and the separation phobias only at another. Sometimes agoraphobia is used in a narrower sense, to refer to the fear of leaving home. This dual or multiple usage will undoubtedly continue, so it must always be made clear whether in a particular passage the writer has in mind "syndrome" agoraphobia or "phobic" agoraphobia (or whatever other particular feature of the syndrome he has in mind).

A Model of Agoraphobia

Agoraphobia is not well understood and all of the theories, including ours, contain a disappointingly high ratio of speculation to fact. In this state of affairs we are in no position to dismiss competing explanations. Our model of agoraphobia selects two facts for special attention—separation phobias and panic attacks. Actually, the model is really no more than a set of best guesses about how phobias and panic fit together to influence the characteristics and course of the disorder. There are two major assumptions contained within the model. One has to do with the nature of the separation anxieties and the other with panic-phobic interactions.

To begin with, we referred to the separation anxieties as being phobias. But are they, or are they the product of the agoraphobic's beliefs that if he travels or separates from support figures he may be rendered helpless in a panic attack? This is how travel and separation avoidance is interpreted by Weekes (1977, p. 13). On her reasoning they would be more appropriately labeled cognitive and not phobic in nature (if the effects of panic are truly incapacitating, then the separation and travel avoidance could be regarded as fearful estimations which are quite in accord with reality).

Weekes' (1977) assertion that the fear of leaving home is a logical sequence of the patient's painful knowledge of his limitations (p. 18) has an element of truth in it. Agoraphobics learn that under the "whipping lash of panic" (p. 13) they can be overburdened and bewildered by the simplest social transactions. But there is more to avoidance than a well-founded fear of panic effects. Travel and separation avoidance continue unabated in simple agoraphobia. With panic attacks a thing of the past, along with worry about their possible occurrence, it should be expected that separation anxieties would dissipate.

The fact is that they do not. Exposure treatment is required (or the informal equivalent thereof). By comparison, cognitive therapies are notably ineffective (Ellis, 1979). Together, these two facts, plus the self-report data, suggest that the separation–travel anxieties are indeed phobic in nature. As an example, when agoraphobics try to venture away from safety, it is not only the absolute distance but also interference with visual access to home or car that disturb them. As one doctor-patient said: "When I go 'round the corner and loose sight of the car, the worry begins; I *know* the car is still there but that still doesn't help me." The instant he lost sight of it, his pulse rate would climb from the 70 to 80 range to above 110 beats per minute. A walk in the opposite direction which took him twice as far from the car while still leaving him within sight of it was always easier. Similarly, the attachment figures "selected" by agoraphobics are not necessarily those who can give the greatest assistance. Another patient of ours, a widower, tolerated travel with less anxiety when his eight-year-old son (who had been told nothing about his father's agoraphobia) was with him. Yet, as the man said, "My kid couldn't do a thing to help if I blew up in a panic." He expressed the same perplexity that all phobics do when they are unable to fit what they know (there's no danger) with what they feel (anxiety). Hence, we conclude that the separation anxieties are of the phobic variety.

The more difficult task is assimilating the separation phobic anxieties to our general model of phobias. The principle thesis in our model is that phobic anxiety occurs in reaction to a small and specific subset of environmental triggers (or their imaginal counterparts) which have evolutionary significance as "natural clues to danger" (Bowlby, 1975). Adaptation and not psychopathology is the starting point in this explanation of phobic anxiety. A phobic anxiety becomes a phobic *disorder* when it persists into adult life past the point when habituation should have occurred and/or when environmental conditions act to deepen instead of lighten the hold of the phobia.

From this perspective the most salient facts are the ubiquity of these reactions and their onset in early childhood and infancy (Bowlby, 1975). On these two counts the separation anxieties of agoraphobia appear to fall outside the explanatory range of our model: Agoraphobia is not a universal phenomenon and, in all but a minority of patients, develops *de novo* in adulthood.

We have added two further assumptions which are necessary to clarify the mechanisms of agoraphobia and fit the phobic components into our general model. We begin by returning to a distinction we drew earlier, between syndrome agoraphobia on the one hand,

and the phobic components of that syndrome on the other. It is the syndrome, as a unit, which appears suddenly, and for the first time, in adulthood. The separation phobias themselves, we believe, are *not* new. Our contention is that they can be better understood as reactions related to the separation phobias that appear for the first time in early childhood. These occur in all infants and are adaptive in that they operate to keep the young within range of familiar adults who can protect them (Bowlby, 1975). In order to explain the *reappearance* of separation anxieties, we must now bring forward our second assumption: the panic attacks that are correlated with the onset and intensification of separation phobias (Emmelkamp, 1979; Marks, 1969; Zitrin, 1981) function as *dishabituating* events that reevoke the long dormant separation phobias. We cannot say why panic attacks emerge in the first place, nor can we say why they potentiate separation phobias more than the other previously mastered phobias of childhood. Bowlby's (1975) answer is that attachment behavior always has been *and still is* fundamental to our survival. He presents a number of interesting findings which reveal that, for young *and* old, separation anxieties can be reawakened in times of natural catastrophes or by other superaversive stressors. It may be that a panic attack is the "internal" equivalent of these and in the same way potentiates attachment behavior. (See Figure 11.1.)

The present account of agoraphobia still leaves much to be desired as a complete account or explanation of this complex disorder. In this form, its greatest value is in the clinical sphere as a reminder to the therapist, and the patient, of the interplay between phobic and panic anxiety. This has a number of implications for therapy. It identifies panic attack assessment as an indispensable requirement in the treatment plan. Second, in focusing on the interplay between panic attacks and separation phobias, it warns the therapist against the incautious use of exposure procedures, which may generate high levels of arousal. Finally, and most important, it gives first priority to the treatment of panic attacks.

Therapies for Agoraphobia

Because agoraphobia is a multifaceted disorder, it is essential to develop a treatment plan for the syndrome which assigns each of the problems to its place in a hierarchy of priorities. We have put together our suggestions for the treatment plan offered in this section in accordance with the model of agoraphobia that we hold.

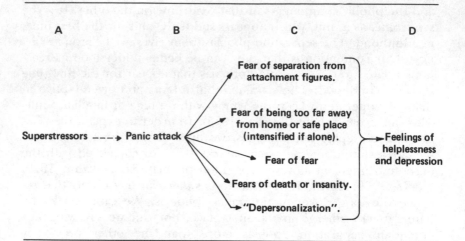

Figure 11.1   Schematic presentation of the origin of sudden-onset agoraphobia (the commonest mode of onset). A "superstressor" of a physiological or psychological nature (these can vary from physical disorders such as an attack of Ménière's disease or a very difficult childbirth, to the sudden death of a significant person in the patient's life) leads to the first, "out-of-the-blue," panic attack. The attack elicits a collection of fears (C), which in their turn are followed by feelings of helplessness and depression. The line between A and B is to indicate our ignorance of the specific environmental and biochemical conditions that lower the threshold for the first panic attacks.

The emphasis in the plan is on the treatment of panic attacks. They are the obvious target for first intervention. Panic attacks sensitize the patient to separation anxieties and impose the greatest strain on the patient and those around him. In "simple" agoraphobia, panic attacks will no longer be a part of the clinical picture. Where they are rare, or absent, the primary task in therapy is then to build a program of exposure exercises for phobic separation anxieties. Exposure therapies ("desensitization," "flooding") are required for complex or simple agoraphobia (i.e., with or without panic attacks, respectively) as indeed they are for all phobic anxieties. The principles and procedures for circumscribed phobias covered in chapter 9 apply in agoraphobia. Inasmuch as agoraphobia presents certain unique problems, however, some modifications to these techniques are indicated, as will be outlined later in the chapter.

We have one last recommendation to make in this preamble and that is for the inclusion of information/rationale early in the implementation of the general treatment plan. Agoraphobics make considerable trouble for themselves by their overabsorption in maladaptive defensive anticipations. These catastrophic cognitions are rooted in misinformation and misinterpretation, the correction of which is the *first* item of clinical business. As we often have to point out to our students, knowing how to apply powerful exposure therapies will count for nothing with patients who are still captured in erroneous beliefs like the common one that they are suffering from a rare, progressive, and incurable "mental illness." Until patients are able to change their thinking, they will not enter into activities which, to them, appear pointless or puzzling.

Rationale Therapy

The elements of rationale therapy are the facts and explanations given to the patient in the beginning about the disorder and about the different techniques when they are introduced. Making a case for rationale therapy, although it is often overlooked in practice, is an easy thing to do; making it work to best advantage is another matter. It will not work if the therapist's vocabulary is replete with technical terms and jargon. It may not work if the therapist assumes, but does not check to ensure, that the patient has an adequate grasp of the information. By "adequate" we mean that the patient is equipped to give an account of agoraphobia, and treatments for it, to others and to (re-)explain it to himself as needed during times of crisis or daily practice routines. Finally, the therapist must be prepared to encounter a clash of perspectives with patients who have developed their own "theories" of agoraphobia which do not match the facts. It is easier to weaken the hold of "home grown" theories than ones which have come from authoritative sources. Usually this is not too much of a problem when agoraphobia is misidentified as depression or a generalized anxiety state. When a patient says to us, "But the last therapist I saw said my problem is 'depression'" (or "anxiety"), we reply, "Yes, that is certainly *part* of the problem, but as you said yourself, you seldom find it easy to do the shopping on your own and from time to time you get these panic feelings. The name for all of this—depression, panic, travel worries, and all the rest— is 'agoraphobia.'"

We do not believe in spending valuable clinical time challenging the incorrect assessments of previous therapists if it is at all possible to accept them as a part of a more comprehensive explanation. Some of the explanations gleaned by the patient, however, have such potential for diminishing his self-regard that they may require more than perfunctory dismissal. The two that we have in mind are long-lived bits of clinical lore that pass for explanations of agoraphobia. Our only reason for mentioning them is that, as they almost always come from a clinical source, the patient may mistake them for the truth.

The first has a psychoanalytic flavor, although we know of its use by therapists who would disavow any commitment to Freudian thinking. In the usual (psychodynamic) manner, the theory discounts the importance of the patient's complaints and treats them as mere "symptoms" of deeper underlying problems. Specifically, the patient's travel and separation anxieties are interpreted as a mask for unconscious psychosexual conflicts. Thus, the patient avoids going out, the more so if "unchaperoned," because she, unconsciously, fears that powerful erotic urges will break free and lead her to indiscriminate sexual behavior. We have not found it difficult to alter patients' views on the "prostitution behavior" theory, as it has been called. Its weakest point is its sheer implausibility. For example, how it would explain agoraphobia in males is not at all clear.

The other "theory" has a certain face validity and requires more attention if it is to be overturned. It has no one name but in all of its varieties it makes the same assertion: patients choose agoraphobia for its instrumental value. The constant demands for support and companionship are attention-getting devices which the agoraphobic uses to gain control over the lives of people around him. This is the "secondary gain" theory dressed up to explain agoraphobia. Unlike the "prostitution behavior" theory, it cannot be dismissed out of hand. Agoraphobic individuals *do* plead for, or demand, assistance from significant others, and serious tensions can develop whenever these others try to evade the constant requests for support. The "secondary gain" theory has the merit of drawing attention to interpersonal problems overlooked by orthodox conditioning explanations. Apart from this, the theory has little to recommend it. Its most serious defect is that it begins with effects and not causes. The patient's "cries for help" during panic and separation episodes are better interpreted as *reactions* to these disruptions and not the reverse. What the secondary gain theory asks us to accept is that the agoraphobic can manufacture the extreme autonomic upheavals which occur during panic attacks and, when needed, produce the intense psychophysiological changes which are evident in phobic avoidance. Worst of all, the secondary gain explanation can have a disastrous effect on the attitudes of the attachment figures; patients themselves are not as drawn to it, for they have a good appreciation of the involuntary nature of panic and phobic reactions. Accordingly, the therapist is well advised to discover the degree of acceptance given to it by those close to the agoraphobic patient. If they take it seriously and feel that they are being "manipulated" by the agoraphobic in the "games" he is playing, then the correct and corrective information should be given.

Before we leave the information-giving stage, we try to be sure that all of the following matters have been covered.

1. *The name of the disorder.* It is true that psychiatric labels can produce undesirable effects on the individual's self-concept and on the way others react to him. This is a real risk when the label is presented as an explanation and, worse still, as one that locates all of the causes "inside" the patient. When used correctly, it tells the patient that his problems are not unique (a common fear) and that something is known about their management ("no one will be able to help me" is another of their fears). Patients experience great relief when we tell them that there are twenty thousand agoraphobics in Sydney alone.

2. *Variability and prognosis.* If at the outset the patient does not know which factors influence the course of agoraphobia (for example, panic attacks, certain illnesses), he must be made aware of these before therapy begins. Allied to this is what the patient expects to happen once therapy commences. The patient's expectations about the rate of change are seldom realistic. There are three frequently encountered but incorrect models which must be disconfirmed: the "no change," "all-at-once," and "straight-line" models (see Figures 9.1 and 9.2 for a full discussion of these).

3. *Relationships with attachment figures.* Nothing in our clinical experience or in the experimental literature gives reason to believe that the spouses of agoraphobics, or those in their families, conform to certain personality types characterized by neurotic needs to keep the agoraphobic in a dependent position. The spouses of agoraphobic patients do not appear in any way to be different from those married to "normals" (Buglass, Clarke, Henderson, Kreitman, & Presley, 1977). (This is the mirror-image theory to the secondary gain explanation described earlier, and it is no more convincing in

its validity.) Once agoraphobia develops, however, one of its likely results is the creation of serious stresses within the patient's family. The amount of "clinging" and the constancy of the demands will vary according to the severity of the condition. It reaches its most extreme level in housebound agoraphobics, who become profoundly dependent. Their strenuous efforts to keep trusted companions at hand or, if these are away, to make them "report in" as often as possible, are taxing in the extreme. When these calls for support are not honored, as sometimes must happen, agoraphobics become anxious during separation and, not infrequently, *very angry* when the attachment figure returns. The anxious demands and angry recriminations provoke conflicting emotions in them. The mixture of guilt and anger that the spouse or family members report feeling is understandable but only deepens the predicament of all involved. From this brief account it is obvious that not only must the patient be given information about the nature of agoraphobia but so also must his support figures.

Panic Attack Therapies

The pivotal role played by the panic attacks of complex agoraphobia makes the search for their mechanisms and causes a target of the first priority. It is a matter of some concern to us that research data do not yet exist to give a solid foundation to clinical practice. The available data are more suggestive than conclusive. The existing management methods make up a collection of *ad hoc* techniques which have yet to be tested rigorously. They fall into categories: pharmacological; cognitive-hypnotic; and behavioral.

Pharmacological Methods

From its long association with learning theories, behavior therapy has always been biased toward the assumption that the origins of maladaptive behavior and the sources of change would be found in the eliciting and reinforcing effects of environmental stimuli. In this climate, scant attention was paid to the role of physiological dysfunction in behavioral disorders. There are signs that a broadening of outlook is replacing the narrow perspective of earlier days (Liberman & Davis, 1975). The change is long overdue but is not yet well developed; we are still a long way from a fully adequate behavioral pharmacology of agoraphobia. Nonetheless, there are some very promising results from experimental investigations into the use of imipramine.

In one of the first studies of any kind of psychotropic drugs for agoraphobia, Klein and Fink (1962) were able to get a complete cessation of panic attacks with imipramine. It will help to put these results into the proper context by noting that Klein and Fink (1962) were working with chronic, hospitalized agoraphobics who had failed to improve after psychotherapy, milieu therapy, and drug (phenothiazine) therapy. The second finding of interest from this study was the selective action of imipramine: panic attacks eased but *phobic* anxiety and avoidance did not. These data and others (Klein, 1964; Zitrin, 1981) are fully consistent with one of the central arguments in this book: panic anxiety and phobic anxiety work through different processes and respond to different treatments. Note too that imipramine seems to work directly on the arousal system and not indirectly via the reduction of depression (Zitrin, 1981, p. 146).

This is the positive side to the results. The negative side is that many of the agoraphobic patients treated in these studies complained of strong, disturbing side-effects (insomnia, irritability, "jumpiness") and some dropped out of the drug therapy conditions. Zitrin (1981) and her co-workers found that they had to cut back the medication to as low as 2 mg per day in such patients. Surprisingly, therapeutic changes in panic anxiety were evident even at these low "homeopathic" dosages. This could be interpreted as a "placebo" reaction but for the fact that moderate or higher intakes of other medications do not seem to do what even very small amounts of imipramine can (Zitrin, 1981).

Phenothiazine drugs have also been tested as a medication for panic attacks. The results have not been encouraging. Klein (1967) found that one of these "major tranquilizers," chlorpromazine, was associated with significant clinical deterioration. As for the "minor tranquilizers," they are routinely prescribed (especially diazepam) but are of no proven value for *panic* anxiety. The judicious use of these drugs has its place, and the relief they provide (for example, from the relief of excessive levels of muscle tension) may encourage the patients to undertake exposure exercises. The beneficial effects, however, are not great (for example, Hafner & Marks, 1976) nor long-lasting. A recent report by the British Committee on the Review of Medicine (1980) concluded with the finding that no evidence existed to show that diazepam conferred any benefits at all after four months of continuous usage.

Cognitive Techniques

We have seen nothing in our clinical practice to suggest that panic attacks are directly triggered by cognitions. At best there may be an indirect connection mediated by the physiological arousal linked to excessive preoccupation with anxiety-laden anticipations. Helping the agoraphobic to dismiss or to gain distance from these thoughts may lower the average level of arousal. Useful techniques in this regard include everything from imparting information about panic attacks to daily practice at meditation. Right now, though, we are concerned with cognitive changes which go on *during* panic attacks. The value of the correct attributions and noncatastrophic cognitions is in causing an attenuation of the distress and possibly even the duration of panic attacks.

Cognitive therapies have a place in the management of panic attacks but only if they are simplified and adapted to meet the severe limitations imposed by the attacks. When trapped in the behavioral stereotypes and internal chaos, there is little scope for complex cognitive strategies or RET-like elaborations. By far the most practical course is to base the cognitive intervention on a small number of therapeutic reminders and simple assertions, such as the ones listed below. These should be used as soon as possible after the onset of the attack:

1. "Just let it happen. It'll pass in a few minutes. I musn't fight it. I'll be all right if I just let it happen. No need to struggle." With these words the patient reminds himself of the paradoxical effects of "struggle" and "capitulation." By coming to terms with the attack ("just let it pass") the impact is diminished (Weekes, 1977). Second, for any patient the duration of panic attacks will not vary a great deal around an average value. Strangely, they rarely notice this. Once it is pointed out, patients can use this information to "bind" the time.

2. "I really feel awful, but all that's happening is that my fear system is working overtime. That's all. Just my fear system. I have had this happen before; I know what it's all about." The words direct the patient toward the right attributions (Schacter & Singer, 1962). Notice that the patient is not advised to say to himself "I'm *not* going crazy" or "I'm *not* going to die." We have discovered that self-statements of this sort have the unhelpful and unintended effect of put-

ting the attention back into highly feared outcomes. Once these extremely upsetting themes are revived, the patient is at risk of being overpowered by "runaway" cognitions.

3. "I'll move slowly and breathe easily. Go slowly. Not too fast. That's right. I'll keep my hands away from my head and my face. I can go to the car in a moment [if outside] but first I'll *stop . . . stop* and go slowly. I'll *slow down* my breathing now." In panic attacks coordinated actions are supplanted by half-completed, fragmented behaviors. Fidgety and disorganized behavior heightens the sense of helplessness and produces a fast, shallow pattern of breathing which merges into hyperventilation, considerably augmenting the process of panic.

In general, self-control self-statements should be brief, phrased in a positive voice and slowly repeated as often as necessary. Once the fears begin to mount, it may be helpful to have the patient rehearse them beforehand and write them down on cards from which they can be read in a panic attack or at other times. They are designed to contain the forces unleashed in panic attacks and, if used by the patient, stem the impulses to hyperventilation and behavioral flight. As simple as they are, when panic hits, patients often forget these self-directions. In these circumstances, additional techniques and special training should be undertaken to enable the patient to get sufficient control so that adaptive cognitive processes will be employed and have the desired effects.

Behavioral Techniques

As they enter the panic state, agoraphobics begin to hyperventilate. After a minute or two of deep and rapid breathing, blood carbon dioxide levels fall and dizziness follows; in some cases there is syncope and tetanic spasms in the hands and feet. The patient may come close to fainting, and this, by itself, can provoke a sharp jump in the level of panic.

Patients are likely to be aware that they breathe too rapidly when in panic. Very few appreciate the role of hyperventilation in "locking" them into the panic. A direct method of treatment is to get the patient to *stop* breathing for about five seconds, then breathe out, slowly for five seconds, pause for three seconds, breathe in for five seconds, and to repeat the cycle until the anxiety subsides.

Some patients have a sharply diminished capacity to bring respi-

ratory processes under conscious control, and directions for measured breathing will achieve little. Wolpe (1969) has these patients
breathe into a paper bag. The inspiration of carbon dioxide for a
minute or more in this way can terminate an attack. Though the
changes come quickly, patients unfortunately fear that it looks
"crazy" or "silly" and are reluctant to use the "bag technique" outside
the home or when others are present.

Once patients have acquired a degree of control with cognitive
or breathing techniques, we ask them to deliberately evoke the early
stages of a panic attack. Hyperventilation and the rehearsal of
alarming outcomes should be sufficient to bring about most of the
precursors to panic within one minute. Immediately, the patient is
instructed to go into the correct breathing routine and to get out his
"panic cards" and read them. This teaches the patient that panic
attacks do have causes. It also gives him the opportunity to practice
control techniques when the problem is "hot" (cf. Beck et al., 1979,
p. 33). These suggestions bear an obvious resemblance to Frankl's
(1970) "paradoxical intention" with one important difference. Unlike paradoxical intention, where the patient describes what he fears
most, attempts to do it, "fails," and rids himself of that fear, agoraphobics *can* produce panic. It goes without saying that the training
should consist of very brief instances of panic provocation.

Hypnosis

Hypnotic techniques can be programmed for anxiety reduction,
anxiety *in*duction (see above), scene enhancement in vicarious exposure, and a variety of other purposes (see chapter 4). The use of
hypnosis with agoraphobics does not call for a contradiction of the
basic principles and procedures. However, the special problems of
agoraphobia call for certain important modifications to standard
practice.

Eye Closure

Direct requests for eye closure may prove threatening and are to be
avoided. Agoraphobics prefer to relinquish visual contact with the
environment only when they feel it can be reestablished quickly. A
good way to begin the induction is to have the patient focus on a
spot that is just out of easy visual reach and proceed with suggestions

of "eye heaviness," making sure to tell the patient that he may close his eyes whenever he wishes: "Your eyes can get very heavy . . . very heavy . . . you may keep them open if you wish, but it will be so much easier just to let them get pleasantly heavy . . . and then to close . . . so restful to close them. You can open them whenever you want to but it will be so much more restful to allow them to close."

Counterproductive Suggestions

Agoraphobics exist in constant readiness to respond to threat. They make an excessive number of orienting, "What is it?" reactions (Marks, 1969). One source of perceived danger emanates from within their own bodies. Therefore, requests from the therapist to focus on inner feelings and suggestions that refer to "strange" reactions may cause alarm. Specifically, suggestions of "tingling," "floating" feelings, and "dreamy" states can precipitate trouble because of their similarity to the early stages of depersonalization and panic. They return the agoraphobic to the incessant round of self-scrutiny and anticipation. Especially to be avoided are rapid-induction techniques that involve rapid breathing. Visual imagery must also be given careful thought. For example, while most people find scenes of quiet country walks or strolls on long stretches of unoccupied beach quite relaxing, agoraphobics obviously will not. Such standard "pleasant scenes" are more likely to cause a quantum *increase* in arousal and flight tendencies.

Counter-Anxiety Measures

At any time during the induction or thereafter, the therapist may observe a sudden increase in restlessness, fidgety behavior, or more florid anxiety reactions. Unplanned eruptions of anxiety or arousal must be closely watched. Where they threaten to culminate in a panic attack, steps should be taken to help the patient feel safe again and at ease. One way that this can be done rapidly is by making physical contact with the patient. The touch or stroke should be to the skin and not the patient's clothing. Evidence from primate research indicates that highly excited and frightened subjects find physical contact with others very soothing (Bowlby, 1975). Care should be taken to announce the intended contact beforehand; always avoid inflicting "surprises" on agoraphobic patients. Be sure not to encircle the body part (for example, the wrist) which is being touched. This produces a sense of restriction which is highly aversive. Verbal reassurance can be given at the same time: "I'm right here beside you . . . you can hear my voice . . . you'll always be able to hear exactly what I'm saying . . . and the anxiety will soon pass." Passages of this sort, containing reminders of the therapist's presence, can be interpolated within imaginal exposure scenes. One might imagine that this would be a troubling contradiction between the two messages (you're here . . . you're in the scene); actually, it is easily tolerated and not at all disturbing.

The literature on agoraphobia is growing at a rapid pace, but there is still very little in it touching on the use of hypnosis. We listed a number of ways (for example, in vicarious exposure therapies) in which it can make a contribution, but the main one would have to be the control of arousal—and thus, panic. Consequently, teaching the techniques of cognitive and behavioral control is vital, but this is no easy task with agoraphobic patients. Few possess the skills of self-relaxation. Most are "slow learners." The widespread practices of giving taped relaxation suggestions and/or "pleasant imagery" exercises to be used at home are to be questioned. These tend to be used on a few occasions and then discontinued. Furthermore, audiotapes cannot be used conveniently outside of the home.

In many ways, relaxation induced in heterohypnosis is the ideal way to begin. As a rule agoraphobics will have fewer self-direction and self-control skills at their disposal than patients with circumscribed phobias but, paradoxically, have a greater need for them. Deep muscle relaxation techniques (see Appendix A) can give relief, but patients who can get temporary respite report that their "mental" worries quickly rearouse them. It is, therefore, essential to help the patient to acquire the appropriate control strategies of relaxation *and* cognitive control. In saying this, we are not downgrading the value of physical relaxation exercises. Even well-learned relaxation techniques may not always give relief or terminate panics each and every time. The next best thing, then, is for the patients to use mental (cognitive) exercises to achieve some disengagement from the physiological arousal that plagues them. After all, it is, strictly speaking, not the physiological changes alone that lead to psychological distress. What must be added is the obsessive attention to and misinterpretation of these peripheral reactions which propel patients so forcefully to the agoraphobic "conclusions" they draw: "I must get home; I must get help; I'm going to die" and the like (Mandler, 1975; Schacter & Singer, 1962). Eventually, self-hypnosis and meditation will be even more important than heterohypnosis. Initially though, the therapist should set up the best conditions for practice. For an agoraphobic any journey with a trusted guide is one they are most prepared to take.

Exposure Therapies

The treatment of choice for any phobic anxiety is exposure to an environment containing those stimuli. The therapist has to decide on the relevant dimensions of the phobia and the rate and conditions of this exposure. The relevant dimensions in agoraphobia are separation from security figures and traveling away from safety, plus the stimuli originating from within the patient's own body (a very important but rarely examined dimension). The rate at which exposure is carried out will depend on the severity of the problem and the resources of the patient. Where the patient is psychologically strong and/or the problem is not incapacitating, the therapist may move quickly to reintroduce him to the situations and places he avoids. For those who are chronically disabled and who have established only tenuous self-control, the therapist must move more cautiously and take special care not to ask the patient to attempt tasks that may overwhelm him. The best guide to the category in which the patient belongs is the presence or absence of recent or recurrent panic attacks. *In vivo* exercises (see Appendix A) are absolutely essential for all cases of agoraphobia, whether simple or complex. In addition, for those in the more serious category, imaginal exercises are very useful for presenting scenes with content to which it would be difficult or impossible to arrange real-life exposure. Losing control of bladder functions, falling to the ground in a fit of terror, or screaming out loud are typical sorts of worries. It matters not that the patient will not ever have done this or anything remotely like it. Despite its status as an improbable or unlikely outcome, this sort of dread can contribute to escape and avoidance behavior. The only "exposure" contact possible with such terrors is in the use of imaginal techniques. This, or any, vicarious exposure can be given greater affective impact, made more vivid, and made to approximate *in vivo* exposure through the use of hypnosis. Examples of scenes and hierarchies are presented in Appendix B. In addition, the following points require special attention:

Visual Contact Problems

Agoraphobics and therapists may be puzzled to discover that the difficulty in separation from places or persons is not a simple function of the physical distance from security. As a very typical example, a patient may be able to get as far as 300 yards away from home up or down the street but no more than 50 yards around the corner. As soon as he loses visual contact with home, anxiety levels climb. This troubles patients because they believe, as do many clinical writers, that anxiety can be explained solely in terms of distance from home or the duration of exposure to this particular distance of separation. In fact, the distance/duration parameters interact with a variety of cognitive and noncognitive variables. The patient *knows* that at 50 yards he is a lot closer to home than at 300 yards, but his knowledge is not enough to lessen the anxiety. Or patients may be able to drive 5 miles in any direction from home but be unable to walk out of visual contact with the car without suffering.

The Location of the Therapist

Research reports never mention the whereabouts of the therapist on *in vivo* exposure trials. This is indeed odd, because this is a fact that agoraphobic patients want in their possession. The presence of the therapist or the knowledge that he is within range is what patients feel they *must* know. Consequently, during vicarious exposure, this should be made more clear in the easier scenes and less so in the ones further up the hierarchy. In the concluding scenes (and, naturally, *in vivo* situations too) the patient should also be unable to forecast the return of the therapist or other attachment figures.

Final Comments on Exposure Therapies

Nowadays, *in vivo* flooding is promoted as the exposure treatment of choice (Marks, 1975). We are not convinced that *in vivo* flooding is actually the best name because it suggests that the therapist can disregard the level of anxiety experienced, whereas, in fact, high anxiety gives no advantage in exposure and may even be detrimental. Second, the term *flooding* implies full unprotected exposure to the most stressful situations. Anyone who has seen an agoraphobic patient carefully and cautiously begin his travel exercise will prefer the term *graduated exposure*. In any case, debates over labels take our attention away from the processes of change.

Another widely held belief is that *in vivo* exposure is always to be preferred to imaginal exposure. We wonder about the validity of this, too. The trouble is that some patients will not attempt *in vivo* exposure at first. Zitrin's (1981) remarks on the apparent suitability of *in vivo* exposure are worth recalling: "There are certain patients who simply will not tolerate *in vivo* exposures. . . . In our experience patients who opt for [this] . . . must be considered a high self-selected group" (p. 170). We agree and we do not see why *both* imaginal and *in vivo* techniques cannot be used.

All of the therapy procedures recommended in this chapter have been aimed at building the skills that the patient needs in order to overcome the restrictions and discomforts of agoraphobia. Achieving this does not bring therapy to a close.

Agoraphobia is a relapsing disorder. The patient must be aware that getting over the problem is not the same as getting rid of the predisposition. Thus, he must learn how to identify, as early as possible, stressful precipitators and how to cope with them. We supplement the final counseling sessions with "relapse therapy"—in which the patient is hypnotized and put into contact with future "outbreaks" of panic and avoidance. Then he is asked to see himself recovering his poise and putting into action the skills he has acquired.

We have yet to gather long-term follow-up data on relapse therapy. Thus far the reports have been encouraging. Patients take setbacks as a cue to recommence the exposure, relaxation, self-hypnotic, and other exercises that served them well earlier.

A Note on Record Keeping

There are a number of good manuals (for example, Mathews et al., 1981) available for a guide to the patient's record keeping. These are easy to construct and use. The point to stress to the patient is that there must be *daily* records (of distance traveled, reactions experienced, time spent in therapeutic exercises—exposure, meditation, relaxation, etc.).

Summary

Agoraphobia is the most prevalent, complex, and difficult of all anxiety-based disorders. It presents the therapist and theorists with a collection of problems which have yet to be overcome. Our model

of agoraphobia gives center place to panic attacks, and our treatment program is built around the separation of panic and phobic
anxieties.

These few statements express the essentials of our analytic and
treatment frameworks. But neither these guidelines nor all that we
have written in the chapter can do more than hint at the cost agoraphobia exacts from the patient.

12

Anxiety
in Sports

As far as possible, sports events should be conducted under the stimulus of pleasant psychological feelings and with a tone of moral enthusiasm. Anything capable of exciting mental pictures of strength, energy, and predominance will give the athlete more strength, energy, and will to fight for victory.

—Gislero Flesch, "What Sports Medicine
Owes to I.P. Pavlov," 1974

In other chapters in this book, we have discussed the use of hypnosis as a facilitating mechanism in the treatment of anxiety and phobic problems in clinical situations. It is clear that hypnosis is a valuable therapeutic aid in the treatment of these disorders, and in other situations that do not, strictly speaking, come under the heading of clinical disorders. Today there is a growing awareness of the use or application of behavioral techniques to minimize the development of physical or psychological problems. This area is sometimes called by the currently popular terms of "behavioral medicine" or "behavioral health management." These areas reflect the extension of behavior therapy practices to promote health, the participation in sensible strategies of living, and the correct and sensible use of leisure time— and not merely to ameliorate pathology. Nowadays, people are being urged, increasingly, to spend a portion of this time in sporting activities, and the escalation in the production of and interest in leisure-time sporting equipment suggests that more and more people are doing just this. The explosion of interest in jogging and squash, for example, demonstrates the prevailing attitude toward exercise and sport.

It is something of a paradox, therefore, that activities that are considered to be sports, pastimes, or leisure pursuits may often create considerable levels of anxiety in participants. From the standpoint of modern-day sports, there is little doubt that participants in both amateur and professional codes of most sporting activities are subjected to considerable pressures to perform consistently at high levels of achievement. These pressures, may in turn, lead to considerable anxiety in an individual.

It would seem appropriate, therefore, to look at some of the factors that underlie sports anxiety, as well as methods of dealing with them. There is a growing awareness among both administrators and players of the need to study behavioral responses of participants in sports so that they can achieve successful results without experiencing adverse physical and psychological strain. Indeed, sports psychology is accepted as a discipline in its own right in the United States and in Eastern Bloc countries. The value of a correct psychological assessment of a sportsperson lies not only in the identification of personal attributes which may aid performance but also of those negative features which may have an inhibitory influence.

Arousal and Anxiety

We know from studies of individuals' performance in their sport and from laboratory studies that arousal is an important ingredient for the achievement of maximal sporting performance. As long ago as 1908, Yerkes and Dodson formulated the, by now, well-known law relating performance efficiency to levels of arousal. This was presented in the form of an inverted-U showing that as arousal was increased to a particular level, so performance improved. If the arousal stimulus was increased beyond the optimal level, however, this, in turn, led to a decrement in performance (Figure 12.1).

The meaning which they and most others give to arousal is the level of behavioral and physiological activity in a particular system, exhibited in response to a variety of exteroceptive or interoceptive stimuli. In spite of rigorous research, the validity of the Yerkes–Dodson hypothesis is still open to question. Some workers (for example, Murphy, 1966; Pinneo, 1961) have failed to confirm the

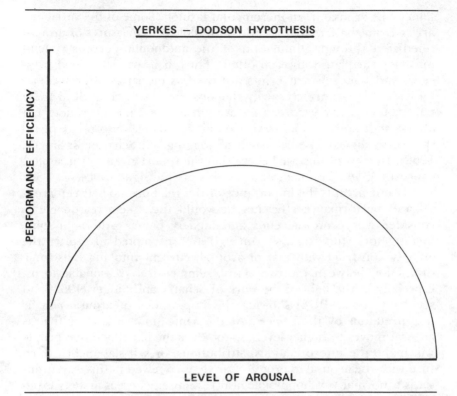

Figure 12.1 The relationship between the level of arousal and performance efficiency known as the Yerkes–Dodson hypothesis (or law) predicts that fluent, effective performance increases with increments to arousal up to a certain, ideal level after which performance declines with further arousal. The hypothesis of an optimal level of arousal is useful as an orienting idea but gives little guidance for specific predictions in particular situations.

hypothesis, while on the other hand, studies by Martens and Landers (1970) on children, Fenz and Epstein (1969) on sports parachutists, and Wood and Hokanson (1965) have validated the Yerkes–Dodson law.

Why is there such a wide divergence of findings among these studies? The answer would seem to lie in the fact that the Yerkes–Dodson hypothesis is more relevant to the performance of skilled tasks in particular, whereas simple tasks are more likely to be enhanced by arousal in an incremental fashion. Some of the variability arises from the fact that accepted physiological measures of arousal (mediated through stimulation of the autonomic nervous system) may not correlate with each other. Thus, if heart rate, blood pressure, and palmar sweat prints are used as measures of arousal, an individual may not necessarily demonstrate changes in all of these parameters. Furthermore, an elevation in these measures does not always indicate a *psychological* arousal, for it may also occur in response to an exercise-task such as jogging (cf. Schacter & Singer, 1962). In view of this, we believe that the report given by the subject concerning *his* assessment of arousal is of vital significance.

If one accepts the importance of the relationship between arousal and performance efficiency, it would then seem reasonable to consider where arousal ends and anxiety begins. Although some investigators (for example, Duffy, 1962) attempted to replace the anxiety construct with that of arousal, current thinking calls for a distinction between the two. This seems entirely reasonable to us, especially in the light of the work of Schater and Singer (1962; and see Isen et al., 1978) showing the importance of arousal *plus* its interpretation by the subject. At the same time, it is clear that as arousal moves to higher levels, so too does the likelihood that people will make the interpretations, attributions, or self-statements which fuse with the arousal to produce "anxiety." Viewed in this way, arousal is a normal psychophysiological response, whereas anxiety is decidedly pathological or dysfunctional in its influence on performance efficiency and psychological well-being. In essence, this is what the inverted-U hypothesis sets out to state, and there is little doubt that this pattern of response occurs quite frequently in competitive sports situations.

In concerning ourselves with the issue of the effect of anxiety on performance in sports, it is relevant to distinguish between state and trait anxiety. State, or impact, anxiety may be considered an overresponse to a particular situation. It fluctuates over time and is "characterized by subjective consciously perceived feelings of apprehension and tension, accompanied by or associated with activation or arousal of the autonomic nervous system" (Spielberger, 1966, p. 17). Obviously, state anxiety is a common experience in individuals who are competing in major sporting endeavors. On the other hand, anxiety that exists on a more or less permanent basis across a variety of situations would be considered trait anxiety. Spielberger (1966) expressed this type of anxiety as "a motive or acquired behavioral disposition that predisposes an individual to perceive a wide range of objectively non-dangerous circumstances as threatening, and to respond to these with state anxiety reactions disproportionate in intensity to the magnitude of the objective danger" (p. 17).

As noted, the relationship between anxiety and performance has been a matter of some interest to experimentalists and clinicians, and it is clear that the investigator is faced by a number of issues associated with the measurement of anxiety. In the majority of sporting situations, competitors are much more likely to experience impact (i.e., state) anxiety, and yet a large majority of studies carried out in this area have used scales that measure trait rather than state anxiety, such as the IPAT anxiety scale (Cattell, 1957) or the IPAT 8 parallel-form anxiety battery (Scheier & Cattell, 1960). For this reason, there is a body of opinion which believes that these scales are not measuring the type of anxiety that the sportsperson really experiences (Martens, 1971). It would appear that it is not possible to be dogmatic on this issue, since the scales would seem, at least, to be partly evaluating impact anxiety. This is borne out by studies carried out in a wide variety of sport situations. Morgan (1970) used these scales when testing college wrestlers and demonstrated that anxiety decreased from preseason to prematch level. Similarly, Hutson (1965) used rating scales to show that anxiety levels decreased and horsemanship improved in novice equestriennes after only three riding lessons. We consider that anxiety rating scales may be of value to the sports psychologist in order to distinguish between impact (or state) anxiety and that which is far removed from the sports situation (trait anxiety).

No discussion of sports anxiety can be complete without recognition of the objectively threatening or dangerous side to sports. It has been our experience that fear occurs far more commonly in sports participants than is generally recognized—even in those who are skilled and who play in major or international competition. In many instances, of course, this fear is not at all unrealistic because of the potential for sustaining bodily injury. This fear may be thought of as a situational fear and is likely to occur, for example, when a baseball batter is standing up at the plate and is facing a ball rushing at him at high speed, or in cricket, when a batsman faces a fast bowler who delivers the ball at speeds in excess of 90 miles per hour. Notwithstanding the realism of such a fear, we have noted that such fears are more prevalent in those individuals who demonstrate trait anxiety.

Attentional Processes

In line with the Yerkes–Dodson hypothesis, there appears to be little doubt that a relationship does exist between arousal and performance efficiency in sporting situations. This being the case, it would seem relevant to consider in what way sports performance is affected by varying levels of arousal. The principal effect would seem to be on an individual's attentional processes, and this effect may have a considerable bearing on performance for "In sport situations involving speed, strength, or endurance, the athlete must be able to focus attention on the important factors relevant to the task" (Landers, 1978, p. 79).

Nideffer (1978) has nicely summarized the attentional styles that a sportsperson may need to call upon in order to perform satisfactorily. He sets out four attentional styles based on whether the individual needs to focus inwardly on his own feelings or outwardly on the factors associated with the sporting situation, and also whether the subject needs to confine (i.e., narrow) his attentional focus or have a wider view of the game. These can best be exemplified by using golf as a model. First, the golfer needs to utilize a broad external focus in order to identify and react to changing environmental conditions. These may include a variety of factors such as wind direction, the presence and position of fairway bunkers, the direction and slope of the fairway, and the flag-placement on the putting green.

Second, a golfer needs to draw upon a narrow external focus when setting himself up to hit the ball. Here, the individual confines his attention to grip, stance, and alignment. The third attentional style is the narrow internal focus. Nideffer (1978) discusses this as being important for rehearsal of tasks, reflection and preparation for a game, and the development of endurance. The last-named effect is best exemplified by distance runners, who direct their attention toward their running style and in this way develop a pain tolerance by not attending to the painful cues. Finally, a sportsperson needs to utilize a broad internal focus in order to plan strategies and develop means of coping with opponents.

As has been alluded to earlier in this chapter, arousal may influence performance by dividing a subject's attention, thereby interfering with all of the four modes or styles just described. Initially, arousal narrows the individual's attention and may be thought of as being a direct influence on cognition. If arousal levels are increased beyond a certain optimal level, then anxiety supervenes and attentional processes are narrowed still further. The subject starts thinking of the past or the future rather than maintaining the essential "here and now" attentional style (Broadbent, 1958; Neisser, 1967). Although anxiety may occur as the result of excessive arousal (Duffy, 1962), it may often be the case that anxiety is the cause of excess arousal. Thus, in such situations, a cycle of arousal–anxiety–arousal is established which invariably will produce a significant performance decrement.

The importance of attention in performance, all would agree, is beyond dispute. The next concern is the relationship between arousal, anxiety, and attention. There is abundant experimental evidence to show that arousal and anxiety interfere with attentional control (Callaway & Dembo, 1958; Wachtel, 1968). An explanation for this has been proposed by Easterbrook (1959), who suggests that it occurs because of the subject's loss of sensitivity to peripheral cues. The basis of Easterbrook's theory of cue utilization is that in performing any task, a subject is exposed to both relevant and irrelevant cues. Since "emotional arousal acts consistently to reduce the range of cues that an organism uses" (p. 183), the first effect of arousal is to reduce the individual's attention to irrelevant cues. Consequently, relevant cues predominate, and this leads to an increment in performance. As arousal levels continue to rise (and anxiety supervenes), however, this has the effect of also eliminating relevant cues, and in that way, performance is diminished. Peripheral narrowing of attention may also occur as the result of fear of personal injury (Berkun, 1964), and this suggests that a subject who fears injury in competition may narrow his attention to a point where he is no longer able to perform satisfactorily.

The Influence of Stress

Individuals who compete in sports are often called upon to face situations that are, for them, especially stressful. How a sportsperson responds to this stress may depend upon a number of factors. These encompass such things as his emotional stability, familiarity with the task at hand, his degree of expertise, situational factors such as the importance of the occasion (Sells, 1970), and fears of particular opponents. For the purpose of present discussion, we view stress as arousal and/or the cognitive environmental stimuli which lead to anxiety or fear.

One of the most striking and valuable *in vivo* studies demonstrating the effects of competitive stress was that of Naruse (1965).

One of the aims of the study, which was carried out on 125 Japanese athletic champions who performed at the 1960 Rome Olympic Games, was to determine the effects of anxiety arising in competition. Naruse viewed the anxiety that arises in competitive sports as being a form of stage fright. The athletes were questioned as to whether they had experienced stage fright; how it was manifested; its effect on their performance; and their success with self-management techniques.

The results of the study showed that the greater majority experienced stage fright, and only 20 percent utilized a psychologically oriented technique to relieve it. Furthermore, Naruse determined that stage fright occurs not only during actual competition but also during the weeks leading up to and immediately before the event. These findings are in agreement with our observations that anticipatory anxiety may play a significant role in diminishing performance efficiency.

Hypnotic Management

From the foregoing discussion it is clear that competitive stress is a significant problem in sports and that many participants have little knowledge of how to cope with this ever-present problem. Hypnosis and hypnotic-like techniques (for example, autogenic training) have been widely and successfully used in the treatment of psychological problems associated with sports (Naruse, 1965; Unestahl, 1979). In line with our delineation of the processes and problems in sports performance there are a number of areas in which hypnosis can be employed:

1. To manipulate arousal through hypnotic suggestion and imagery.
2. To control attentional problems by means of hypnosis, self-hypnosis, and meditation.
3. For the alleviation of anxiety by the use of "conditioned relaxation" and desensitization procedures.
4. By influencing the motivated behavior of a subject.

It becomes clear, therefore, that in order to use hypnosis effectively in the treatment of sports anxiety, the particular area(s) of difficulty must first be clearly defined.

Arousal: Treatment Considerations

Although maximum performance efficiency is dependent on optimal arousal levels, in practical terms, their achievement and maintenance is not always as straightforward as the Yerkes–Dodson hypothesis would suggest. This hypothesis, though substantively correct, does not take into account the complex arousal pattern that some athletes experience. Some individuals, for example, have a high level of arousal pre-competition, but experience a precipitate drop during performance. The therapist, in treating these athletes, has a twofold problem. First, he must utilize techniques that reduce *anticipatory* anxiety and, second, must teach the individual techniques of inducing arousal during actual competition. On the other hand, other athletes may exhibit excessively high levels of arousal—both before and during performance. These individuals have to be taught techniques that will decrease their arousal to a point where they can maintain maximal efficiency. Thus, the uses to which hypnosis can be put will depend on whether the need is for arousal reduction or *induction*.

It is clear from what we have said thus far that hypnotic techniques may be of great value in correcting problems of arousal in sports (always assuming that the problems do not stem from an inadequate skills repertoire). Sports involving speed and endurance (for example, swimming and running) lend themselves especially to these procedures. As an example of this, consider a swimmer whose best performance time for swimming a 100 meter butterfly race is 73 seconds, and who consistently performs close to that figure. Irrespective of what peaks of fitness he achieves, the swimmer's time is guided by the timing on his psychological clock (in this case, 73 seconds) until active steps are taken to alter this. Thus, if the subject believes that he is capable of swimming the same race in, say, 68 seconds, then the psychological clock will have to be speeded up; otherwise he will continue to swim to *his* clock. This is obviously important where hundredths of a second may mean the difference between winning and losing a race. It follows, therefore, that arousal levels must be increased, and suggestion and imagery in hypnosis may prove beneficial in achieving this goal. The point we wish to make is that the general public and perhaps most practitioners think of hypnosis as a tool for relaxation. While this has certainly been demonstrated (Benson, 1975, 1981), it is also possible to use suggestion in hypnosis to augment arousal (Bower, 1981).

The Hypnotic Management
of Attentional Problems

Early in this chapter we discussed the four attentional foci which
sports participants draw upon when achieving optimal performance.
The treatment of attentional problems hinges on the identification
of the particular focus which anxiety is influencing. It is not sufficient, for example, to label a sportsperson as having "poor concentration," for this does little to clarify the particular attentional process needing treatment.

One should not, however, think of these attentional processes
as being rigidly compartmentalized. Instead, a player usually finds
that the type of focus needed (for example, broad or narrow external) changes continuously to suit the needs of competition. Anxiety
may interfere with these changes in attentional style by inhibiting a
subject's ability to constantly and rapidly adapt to "here and now"
situations. In such individuals, imaginal rehearsal in hypnosis and
self-hypnosis is an effective method of correcting these attentional
difficulties.

A technique that can aid the rapid change in attentional style
needed in competition is the use of a cuing mechanism. In long-
duration sports such as golf, the player is involved in actually hitting the ball for a relatively short time. It has been calculated that a
professional golfer spends seven and a half minutes actually hitting
the ball over four rounds of a tournament (Patmore, 1979, p. 74).
The maintenance of a narrow external attentional focus throughout the whole round of golf is obviously unattainable but must be
restricted to the phase of actually hitting the ball if success is to be
achieved. The player must then be able to revert to the broad
external focus. It is in this process of changing attentional style that
cuing mechanisms may be utilized, especially in those players who
note a "loss of concentration" during some phase of their game.

The process of changing attentional style to meet the needs of
the moment often proves difficult for many competitors. These difficulties can be corrected by the introduction in hypnosis of an appropriate cue (a word; breathing; touching some part of the sports
armamentarium). Reinforcement of this cue through imagery and *in
vivo* practice is necessary for it to become an involuntary response.

Hypnotic Techniques and Sports Anxiety

An athlete who is anxious in competition will often manifest this in a
variety of ways (for example, somatic tension, excessive concern

about a forthcoming event, difficulty in sleeping, loss of confidence and self-esteem, and a fear of injury). Somatic tension in particular (and this is usually first experienced in the hands and arms) may lead to a loss of integration and synchrony of movements—especially those involving fine coordination.

Treatment in hypnosis must be aimed at reducing anxiety levels, inculcating feelings of relaxation while participating, and in the development of self-confidence and self-esteem. Suggestive therapy may go a long way to reestablishing self-confidence and self-esteem and also provide a means of reinforcing positive self-statements. These suggestions should be "tailored" to the individual's particular difficulties rather than be of the stereotyped "ego-strengthening" variety proposed by Hartland (1971), which we view to be excessively general.

Exposure Techniques

In chapter 8 we recorded the voluminous data supporting the value of techniques which lie along the exposure dimension (systematic desensitization through to flooding) in the management of anxiety. In that discussion, we paid special attention to the needs for putting anxiety-inhibiting control techniques (hypnosis, meditation, relaxation) into the hands of very anxious patients. The reason for this is to counteract possible sensitization episodes. We also pointed out that the *total* elimination of anxiety is not an easy, nor probably a desirable, goal. Rather, we emphasized the value of teaching the patient to use anxiety and stress as signals for the use of self-control techniques. With athletes, the same advice holds true but with two exceptions: First, in nonpatient populations, anxiety reactions are likely to be more circumscribed and less pervasive. Thus, the need for spending valuable clinical time teaching anxiety-inhibiting strategies is not as apparent. Second, for athletes, anxiety at moderate levels can contribute to better performance. In a manner of speaking, then, we tell the patient to do the best he can with moderate levels of anxiety, and we tell the sportsman that he *can* do the best he can with moderate levels of anxiety.

The techniques used in treating sports anxiety and fear are systematic desensitization and flooding (the reader is referred to chapter 9 for a detailed description of these). In that chapter, we expressed the view that exposure techniques lie along a continuum—bounded at one end by classical systematic desensitization and at the other by the most extreme flooding procedures. In the treatment of sports anxiety, athletes tend to be more responsive to a technique which moves more toward the flooding end of this continuum. This is especially the case in those individuals whose anxiety is associated with a fear of failure or poor performance.

Hypnosis and Motivated Behavior

There is no doubt that a great deal of experimental and ecological research is being conducted in an effort to increase man's ability to perform better in a great number of areas of life, including sports. People are constantly endeavoring to run faster, jump higher and longer, throw a ball further—in short, to surpass standards of performance which hitherto have appeared to be "the ultimate." Many people still view hypnosis as having a magical flavor which will enable them to perform sports tasks that would otherwise be unattainable. Such concepts are naive and untenable, for they fail to take into account the genetic capacity of an individual and his physiological potential. Thus, hypnosis will not convert a runner who lacks the correct proportions of long and short muscle fibers or who does not possess the necessary cardiovascular resources into a champion sprinter or distance performer. Again, if a sprinter has the performance *capacity* to run 100 meters in 11.2 seconds, he will be unable to run that distance in, say, 11 seconds, either as a result of hypnotic intervention or because of any other approach. It would be akin to giving a short-sighted person suggestions that he is going to have perfect visual acuity.

Perhaps the unanswered (and unanswerable) question in the minds of all sportspersons is whether they have actually reached their maximum performance capacity. It would seem that this doubt must lie largely unresolved in the sporting arena, although it *is* possible to clarify certain aspects of it in an experimental setting. Jackson et al. (1979) assessed the influence of posthypnotic suggestion on endurance performance in a group of 55 physically trained male subjects. These subjects were assigned to five groups: control, hypnosis alone, motivation alone, low-susceptible hypnosis subjects given motivational suggestions, and high-susceptible subjects given motivational suggestions. Each subject was required to perform two runs to his maximum capacity (exhaustion), on a treadmill which was moving at a constant speed of 200 meters per minute. Maximum endurance capacity was measured by oxygen consumption, blood lactate concentration, and respiratory quotient. It was necessary for the subjects to fulfill at least two of the criteria for maximum capacity (Astrand & Rodahl, 1977).

The findings of the study revealed that high-susceptible subjects, through the motivational suggestions given in hypnosis, were able to *maintain* their maximum endurance capacity for a significantly longer time than in their control run. It should be noted here that the subjects did not exceed their control performance after hypnotic intervention. This finding, in our view, supports our proposition that it is not possible through the use of hypnosis to add anything that will cause a person to exceed those limits of performance which are imposed by his own physiological or psychological barriers. Although this would, at first sight, appear to be an argument against the use of hypnosis in increasing endurance in sports, further consideration would indicate that it is a fortunate state of affairs. If, indeed, it were the case that hypnosis could induce a person to exceed his maximum capacity, then it would not be too hard to imagine the possibility of serious physiological and/or psychological damage occurring as the result of these changes.

In line with the work of many previous researchers (for example, Barber & Calverley, 1964b; Collins, 1961; London & Fuhrer, 1961; Orne, 1959), the study also showed that the subjects who were not hypnotized but given motivational suggestions alone also achieved a significantly longer endurance time on the treadmill runs. These findings add further weight to our argument (see chapter 2) that responses achieved in hypnosis may also occur in the nonhypnotic state.

In light of these findings, is there anything to be achieved by using hypnosis as a method of increasing motivation in sports? From our experience based on the treatment of a considerable number of sportspersons, we would give an unqualified "yes" to that question. Hypnosis may be used to increase motivation in three ways. First, it may be utilized to produce a change in attitudes in an individual (i.e., to change the hedonic valence of a stimulus or situation). There is a body of opinion (Bem & Allen, 1974) which believes that in order to change attitudes, it is first necessary to change behaviors. We have, throughout the book, stressed the close relationship that exists between hypnosis and behavioral changes, and it would seem entirely reasonable, therefore, to view hypnosis as an ideal way of eliciting these responses.

Second are its effects on increasing a sportsperson's output. In a sports situation, many individuals are unable to collate the cues around them. This is especially so in highly competitive situations and inevitably leads to diminished performance efficiency. Hypnosis (especially through the use of imagery) can help the person more effectively utilize *input* stimuli by making him more aware of the world around. In this way, he is better able to recognize and respond to environmental cues associated with the sporting situation. Finally, hypnosis enables the therapist to instill or add to the repertoire of a subject by the further refinement of existing skills. An apparent loss of skill may be a potent factor in reducing a person's motivation, and the correction lies in the building-in of new responses or by the rearrangement of established ones.

The Role of Self-hypnosis and Meditation

In the chapters on meditation and self-hypnosis, we began by underscoring the limitations of hypnosis and hypnotic-like techniques when the use of these is tied to the clinical application by the therapist. The need to avoid unfortunate dependency problems and the therapeutic utility of enhancing self-direction and self-control led naturally to the matter of self-hypnosis. From there, we cited the evidence for meditation as a self-control technique in its own right and as a way to lower the threshold for receptivity to self-suggestion. Our discussion in those chapters centered around meditation and self-hypnosis as tools to combat clinical anxiety in all of its forms. In contrast to that, the central interest in this chapter is anxiety and sports. Anxiety in sports does not justify erecting still more conceptual categories of anxiety. Nevertheless, there are important differences in the person's, and hence the clinician's, focus. The sports performer has uppermost in his mind the need for a smooth and well-integrated performance. He may, of course, be eager to eliminate subjective distress, but mainly because that interferes with the supple and forceful execution of his skill. Precision performance is likely to be a secondary concern to the patient who first of all wants to "feel better and stop worrying."

The rationale for using self-hypnosis for the development of self-mastery and self-direction in sporting endeavors is no different from that described in the treatment of clinical disorders. It is important, for example, that the therapist provide a detailed explanation of the nature, purposes, and ways of using self-hypnosis (see chapter 7). This should always be couched in phraseology that the individual understands:

"After all the training and skills-learning that you have to do for your sport, I guess you must be wondering why I am asking you to spend another 20 minutes or so each day using these relaxation and hypnotic techniques. Well, it is simply this: relaxing in the way that you have been shown today makes your mind very sensitive to thoughts and suggestions. In fact, any positive thoughts relating to your sport that you instill into your mind when you are in this very relaxed state will have considerable effect on you when you are actually playing. But more than this, you can also imagine yourself doing things in your sport just the way you want them. If you go on practicing these things in your mind each time you use your self-hypnosis, you will find that when you participate in that sporting event, then you will be more likely to play just as you imagined. Some people call this 'mental rehearsal,' and it can be a very powerful means of ensuring that your responses are not only just as you want them to be but they are also, in a sense, involuntary. Practice these each day as I suggest, and you will notice these desired patterns of change happening to you. They may not all happen in the next match in which you play, but you will notice that they develop more and more over successive matches."

Meditation is also of demonstrable value in the mastery of clinical anxiety. What has it to offer the sportsman or contestant? Do the benefits of meditation extend to sports behavior? The answer would appear to be "yes." The basketball great Bill Walton is an enthusiastic supporter of meditation as preparation for top-level performance. In her excellent book on meditation, Dr. Patricia Carrington (1978) reviews the literature showing the performance benefits on a variety of tasks which could be attributed to regular meditation: "It seems worth investigating what elements of meditation make it particularly useful for people engaged in sports" (p. 119). Her conclusion based on this evidence is that it is useful for participants to engage in regular daily meditation, and especially to meditate for at least a few minutes immediately before the start of a contest or a performance attempt. We agree with Carrington and strongly recommend the strategic use of meditation just before getting under way with the task at hand.

Summary

From the issues we have raised in this chapter, it is clear that the behavioral responses of sportsmen are inextricably intertwined with performance efficiency. As obvious as this may appear, the relationship is not always recognized, especially by sports participants themselves. We have utilized research and anecdotal findings to emphasize the influence of anxiety on attentional processes and its behavioral and hypnotic management. The control of attention is of *major* importance.

Appendix A
Techniques of
Progressive
Relaxation

Rationale

In chapter 8 we presented a summary of the debate between those who see no point in relaxation procedures and those, like ourselves, who believe they have a place in clinical practice (for a good recent review of this area, see King, 1980). Our interest at this point is in the patient's attitude toward progressive relaxation. In the main body of the book, we mentioned repeatedly the crucial place of a coherent and persuasive rationale in raising levels of compliance. For the *clinician* to know that technique *x* or *y* has solid support in evidence is only half the story; the other half is transmitting this to the *patient*, clearly and in a nontechnical language. These presentations, if properly done, can have a motivating as well as an educational effect. The rationale plus the diary record of homework exercises can significantly increase compliance rates and, thereby, therapeutic results.

The following is the justification to be given to the patient before embarking on relaxation training. For the most part, patients accept the value of relaxation as a general aim. But if they take this as self-evident, the particulars of the muscle relaxation procedure may, nonetheless, lack face validity if the presumed mechanisms are not outlined. In particular, patients often wonder how their needs will be served by a technique which is said to aim at relaxation but which begins with an *increase* in muscle tension. Second, patients may appreciate the desirability of relaxation but be unaware of the psychological costs of chronic tension. Consequently, the introduction to progressive relaxation should incorporate clarifying remarks on both.

"We all appreciate that relaxation is probably a good thing, but most of us may not realize that what is happening with our muscles can make the difference between being 'up-tight' and being comfortably relaxed. The first thing to remember is that when we contract our muscles [the therapist can demonstrate this by tensing his hands and shoulders], we are doing *work.* This means that energy is being expended, lost. Note that whether or not this work achieves a useful purpose is beside the point. For instance, take the example of two men, Mr. A and Mr. B. Mr. A 'spends' a certain amount of energy painting his house. Mr. B spends exactly the same amount of time and energy, but all he is doing is sitting at work unnecessarily tense all day long. As far as the first person is concerned, the muscle contractions which Mr. A performed in the work of getting his house painted were productive; in the second, Mr. B sitting tense at his desk, the work was wasted. But the decline in energy levels was the same in the two cases. As another example, we have Mr. C and Mr. D, who work side by side at the same job. Mr. C's levels of muscle tension are exactly what he needs to get the job done properly. Mr. D is twice as tense. In one way, it would be correct to say that because of that Mr. D works a 16-hour day, or a 10-day week. But, of course, the company is not going to pay him twice as much or double his vacation period. Actually, in this example, Mr. D would not only be more up-tight than his less tense work-mate but his job efficiency would probably suffer as well. So the first reason to learn to control muscle tension, all over the body, is to get free of *avoidable* fatigue. As you know from your own experience, the more fatigued and worn out you are, the more easily you can become emotionally upset.

"There is a second reason for practicing and learning the skills of muscle relaxation: anxiety 'feeds' on muscle tension. I don't mean to say that being tense is the same thing as being anxious. Look, I can make my right hand and arm *very* tense [demonstrate] but I'm no more anxious now than I was 10 seconds ago. However, had I been anxious before I did that, for whatever reason, then muscle tension could have added to it, especially if I had kept it up for a long time, as anxious individuals often do. One way it can do that is by making worse the physical changes which go along with the feeling of being anxious. To give one example, when we tense our muscles, we can increase the speed and intensity of cardiovascular activity. People often report that when they are anxious they are aware of their heart pounding; muscle tension can play a part in this by increasing the bodily systems that are at work in anxiety. And just as important, using muscle relaxation exercises during such bad times can help to slow down these unpleasant reactions and, through that, help to reduce anxiety. There are other reasons, too, why excessive muscle tension can be a problem: it can interfere with our efforts at meditation and hypnosis (in the clinic here or at home); also muscle tension creates a lot of inner 'noise' which, as I've already said, can make it harder to be efficient at our jobs and happy in our play.

"Well, if all of this makes the case against excess tension and for muscle relaxation, it still doesn't tell us what to do about it. The first thing I must say is that there is no one method alone by which relaxation can be achieved. In fact, there are a number of widely used relaxation methods. These can be divided into two types—those which emphasize techniques of producing 'mental calm,' where it is expected that physical relaxation will automatically follow, and others which begin with physical relaxation training in the hope somehow that mental calm will also happen. Our practice is to teach both, which is why I showed you the meditation technique earlier [see chapter 6]. Each of these can help the other. The one we're going to start with right now is called progressive muscle (or sometimes 'deep muscle') relaxation and it is a widely used method for eliminating physical tension.

"In general terms, the exercises are simple to teach and learn and involve only a sequence of tensing and relaxing movements in various parts of the body. Now it may seem odd that we should begin with tensing the muscles. After all, isn't this all about *relaxation* training? Many people wonder about that. The answer is that when we are under stress, muscle tension can be fairly high and go on and on and on without our being aware of it. By first making the muscles tense, we learn how to develop a kind of automatic 'tension detector.' "

Patient Estimates of Muscle Tension: Quantitative or Qualitative?

All of the relaxation methods with which we are familiar call upon the patient to make distinctions between higher and lower levels of tension, but the requests are communicated and assessed in qualitative terms ("I was fairly tense yesterday when I was called upon to speak in class" or, from the therapist, "make your right hand very tense," etc.). We see this practice as inefficient if the clinician wants to know more about the levels of tension or if he wishes to request the production of tension within a given range (see below). The problem we are addressing here is exactly like the one that led to the use of SUDS (subjective units of discomfort) scales to get more precision into therapist–patient communication about anxiety (Lang, 1969; Wolpe, 1969). Tension levels can and, we feel, should be assessed in exactly the same way. Thus we say to the patient:

> "In our practice I'll be asking you to 'turn on' different amounts of tension in various muscle groups, or I may want to ask you *how* tense you are at a given time—or to rate how much tension you felt at some other time [in the elevator, leaving the house, or whatever the patient's stress situation]. Words like 'a lot' or 'a little' or 'terribly high' may not mean quite the same thing to you as they do to me, and what I mean by them may not be clear to you. To get around that communication problem we can use an imaginary measuring scale to measure tension. The scale has 100 points on it. At the bottom is zero, which means no tension in *that part of the body* [be sure that the patient realizes that here specific and not global ratings are requested] and 100 means as much tension as you could make in that part. I'll show you what I mean. Look at my right hand. See how relaxed it is? I'd give it a number somewhere between 0 and 10 [point out that numbers are to indicate the amount of tension within a 5 to 10 point range]. Now [therapist makes a loose fist] it's not much higher—I'd say about 10 to 15 on the tension scale [by modeling being at ease with an *estimate* of tension levels, the therapist can forestall worries in the patient that he must be *exactly* precise in the numbers he uses]. I'll increase it up to about 30. See the difference? And now up to 50 . . . now its at 90 to 100 [fist and arm shaking with the effort]."

Tension Changes: Gradual or Abrupt?

All of the manuals we have consulted agree on the *timing* of tension release—to be done during exhalation—but not on the amount to be released. There is a slight, unconditioned, reflexive, easing of tension when we exhale and, conversely, a slight tendency to increase muscle tension as we inhale. By pairing relaxation with the outflow of breath, we can capitalize on this natural contingency. But how much tension is to be let out during exhalation? In some systems the patient is asked to release a barely perceptible amount with each breath, while others request the patient to "let it all go at once" (for example, Rimm & Masters, 1979, pp. 36–39). Despite the popularity of the two different methods, there has been little debate over the advisability of one over the other. We find the general indifference to the question puzzling, for patients usually report a strong preference for the "all-at-once" release. Quite apart from the greater satisfaction, there are other reasons for the abrupt-decrease method. Chronically tense individuals typically show a poor awareness of tension levels and a corresponding difficulty in detecting small changes in these. Beginning with the general principle that discrimination learning will always proceed most rapidly when training begins with large differences before the subject is called upon to discriminate more subtle differences (Terrace, 1966), it makes good sense for tension-release instructions to emphasize the quick, abrupt mode of release in the target areas. In discussing the merits of the two, Malmo (1975) referred to a number of EMG reports of muscle tension (EMG stands for electromyograph, a procedure for measuring changes in the activity of specific muscles). He wrote that "the rate of terminal fall also seems of psychological significance. A *prompt, large* EMG drop generally coincides with successful completion of a task, giving the person a 'feeling of closure.' A much slower fall in muscle tension, on the other hand, is usually associated with something not quite complete or not fully satisfying about the performance" (p. 57, emphasis added).

This is not to say that the therapist should always ask the patient to generate and sustain maximal (i.e., "100") levels so as to get the greatest possible drop on the release phase. Indeed, we can see two reasons not to ask for the maximum possible amount of tension at the beginning of each subroutine. First, achieving and holding "100" levels is very fatiguing, and some patients feel the disturbing after-effects of such efforts well after the signal to "return to zero." Second, even chronically tense patients rarely experience maximal tension in their everyday lives. The problem is not that they become *that* tense. It is that they get up to and stay at intermediate levels for long periods of time (Malmo, 1975). Thus, we spend most of our time working in the 40 to 70 range with the aim of maximizing transfer and increasing the "ecological validity" of progressive muscle relaxation therapy.

Duration

There are a number of related questions to consider under this heading. First, there is the duration of a given tension—release cycle. The ideal length is not known, but most manuals that offer a recommendation on this point advise 25 seconds or less. We have found it helpful if the patient can hold the requested level in the nominated muscle group for two breathing cycles (i.e., between 15 and 20 seconds). Much shorter durations than that do not permit the patients to "tune into" and study the tension-related sensations, and ones longer than that can be tiring and unpleasant.

Second, we can ask about the number of repetitions in any given target muscle group. Once again we lack a good data base on which to form a decision. It is probably desirable to have more than one trial with a particular muscle group, but just how many more than that will depend on the patient's ability to get down to and stay within the 0 to 10 range following release. Most important of all, it will depend on the sites where the individual experiences the worst tension in stress situations. Some people may be predominantly "face responders," others back or arm responders, and so on (Lazarus, 1965; Malmo, 1975). The greatest attention and the most practice should be given to these trouble spots. So, if the therapist elects to do all of the major voluntary muscles (a standard sequence is: hands, biceps and triceps, shoulders, neck, forehead, eyes, lips, tongue—pressed into the roof of the mouth, back, midsection, thighs, calves, feet, and toes; see below for detailed instructions to the patient), extra practice should be scheduled for the *individual's* problem areas (which are often to be found in: the hands, face, lips, forehead, eyes, arms, and neck and shoulders). Finally, the duration of training overall is an issue. The range extends from a few minutes to many sessions. Our experience, which is in line with the available research (Borkovec & Sides, 1979) indicates that at least one (40 minute) session will be required. How many more than that will depend on the extent of the problem and the goals in therapy.

Problems

1. Although patients are instructed to isolate the requested tension to the target areas, the "migration" of tension to other muscles is to be expected. Patients will need many reminders, *during training*, to keep the tension localized. One way to inhibit this spread is to give repeated emphasis to the importance of maintaining the integrity of

the breathing rhythm. We have never seen it to fail that anxiously tense patients either stop breathing altogether or breathe too deeply and strenuously during tension induction.

2. Certain muscle groups appear to be more prone to cramping (for example, the shoulder–neck area when hunched, the underside of the thighs, and the arch of the feet when the toes are tensed). Care must be taken in these areas to keep the tension below 70 in individuals who show any tendency to experience muscle spasms and cramps.

3. Most relaxation procedures begin with the tensing of fists, often more than once. If the patient is not told to keep his (and especially her) fingers flat against the palms, the tensing will result in the nails digging painfully into the palms.

Sample Exercise

The one sketched out below is the "hand exercise," but the same delivery is used for all of the other muscle groups. The first set of instructions in any area will always be more lengthy than they will need to be on repetitions of the cycle.

"Now that you have a nice easy breathing rhythm be sure that you don't let the tension which you will be producing interfere with your breathing. I'd like you to continue as though your breathing didn't 'know' anything about the tensing or relaxing. Good. All right, in a minute or so I'm going to ask you to make your right hand into a fist, fingers flat against your palms so your fingernails don't dig into them. I'm going to ask you then to go up to 70 [or whatever level] and hold onto it until I ask you to let it go. One more thing: As I said earlier, make certain that you get up to the 70 level before you finish inhaling the breath on which I ask you to begin. By the time you get to the 'top of the breath,' so to speak, you should be 'at' 70. After two cycles of in and out breathing I'll ask you to let all that tension go *as you are breathing out.* And it should all be gone before you complete the outbreath on which I ask you to release the tension. In other words before you get to the 'bottom' of that breath, and certainly before you begin the next breath in, the tension level in you hand should be as close to zero as you can let it be.

"OK, let's start. The next breath *after* this one, make your right hand into a fist and go up the tension scale until you get to 70 or thereabouts . . . good [if the patient stops breathing or starts breathing too deeply remind him to 'return to the steady breathing'] . . . don't let the tension start anywhere else . . . now study the sensations you feel in your hand and up to your forearm, pay attention to them . . . good . . . next breathe out, let it *all* go . . . that's it . . . notice the difference between the tension you felt a few seconds ago and what you are presently experiencing in your right hand . . . if you notice any residual or 'leftover' tension just let it slip away the next time you exhale." [The therapist can also ask the patient to notice the quiet and the calm he feels, and "how much nicer it is" in the absence of high tension levels.]

Additions and Variations

After going through the complete cycle (hands, arms, etc.), the therapist can have the patient superimpose the word "tense" whenever muscle tension is increased (i.e., as he breathes in) and the word "relax" to accompany tension release (on exhalation). This is known as *cue-controlled relaxation* (Russell & Sipich, 1973). This gives the patient cognitive control over muscle tension and can deepen his awareness of what is going on in his body. (After constant practice with the use of these cues, patients tell us things like: "It was surprising the other day when I was held up in a traffic jam; I started to get pretty wound up and then I 'heard' the word 'tense' in my head and it reminded me to relax.")

When patients are accomplished in the use of progressive relaxation in the clinic and during daily home practice (i.e., in optimal conditions), we ask them to do daily (and short—less than 3 minutes) exercises in the face of self-imposed stressors (for example, making the shower colder; deliberately driving in the slower lane; or turning on the radio so that the station selection device gets two programs at once, or static). This is a kind of "stress inoculation" (Meichenbaum & Tuck, 1976) which can, in addition, promote generalization from the safety and security of the practice situation to the rigors of their real-life encounters with tension and stress.

Finally, a reminder: with progressive relaxation as with all of the other techniques mentioned in this book, daily home practice and the associated record keeping must be built into the program and reviewed at each clinical meeting.

Appendix B
Sample Hierarchy
Scenes

In this appendix we are presenting, in outline form, a number of standard hierarchies. Within each, items are arranged so that the easier scenes are at the top and the more difficult ones at the bottom. The amount of time on each item and the rate at which the therapist and patient progress through the list of scenes will be a function of the severity of the problem and the patient's ability to recover from anxiety. As a rule of thumb, if the patient signals that the anxiety is still at or above 50 (out of 100) on the SUDS scale, it indicates that more time must be spent on that scene (or more coping/counter-anxiety imagery must be added). In compiling this list of hierarchies we have not attempted to draw black-and-white distinctions between scenes of phobic as contrasting with nonphobic anxiety. Most clinical cases will contain elements of both. Where the phobic content predominates (as in claustrophobia), the stress should be on prolonged exposure. The duration of exposure is extremely important, and where little in the way of anxiety-competing images and responses is utilized, the exposure probably should be at least of ten minutes' duration (Levis & Hare, 1977). The best policy, however, is not to adhere rigidly to a preset time but to make offset of the scene contingent upon a reported decrease in anxiety (Marshall et al., 1979). If shorter exposure times are used, then these should probably be accompanied by some sort of training to inhibit excessive (in our view, above 50 SUDS) anxiety (Watt, 1979; Wolpe, 1969).

Where the presenting problem indicates a more cognitive form of anxiety (connected to performance anxiety and maladaptive cognitive reactions, as in worries associated with sexual situations), more attention should be devoted to the detection and modification of negative sets and self-statements.

A distinction that we have chosen to overlook altogether is the one between systematic desensitization and flooding. We see these "brand names" as referring to no more than the anchor or end points on the continuum of exposure. In reality, there exists a family of such techniques which differ in degree with respect to the conditions and rate of exposure (see chapter 8). The place on the continuum at which we begin is a matter of judgment, and it will be determined in large part by the patient's psychological resources and the therapist's estimate of the risk of sensitization or other iatrogenic effects.

The first problem listed is agoraphobia. This is because it is the most prevalent (clinically) and the most difficult of all of the anxiety-related disorders to treat successfully (social phobia—not to be confused with social anxiety—is a close second on the list of "difficult phobias" and it, too, has been outlined in some detail). For this reason, the agoraphobia hierarchies are set down in greater detail than are those connected with the other problems. In fleshing out the other hierarchies (and even the agoraphobia hierarchies are presented only in skeletal form), the therapist must consult the patient for precise details about the visual, auditory, olfactory, *and* internal (cognitive and physiological) stimuli which are relevant in the *in vivo* situation. It is probably a good practice to conclude each scene, or, if that is not feasible or necessary, the last scene of the session, with coping thoughts and imagery. So, for example, in item number 4(b), we ask the agoraphobic patient to engage in the correct (i.e., slower) style of breathing despite the existence of disturbing cognitive, affective, and physiological responses. Through this (vicarious) contact with anxiety and the reestablishment of task-relevant activities, the patient can develop a valid set of expectancies ("I won't find it all that easy and pleasant to do at first but I'll be able to carry on") and a therapeutic set of coping skills ("now, let's see, I must remember to keep muscle tension below 50, breathe slow, and keep my mind on the job at hand"). This is essential whether or not the patient's anxiety is largely phobic in nature.

Last, there is the debate over the number of steps, or scenes, in the hierarchy. Much used to be made of the need for carefully scaling procedures to ensure that the psychological distances between each item are of the same magnitude (the same number of just noticeable differences—j.n.d's). There has yet to appear a study that supports the need for such special care to quantitative detail in the construction of anxiety hierarchies (and the results from the "one-item" flooding studies indicate that all of the time and effort required in this work does not lead to a clinical payoff). The core of the hierarchy can be developed out of 5 to 19 scenes ranging in SUDS levels from the 0 to 10, all the way up to 90 to 100 scenes (we have presented 7 such scenes). At any given level where progress is slow or the jumps appear too large, the therapist can elaborate additional material and, in so doing, generate a hierarchy of 15 or more scenes. The real issue is not the number of items but the patient's reaction to them. The therapist's job is to obtain the most rapid progress possible while at the same time keeping cognizant of the risk of sensitization.

Another question that troubles practitioners is the best way to arrange exposure when the phobia has two or more dimensions. As a case in point, take the hierarchy for social phobias. If the patient is afraid of eating *and* writing in public, should these be taken separately or should complex scenes (containing progressively more exposure to both) be employed? We have always found what the patient finds most believable to be the deciding point. The social phobic who finds it implausible to visualize himself writing and eating in the same (extended) scene will require a unidimensional hierarchy. Some problems, however (for example, public speaking anxiety), must be treated in all dimensions simultaneously.

Agoraphobia

Major Themes and Dimensions

1. Distance from safe areas (for example, home, car).
2. Access to or support from attachment people (for example, spouse, therapist), especially when away from an area that is perceived as safe.
3. Concern over possible extreme reactions (for example, panic, feeling "giddy," or losing consciousness).
4. Being observed by others when extremely anxious.
5. Being held up when wanting to get to safety and/or having to tolerate incompletion in task performance.

HIERARCHY SITUATIONS.   (For a moderate to severe case where panic attacks are a risk and an unaided *walk* of more than 200 feet from home or car is very difficult.)

1. a.   Standing at the door of your home (or next to the car), next to your (husband, wife, the therapist) and ready to leave. There is a slight amount of distress coexisting with feelings of confidence.

   b.   Your (husband, wife) is getting ready to leave on a short errand. You will be alone for that time. You wish she was not going but you do realize the need for this and you can see that, in the long run, it will benefit you in overcoming agoraphobia.

2. a.   You leave the house (or car) with the other person and walk down the street for 20 yards or so. You can feel the anxiety beginning to rise but, by breathing quietly, you regain your composure.

   b.   Your spouse leaves the house and your first reaction is to call her back. You don't do this. Instead you start on your relaxation and meditation exercises, all the time reminding yourself that until recently you could never have done this.

3. a.   You are well down the street, the other person is still at your side, but the house (or car) is 50 to 70 yards away and you wonder whether you should turn and walk back to it. You keep on walking, but more slowly now, filled with conflict. "Do I go forward or back to safety?" It is getting more difficult to keep your breathing in check.

   b.   You walk quickly to the door in the hope of catching sight of your wife only to see the car turn the corner and pass out of sight. You wonder: "How am I going to cope, alone, for the next (hour, or longer as appropriate)? Will the panic come? What will I do if it does? Who can I contact? These are the thoughts that plague you. The anxiety and tension levels are up to 50 to 60 on the scale.

4. a.   You turn to look at the house and to your surprise you discover that you're further from it than you would have guessed—perhaps 300 yards. As you try to continue your walk you feel even more intensely the desire to go back. Your worries are now about evenly divided between the distance back to the house and the fear that you may become panicky.

   b.   The time for the return of your wife is approaching. Will she be on schedule? Is she all right? Suppose something has happened to her? The relaxation exercises are helping but its difficult to concentrate on them. The instant you stop, your thoughts are taken up with how bad you feel. Your breathing is going on a little too quickly and you remember to slow it down.

5. a.   You turn the corner and you can no longer see your house. The anxiety jumps suddenly and your palms start to get wet. "Will I panic?" You tell yourself, "Let's see what'll happen if I carry on. Just get anxious, that's all. I can cope with that." Nevertheless, you have become very aware of your heart thumping in your chest. You are grateful that your companion is with you. But when he talks to you it is difficult to concentrate on what he is saying. So you give your full attention to his words.

   b.   Your wife should have been home 15 minutes ago. You wonder where she is. If only she would return. You start to get angry at her and then quite anxious as you experience the feelings of loss and isolation. Coming in on top of this is the worry that you might be heading for a panic: You sit down and try to calm yourself. "Where *is* she?" you ask yourself. You find it difficult to control your breathing. It is only with effort that you manage to slow it down. The phone rings and startles you. When you answer it you discover that it is an acquaintance who is rather difficult to stop once he begins a phone conversation. In a way you are happy for the distraction, but you are also worried that he'll think your reactions are a little odd. Then you change your mind and decide not to stay on the phone because that is just a way of hiding from your worries by distracting yourself.

6. a.   You and your companion arrive at the store and go in together. Then, by prearranged plan, he walks away and leaves you by yourself. The *instant* he moves off, your anxiety levels jump and your fears of fainting come back. As you stand there, you can imagine what it would be like were you to lose control of yourself in every possible way and fall over screaming for help [we advise the use of "embedding" a potentially very stressful scene with a daydream *within* the scene]. You find yourself getting extremely jumpy and restless, and you commence the abbreviated meditation and relaxation.

   b.   It's more than an hour now and no news from your wife.

You make a few phone calls to places where she might be, but you find that she is not there and your fears threaten to overpower you. You picture yourself running outside, frantic to get help. This stimulates you to the edge of a panic attack, and your breathing accelerates. Dizzy feelings come on. The physical signs of anxiety act as a cue for you to start right in on the relaxation exercises and the self-reminders for "going with" the feelings.

7. a.   The store grows very crowded and you cannot find your companion, so you walk back to the car. You are getting quick surges of anxiety. When you get to your car you are unable to start it, and you are stuck there a long way from home, all alone. Your hands start to tingle and feelings of strangeness come over you [depersonalization]. You are so tense you want to scream out but people would only think you're odd. You take out the card which has written on it the words, "It's only the fear system, and the panic will pass in a short time" and "Don't fight the fear; just go with it and things will get better."

   b.   A long time has gone by and your worry is so great about your wife's absence that you make another phone call. You find out that she has had a short visit there and plans to spend the rest of the day shopping. This means that you'll be all alone for hours. And then the panic begins. The one thing you have to do now is to slow down your movements and especially your breathing. Instead of getting angry or anxious, you know that you have to use responsible self-talk. ("If I didn't have agoraphobia I wouldn't mind if my wife took some time off to go shopping or see friends.") You think to yourself: "Soon I will be more able to be free of these worries, but only if I see these episodes through, so I must slow down, settle myself, and just let it pass."

Social Phobia

Major Themes and Dimensions

1.   Eye contact.
2.   Speaking with strangers, which is exacerbated by any signs of critical reaction in them.

3. Signing one's name or doing any handwriting under the scrutiny of another.
4. Fear of vomiting (self or others).
5. Blushing.

HIERARCHY SITUATIONS. (Note: All of the above situations become more threatening in the presence of strangers. Another point is that not all of these themes will appear in all cases. We have chosen to illustrate hierarchy development in social phobia in a patient whose major fears are of hand shaking and eye contact, which are common manifestations of social phobia.)

1. You are at home and only your spouse (or most trusted friend) is with you and you prepare to sign your name.
2. You are at home with a few friends and you are holding a cup of coffee (or you are writing your signature on a paper) as they talk about a topic of interest to them.
3. You are at a friend's place with one or two others well known to you. One of these people has an interest in handwriting and asks for a sample of yours. As soon as you hear the request, the blood rushes to your face and the direct looks of the others around you are difficult to meet.
4. At a large party, you are sitting down at the end of the table. The people around your place are not well known to you but seem not to be watching as you start to eat your soup. Your hand shakes a little nevertheless, and as soon as it does your distress rises.
5. The people at this large gathering (or at work) look over at you when someone there asks you a question in a loud voice. You are so startled that you cannot think of what to say and you freeze with anxiety. You take a long slow breath and tell yourself to recall the words of the question. You then deliberately pick up the glass in front of you and have a sip. The people don't seem to notice the tremble of your hand.
6. You become the center of attention when one of the (many) people with you asks you to recount a particularly amusing episode. You blush furiously—but no one seems to care. All of the people looking directly at you makes you terribly ill-at-ease, but you manage to handle it by looking at the person furthest from you as you speak.
7. At a very large party you are met, when you arrive, by the

organizers, who ask you to sign a birthday card for the main guest. All eyes are on you. Your hand trembles terribly and you feel like fleeing to some quiet place where you can be alone. It is made even worse when you are asked to say a few words about yourself and before you do, someone comments quietly, but audibly, that "he seems quite nervous."

Claustrophobia

Major Themes and Dimensions

1. Confinement (as assessed in physical parameters: size of the area and the number of doors and windows).
2. Confinement (as assessed in cognitive parameters: its likely duration and the patient's control over the termination of conflict).
3. The patient's difficulties in breathing in the confined situation.
4. The number of people in the confined area with the patient.
5. The claustrophobic patient's reactions to his fears and the others with him observing his distress.

Hierarchy Situations

1. You are at the threshold of a small room (or elevator) with one other person.
2. You are in the small room with only one or two people but you can leave easily and whenever you wish.
3. You are in the center of a relatively small room with five to ten others between you and the exit (but there are windows on the other side of the room).
4. There are many people blocking your way to the door. You begin to experience some difficulty in breathing [an often overlooked dimension in claustrophobic fears—some individuals cannot tolerate any kind of mask or covering over their face or head].
5. You are *locked* in a small room by yourself for a short interval [this can be varied from having the patient know beforehand, and agree to, the exact length of the interval to his having no prior knowledge or control over the duration].

6. You are in the same situation as above, except for the following changes: the atmosphere is extremely close and this makes your breathing very tortured. Others notice your agitation, as you can plainly see.
7. The room is packed, it is very hot (or the elevator stalls between floors) and you get to the point of panic and want to scream for release.

Test (Exam) Anxiety

Major Themes and Dimensions

1. Self-preoccupation with negative evaluation (by self and others).
2. Emotional arousal and its disturbing influences.
3. Behavior of others in the test situation.

HIERARCHY SITUATIONS. (Note: Exposure therapies can eliminate emotional arousal, but it is not clear that they have any positive effect at all on actual performance. This points to a need for "combination techniques" as suggested by Allen, [1980]. These could include attentional training and steps taken to improve study skills. Thus, by itself, exposure can work only to reduce felt anxiety. The scenes below, to be of further benefit, can be used to set the stage for the changes in self-statements which are more closely tied to performance deficits.)

1. You are at home about to leave for the exam. You wonder whether you have done enough work in preparation for today.
2. You are outside of the exam room. The others waiting are nervous too. You begin to get involved in thoughts like, "I wonder if I'll be good enough to cope; the others seem confident, though."
3. You are sitting in the exam room, fearing that you may panic and go blank, unable to do more than write your own name.
4. The examiner tells everyone to open their booklets. You look at the questions and notice that there seem to be so many and you feel that you hardly know where to begin. You feel your hands gripping the pen too tightly, your mouth is too dry, and your anxiety is too high.

5. You notice that all of the others have already started on their exams and are writing diligently. You ask yourself: "Won't I ever do well on an exam? I must be the worst in the room."
6. After beginning on an easier question, you come to one that puzzles you. You start to doubt that you can answer the question or pass the exam. You begin to have trouble concentrating and your awareness is filled with thoughts of failure.
7. You encounter an even more difficult question which, if you miss it, means that you could fail the exam. You get angry at yourself for not studying and at all the others in the room for appearing to be so alert and confident in their performance.

Public Speaking Anxiety

Major Themes and Dimensions

1. The number of people in the audience.
2. Mastery of the material.
3. The length of the talk.
4. Overt expressions of anxiety detected by members of the audience.
5. An audience reaction of criticism, scorn, or pity.
6. Eye contact.

HIERARCHY SITUATIONS.   (Note: Public speaking anxiety shares a number of features with "test anxiety" with the addition of a "phobic" dimension—see chapter 9—being stared at by many.)

1. You are talking for a brief period on a favorite topic in front of a few good friends.
2. You are speaking on a topic unfamiliar to you, causing you to pause from time to time to gather your thoughts. The audience numbers eight to ten people; most of them are friends of yours.
3. You are in class (for example, adult education, or at a social gathering) and you are scheduled to speak next, in a minute or two. You will be expected to talk for about five minutes on a book which you know well, in front of an audience of about ten (and they all have to speak, too).

4. You are speaking to a neutral audience of ten or so, made up of people you do not know well. Having everyone sitting so quietly, staring at you, is a bit unnerving.

5. As you speak, you become more anxious as your hands begin to tremble [the number in the audience can be increased to make this more stressful]. To control this, you grip the lecture stand firmly.

6. You are speaking too quickly and your voice starts to quaver. This worsens when you lose the thread of your talk, forcing you to stop. In the ensuing (brief) silence, people begin to whisper to each other, probably about your difficulties.

7. You are discussing a difficult topic in front of a large audience of strangers, many of whom are experts in the area of your topic. You attempt a little joke to break the tension. Nobody laughs. Then your hands shake visibly and you drop your papers on the floor. Then you forget your speech and feel the sweat on your face and the blushing. Some of the people are impatient with your faltering efforts while others feel sorry for you.

References and Bibliography

Abramson, L.Y., Seligman, M.E.P., & Teasdale, J.D. Learned helplessness in humans: Critique and reformulation. *Journal of Abnormal Psychology*, 1978, *87*, 49–74.

Adler, M.H., & Secunda, L. An indirect technique to induce hypnosis. *Journal of Nervous and Mental Disease*, 1947, *106*, 190–193.

Agras, W.S., Sylvester, D., & Oliveau, D.C. The epidemiology of common fears and phobias. *Comprehensive Psychiatry*, 1969, *10*, 151–156.

Ahsen, A., & Lazarus, A.A. Eidectics: An internal behavior approach. In A.A. Lazarus (Ed.), *Clinical behavior therapy*. New York: Bruner/Mazel, 1972.

Alberti, R.E., & Emmons, M.L. *Your perfect right: A guide to assertive behavior.* San Louis Obispo, Calif.: Impact Press, 1974.

Alden, L., & Cope, R. Nonassertiveness: Skill deficit or selective self-evaluation. *Behavior Therapy*, 1981, *12*, 107–114.

Alden, L., & Safran, J.D. Irrational beliefs and nonassertive behavior. *Cognitive Therapy and Research*, 1978, *4*, 357–364.

Allen, G.J. The behavioral treatment of test anxiety: Therapeutic innovations and emerging conceptual challenges. In M. Hersen, R.M. Eisler, & P.M. Miller (Eds.), *Progress in behavior modification* (Vol. 9). New York: Academic Press, 1980.

Ambrose, G. Hypnosis in the treatment of children. *American Journal of Clinical Hypnosis*, 1968, *11*, 1–5.

Anand, B.K., Chhina, G.S., & Singh, B. Some aspects of electroencephalographic studies of yogis. *Electroencephalography and Clinical Neurophysiology*, 1961, *13*, 452–456. (a)

Anand, B.K., Chhina, G.S., & Singh, B. Studies of Shri Ramanand Yogi during his stay in an air-tight box. *Indian Journal of Medical Research*, 1961, *49*, 82–89. (b)

Anderson, J.R., & Bower, G.H. Recognition and retrieval processes in free recall. *Psychological Review*, 1972, *79*, 97–123.

Andrews, J.W.D. Psychotherapy of phobias. *Psychological Bulletin*, 1966, *66*, 455–480.

Andreychuk, T., & Skriver, C. Hypnosis and biofeedback in the treatment of migraine headaches. *International Journal of Clinical and Experimental Hypnosis*, 1975, *23*, 172–183.

Asher, R. Respectable hypnosis. *British Medical Journal*, 1956, *11*, 309–313.

Ashford, B., & Hammer, A.G. The role of expectancies in the occurrence of posthypnotic amnesia. *International Journal of Clinical and Experimental Hypnosis*, 1978, *26*, 281–291.

Astrand, P.O., & Rodahl, K. Textbook of work physiology (2nd ed.). New York: McGraw-Hill, 1977.

Ayllon, T., & Azrin, N.H. *The token economy: A motivational system for therapy and rehabituation.* New York: Appleton-Century-Crofts, 1968.

Bakan, P., & Svorad, D. Resting EEG alpha and asymmetry of reflective lateral eye movements. *Nature*, 1969, *223*, 975–976.

Bandler, R., & Grinder, J. *Patterns of hypnotic techniques of Milton Erickson.* Cupertino, Calif.: Meta Publications, 1975.

Bandura, A. *Principles of behavior modification.* New York: Holt, Rinehart & Winston, 1969.

Bandura, A. Self-efficacy: Toward a unifying theory of behavioral change. *Psychological Review*, 1977, *84*, 191–215.

Bandura, A., & Menlove, F.L. Factors determining vicarious extinction of avoidance behavior through symbolic modeling. *Journal of Personality and Social Psychology*, 1968, *8*, 98–108.

Bandura, A., Jeffrey, R.W., & Wright, C.L. Efficacy of participant modeling as a function of response induction aids. *Journal of Abnormal Psychology*, 1974, *83*, 56–64.

Barber, T.X. Experiments in hypnosis. *Scientific American*, 1957, *196*, 54–61.

Barber, T.X. The effects of "hypnosis" and motivational suggestions on strength and endurance: A critical review of research studies. *British Journal of Social and Clinical Psychology*, 1966, *5*, 42–50.

Barber, T.X. *LSD, marihuana, yoga, and hypnosis.* Chicago: Aldine-Atherton, 1970.

Barber, T.X. Suggested "hypnotic" behavior: The trance paradigm versus an alternative paradigm. In E. Fromm & R.E. Shor (Eds.), *Hypnosis: Research developments and perspectives.* Chicago: Aldine-Atherton, 1972.

Barber, T.X., & Calverley, D.S. Toward a theory of "hypnotic" behavior: Enhancement of strength and endurance. *Canadian Journal of Psychology*, 1964, *18*(2), 156–157. (a)

Barber T.X., & Calverley, D.S. Comparative effects on "hypnotic-like" suggestibility of recorded and spoken suggestions. *Journal of Consulting Clinical Psychology*, 1964, *28*, 384. (b)

Bärmark, S.M., & Gaunitz, S.C.B. Transcendental Meditation and heterohypnosis as altered states of consciousness. *International Journal of Clinical and Experimental Hypnosis,* 1979, *27,* 219–226.

Bauer, R.M., & Craighead, W.E. Psychophysiological responses to the imagination of fearful and mental situations: The effects of imagery instructions. *Behavior Therapy,* 1979, *10,* 389–403.

Baum, M. Extinction of avoidance responding through response prevention (flooding). *Psychological Bulletin,* 1970, *74,* 276–284.

Beck, A.T. *Depression.* Philadelphia: University of Pennsylvania Press, 1967.

Beck, A.T. Role of fantasies in psychotherapy and psychopathology. *Journal of Nervous and Mental Disease,* 1970, *150,* 3–17.

Beck, A.T., Cognition, affect, and psychopathology. *Archives of General Psychiatry,* 1971, *24,* 495–500.

Beck, A.T., Rush, A.J., Shaw, B.F., & Emery, G. *Cognitive therapy of depression.* New York: Guilford Press, 1979.

Bem, D.J., & Allen, A. On predicting some of the people some of the time: the search for cross-situational consistencies in behavior. *Psychological Review,* 1974, *81,* 506–520.

Benson, H. *The relaxation response.* New York: William Morrow, 1975.

Benson, H., Arns, P.A., & Hoffman, J.W. The relaxation response and hypnosis. *International Journal of Clinical and Experimental Hypnosis,* 1981, *29,* 259–270.

Berecz, J.M. Phobias of childhood: Etiology and treatment. *Psychological Bulletin,* 1968, *70,* 694–720.

Bergin, A.E. The evaluation of therapeutic outcomes. In A.E. Bergin & S.L. Garfield (Eds.), *Handbook of psychotherapy and behavior change: An empirical analysis.* New York: Wiley, 1971.

Berkun, M.M. Performance decrement under psychological stress. *Human Factors,* 1964, *6,* 21–30.

Bernstein, D.A., & Nietzel, M.T. Demand characteristics in behavior modification: The natural history of a "nuisance." In M. Hersen, R.M. Eisler, & P.M. Miller (Eds.), *Progress in behavior modification* (Vol. 4). New York: Academic Press, 1977.

Blanchard, E.B. A note on the clinical utility of the Rathus Assertiveness Scale. *Behavior Therapy,* 1979, *10,* 571–574.

Boring, E.G. *A history of experimental psychology.* New York: Appleton-Century-Crofts, 1950.

Borkovec, T.D., & Sides, J.K. Critical procedural variables related to the physiological effects of progressive relaxation: A review. *Behaviour Research and Therapy,* 1979, *17,* 119–125.

Bower, G.H. Mood and memory. *American Psychologist,* 1981, *36,* 129–148.

Bowers, K.S. *Hypnosis for the seriously curious.* New York: Jason Aronson, 1977.

Bowers, K.S. Has the sun set on the Stanford Scales? *American Journal of Clinical Hypnosis,* 1981, *24,* 79–88.

Bowlby, J. *Attachment and loss* (Vol. 2). Middlesex, England: Penguin Books Ltd., 1975.

Braid, J. *Neurypnology; or the rationale of nervous sleep considered in relation with animal magnetism.* London: Churchill, 1843.

Broadbent, D.E. *Perception and communication.* New York: Pergamon Press, 1958.

Budzynski, T.H. Biofeedback and the twilight states of consciousness. In G. Schwartz & D. Shapiro (Eds.), *Consciousness and self-regulation: Advances in research* (Vol. 1). New York: Wiley, 1976.

Buglass, D., Clarke, J., Henderson, A.S., Kreitman, N., & Presley, A.S. A study of agoraphobic housewives. *Psychological Medicine*, 1977, 7, 73–86.

Callaway, E., & Dembo, E. Narrowed attention: A psychological phenomenon that accompanies a certain physiological change. *Archives of Neurological Psychiatry*, 1958, 79, 74–90.

Campbell, D., Sanderson, R.E., & Laverty, S.G. Characteristics of a conditioned response in human subjects during extinction trials following a single traumatic conditioning trial. *Journal of Abnormal and Social Psychology*, 1964, 68, 627–639.

Carrington, P. *Freedom in meditation.* Garden City, N. Y.: Anchor Press, 1978.

Cattell, R.B. The IPAT anxiety scale. Champaign, Ill.: Institute for Personality Ability Testing, 1957.

Collins, J.K. Muscular endurance in normal and hypnotic states: A study of suggested catalepsy. Unpublished honours thesis, University of Sydney, 1961.

Collison, D.R. Hypnotherapy in asthmatic patients and the importance of trance depth. In F.H. Frankel & H.S. Zamansky (Eds.), *Hypnosis at its bicentennial: Selected papers.* New York: Plenum Press, 1978.

Collison, D.R. Hypnosis and respiratory disease. In G.D. Burrows & L. Dennerstein (Eds.), *Handbook of hypnosis and psychosomatic medicine.* Amsterdam: Elsevier/North-Holland Biomedical Press, 1980.

Committee on the Review of Medicine. *British Medical Journal*, 1980, 910–912.

Conn, J.H. Is hypnosis really dangerous? *International Journal of Clinical and Experimental Hypnosis*, 1972, 20, 61–79.

Cooper, L.M., & London, P. Children's hypnotic susceptibility, personality, and EEG patterns. *International Journal of Clinical and Experimental Hypnosis*, 1976, 24, 140–148.

Cooper, L.M., & London, P. The Children's Hypnotic Susceptibility Scale. *American Journal of Clinical Hypnosis*, 1979, 21, 170–185.

Coué, E. *The practice of autosuggestion.* New York: Doubleday, 1922.

Council on Mental Health: American Medical Association. Medical use of hypnosis. *Journal of the American Medical Association*, 1958, 165, 186–189.

Crowe, M.M., Marks, I.M., Agras, S.W., & Leitenberg, H. Time-limited desensitization implosion and shaping for phobic patients: A crossover. *Behaviour Research and Therapy*, 1972, 10, 319–328.

Davidson, R.J., & Goleman, D.J. The role of attention in meditation and hypnosis: A psychobiological perspective on transformations of consciousness. *International Journal of Clinical and Experimental Hypnosis,* 1977, *25,* 291–308.

Davidson, S. School phobia as a manifestation of family disturbance: Its structure and treatment. *Journal of Child Psychology and Psychiatry,* 1960, *1,* 270–287.

Deikman, A.J. Bimodal consciousness. *Archives of General Psychiatry,* 1971, *25,* 481–489.

Dember, W.N. *The psychology of perception.* New York: Holt, Rinehart & Winston, 1965.

Deutsch, J., & Deutsch, D. Attention: Some theoretical considerations. *Psychological Review,* 1963, *70,* 80–90.

DeVoge, J.T., & Beck, S.J. The therapist–client relationship in behavior therapy. In M. Hersen, R.M. Eisler, & P.M. Miller (Eds.), *Progress in behavior modification* (Vol. 6). New York: Academic Press, 1976.

Diamond, M.J. Hypnotizability is modifiable: An alternative approach. *International Journal of Clinical and Experimental Hypnosis,* 1977, *25,* 147–166.

Dixon, F. *Subliminal perception: The nature of a controversy.* London: McGraw-Hill, 1971.

Duffy, E. *Activation and behavior.* New York: Wiley, 1962.

Easterbrook, J.A. The effect of emotion on cue utilization and the organization of behavior. *Psychological Review,* 1959, *66,* 183–201.

Ellis, A. *Reason and emotion in psychotherapy.* New York: Lyle Stuart, 1962.

Ellis, A. *Humanistic psychotherapy.* New York: McGraw-Hill, 1973.

Ellis, A. Rational-emotive therapy: research data that supports the clinical and personality hypothesis of RET and other modes of cognitive-behavior therapy. *Counselling Psychologist,* 1977, *7,* 2–42.

Ellis, A. A note on the treatment of agoraphobics with cognitive modification versus prolonged exposure *in vivo. Behaviour Research and Therapy,* 1979, *17,* 162–164.

Ellis, A., & Harper, R.A. *A new guide to rational living.* Englewood Cliffs, N.J.: Prentice-Hall, 1975.

Emmelkamp, P.M.G. Clinical phobias. In M. Hersen, R.M. Eisler, & P.M. Miller (Eds.), *Progress in behavior modification* (Vol 8). New York: Academic Press, 1979.

Emmelkamp, P.M.G., & Kuipers, A.C.M. Agoraphobia: A follow-up study four years after treatment. *British Journal of Psychiatry,* 1979, *134,* 352–355.

Emmelkamp, P.M.G., & Wessels, H. Flooding in imagination *vs* flooding *in vivo:* A comparison with agoraphobics. *Behaviour Research and Therapy,* 1975, *13,* 7–16.

English, H.B. Three cases of the conditioned fear response. *Journal of Abnormal and Social Psychology,* 1929, *24,* 221–225.

Erwin, E. *Behavior therapy: Scientific, philosophical, and moral foundations.* Cambridge: Cambridge University Press, 1978.

Esdaile, J. (1846) *Hypnosis in medicine and surgery.* New York: Julian Press, reprinted in 1957.

Estabrooks, G. *Hypnotism.* New York: E.P. Dutton, 1957.

Evans, F.J. Hypnosis and sleep: Techniques for exploring cognitive activity during sleep. In E. Fromm & R.E. Shor (Eds.), *Hypnosis: Research developments and perspectives.* Chicago: Aldine-Atherton, 1972.

Evans, F.J. Phenomena of hypnosis: 2. Post-hypnotic amnesia. In G. D. Burrows and L. Dennerstein (Eds.), *Handbook of Hypnosis and Psychosomatic Medicine.* Amsterdam: Elsevier/North-Holland, Biomedical Press, 1980.

Eysenck, H.J. The effects of psychotherapy: An evaluation. *Journal of Consulting Psychology,* 1952, *16,* 319–325.

Eysenck, H.J. *Handbook of abnormal psychology* (Chapter 1). London: Pitman, 1960.

Eysenck, H.J., Arnold, W., & Meili, R. *Encyclopedia of Psychology.* London: Fontana, 1975.

Eysenck, H.J., & Rachman, S. *The causes and cures of neurosis.* London: Routledge and Kegan Paul, 1965.

Falck, F.J. Stuttering and hypnosis. *International Journal of Clinical and Experimental Hypnosis,* 1964, *12,* 67–74.

Faria, J.C. di, Abbé. *De la cause du sommeil lucide; ou étude sur la nature de l'homme,* 1819, (2nd ed.), D.G. Dalgade (Ed.). Paris: Henri Jouve, 1906.

Farmer, R.G., & Blows, M. Overcoming the effects of early sexual trauma: systematic desensitization using "guessing." Paper presented at the Annual Conference of the Australian Psychological Society, Sydney, August, 1973.

Fazio, A.F. Implosive therapy with semiclinical phobias. *Journal of Abnormal Psychology,* 1972, *80,* 183–188.

Felipe, A. Attitude change during interrupted sleep. Unpublished doctoral dissertation. Yale University, 1965.

Fenichel, O. *Psychoanalytic theory of neurosis.* New York: Norton, 1945.

Fenz, W.D., & Epstein, S. Stress in the air. *Psychology Today,* 1969, *3,* 27–28, 58–59.

Fish, J.M. *Placebo therapy.* San Francisco: Jossey-Bass, 1973.

Foenander, G., Burrows, G.D., Gerschmann, J., & Horne, D.J. Phobic behaviour and hypnotic susceptibility. *Australian Journal of Clinical and Experimental Hypnosis,* 1980, *8,* 41–46.

Frank, J.D. Restoration of morale and behavior change. In A. Burton (Ed.), *What makes behavior change possible?* New York: Bruner/Mazel, 1976.

Frankel, F.H. Trance capacity and the genesis of phobic behavior. *Archives of General Psychiatry,* 1974, *31,* 261–263.

Frankel, F.H. *Hypnosis: Trance as a coping mechanism.* New York: Plenum Medical Book Company, 1976.

Frankel, F.H., & Orne, M.T. Hypnotizability and phobic behavior. *Archives of General Psychiatry,* 1976, *31,* 261–263.

Frankl, V.E. (Ed.) *Psychotherapy and existentialism: Selected papers on logo therapy.* New York: Souvenir Press, 1970.

Freeman, B.J., Roy, R.R., & Hemmick, S. Extinction of a phobia of physical examination in a seven-year-old mentally retarded boy—A case study. *Behavior Research and Therapy,* 1976, *14,* 63–64.

Freud, S. Analysis of a phobia in a five-year-old boy. In S. Freud, *Collected Papers* (Vol. 1). New York: Basic Books, 1959.

Friedman, J.H. Short-term psychotherapy for "phobia of travel." *American Journal of Psychotherapy,* 1950, 4, 259–278.

Frischholz, E.J., Spiegel, H., Tryon, W.W., & Fisher, S. The relationship between the Hypnotic Induction Profile and the Stanford Hypnotic Susceptibility Scale, Form C: Revisited. *American Journal of Clinical Hypnosis,* 1981, *24,* 98–105.

Fromm, E., Brown, D.P., Hurt, S.W., Oberlander, J.Z., Boxer, A.M., & Pfeifer, G. The phenomena and characteristics of self-hypnosis. *International Journal of Clinical and Experimental Hypnosis,* 1981, *29,* 189–246.

Fromm, E., Lichtman, J., & Brown, D. Similarities and differences between heterohypnosis and self hypnosis: A phenomenological study. Paper presented at the 25th annual meeting of the Society for Clinical and Experimental Hypnosis, 1973.

Gambrill, E.D., & Richey, L.A. An assertion inventory for use in assessment and research. *Behavior Therapy,* 1975, *6,* 550–561.

Garcia, J., Clarke, J.C., & Hankins, W. Natural responses to scheduled rewards. In P. Bateson & P. Klopfer (Eds.), *Perspectives in ethology.* New York: Plenum Press, 1974.

Gardner, G.G. Hypnosis with children. *International Journal of Clinical and Experimental Hypnosis,* 1974, *22,* 20–38.

Gardner, G.G. Teaching self-hypnosis to children. *International Journal of Clinical and Experimental Hypnosis,* 1981, *29,* 300–312.

Gelfand, D.M. Social withdrawal and negative emotional states: Behavior Therapy. In B.B. Wolman, J. Egan, & A.O. Ross (Eds.), *Handbook of treatment of mental disorders in childhood and adolescence.* Englewood Cliffs, N.J.: Prentice-Hall, 1978.

Gibson, E.J., & Walk, R.D. The "visual cliff" (1960). In W.T. Greenough (Ed.), *Readings from Scientific American: The nature and nurture of behavior.* San Francisco: W.H. Freeman, 1972.

Glick, B.S. Conditioning therapy by an analytic therapist. *Archives of General Psychiatry,* 1967, *17,* 577–583.

Glogower, F.D., Fremouw, W.J., & McCroskey, J.C. A component analysis of cognitive restructuring. *Cognitive Therapy and Research,* 1978, *2,* 209–224.

Glueck, B.C., & Stroebel, C.F. Biofeedback and meditation in the treatment of psychiatric illness. *Comprehensive Psychiatry,* 1975, *16,* 303–321.

Goldfried, M. Anxiety-reduction through cognitive-behavioral intervention. In P.C. Kendall & S.D. Hollon (Eds.), *Cognitive-behavioral interventions.* New York: Academic Press, 1979.

Goldfried, M.R., & Davison, G.C. *Clinical behavior therapy.* New York: Holt, Rinehart & Winston, 1976.

Goldfried, M.R., & Sobocinski, D. The effect of irrational beliefs on emotional arousal. *Journal of Consulting and Clinical Psychology,* 1975, *43,* 504–510.

Goldstein, A.J., & Chambless, D.L. A reanalysis of agoraphobia. *Behavior Therapy,* 1978, *9,* 45–59.

Goorney, A.B., & O'Connor, P.J. Anxiety associated with flying: A retrospective survey of military aircrew psychiatric casualties. *British Journal of Psychiatry,* 1971, *119,* 159–166.

Gottfredson, D.K. Hypnosis as an anesthetic in dentistry. Unpublished doctoral dissertation, Brigham Young University, 1973.

Gray, J. *The psychology of fear and stress.* New York: McGraw-Hill, 1971.

Graziano, A.M. Reduction of children's fears. In A.M. Graziano (Ed.), *Behavior therapy with children* (Vol. 2). Chicago: Aldine, 1975.

Grey, S., Sartory, G., & Rachman, S. Synchronous and desynchronous changes during fear reduction. *Behaviour Research and Therapy,* 1979, *17,* 137–147.

Grossman, S.P. *A textbook of physiological psychology.* New York: Wiley, 1967.

Hafner, J., & Marks, I.M. Exposure *in vivo* of agoraphobics: Contributions of diazepam, group exposure, and anxiety evocation. *Psychological Medicine,* 1976, *6,* 71–88.

Hagman, E. A study of fears of children of preschool age. *Journal of Experimental Education,* 1932, *1,* 110–130.

Haley, J. *Strategies of psychotherapy.* New York: Grune & Stratton, 1963.

Hallam, R.S., & Hafner, R.J. Fears of phobic patients: Factor analyses of self-report data. *Behavior Research and Therapy,* 1978, *16,* 1–6.

Hallam, R.S., & Rachman, S. Current status of aversion therapy. In M. Hersen, R.M. Eisler, & P.M. Miller (Eds.), *Progress in behavior modification* (Vol. 2). New York: Academic Press, 1976.

Hamel, P.M. *Through music to the self.* Tisbury, Wiltshire: The Compton Press Ltd., 1978.

Hand, I., & Lamontagne, Y. The exacerbation of interpersonal problems after rapid phobia removal. *Psychotherapy: Theory, Research and Practice,* 1976, *13,* 405–411.

Harlow, H.F., & Zimmerman, R.R. Affectional responses in the infant monkey. *Science,* 1959, *130,* 421.

Harter, M., Seiple, W., & Musso, M. Binocular summation and suppression: Visually evoked cortical responses to dichoptically presented patterns of different spatial frequencies. *Vision Research,* 1974, *14,* 1169–1180.

Hartland, J. *Medical and dental hypnosis and its clinical applications.* London: Baillière Tindall, 1971.

Hatzenbuehler, L.C., & Schroeder, H.E. Desensitization procedures in the treatment of childhood disorders. *Psychological Bulletin,* 1978, *85,* 831–844.

Hebb, D.O. On the nature of fear. *Psychological Review,* 1946, *53,* 259–276.

Hebb, D.O. *The organization of behavior.* New York: Wiley, 1949.

Herrigel, E. *Zen in the art of archery.* New York: Pantheon Books, 1953.

Hersen, M. Complex problems require complex solutions. *Behavior Therapy,* 1981, *12,* 15–29.

Hess, W.R. *Diencephalon: Autonomic and extrapyramidal functions.* New York: Grune & Stratton, 1954.

Hilgard, E.R. *Hypnotic susceptibility.* New York: Harcourt Brace & World, 1965.

Hilgard, E.R. *Divided consciousness: Multiple control in human thought and action.* New York: Wiley, 1977.

Hilgard, E.R. The Stanford Hypnotic Susceptibility Scales as related to other measures of hypnotic responsiveness. *American Journal of Clinical Hypnosis,* 1978/79, *21,* 68–82.

Hilgard, E.R. The eye roll sign and other scores of the Hypnotic Induction Profile (HIP) as related to the Stanford Hypnotic Susceptibility Scale, Form C (SHSS:C): A critical discussion of a study by Frischholz and others. *American Journal of Clinical Hypnosis,* 1981, *24,* 89–97. (a)

Hilgard, E.R. Further discussion of the HIP and the Stanford Form C: A reply to a reply by Frischholz, Spiegel, Tryon and Fisher. *American Journal of Clinical Hypnosis,* 1981, *24,* 106–108. (b)

Hilgard, E.R., & Morgan, A.H. Heart rate and blood pressure in the study of laboratory pain in man under normal conditions and as influenced by hypnosis. *Acta Neurobiological Experimentatis,* 1975, *35,* 741–759.

Hilgard, E.R., Weitzenhoffer, A.M., Landes, J., & Moore, R.K. The distribution of susceptibility to hypnosis in a student population: A study using the Stanford Hypnotic Susceptibility Scale. *Psychological Monographs,* 1961, *75,* (8, Whole No. 512).

Hilgard, J.R. *Personality and hypnosis: A study of imaginative involvement.* Chicago: University of Chicago Press, 1970.

Hilgard, J.R. Imaginative involvement: Some characteristics of the highly hypnotizable and the non-hypnotizable. *International Journal of Clinical and Experimental Hypnosis,* 1974, *22,* 138–156.

Hill, R., & Hansen, D.A. Families in disaster. In G.W. Baker & D.W. Chapman (Eds.), *Man and society in disaster.* New York: Basic Books, 1962.

Hirai, T. *Zen meditation therapy.* Tokyo: Japan Publication, 1975.

Hodgson, R.J., & Rachman, S. An experimental investigation of the implosion technique. *Behaviour Research and Therapy,* 1970, *8,* 21–27.

Hodgson, R., & Rachman, S. Desynchrony in measures of fear. *Behaviour Research and Therapy,* 1974, *12,* 319–326.

Hoenig, J. Medical research on yoga. *Confina Psychiatrica,* 1968, *11,* 69–89.

Hollon, S.D., & Beck, A.T. The cognitive therapy of depression. In P.C. Kendall & S.D. Hollon (Eds.), *Cognitive-behavioral interventions: Theory, research and procedures.* New York: Academic Press, 1979.

Holmes, F.B. An experimental investigation of a method of overcoming children's fears. *Child Development,* 1936, *7,* 6–30.

Horne, A.M., & Matson, J.L. A comparison of modeling, desensitization, flooding, study skills, and control groups for reducing test anxiety. *Behavior Therapy*, 1977, *8*, 1–8.

Horowitz, S.L. Strategies within hypnosis for reducing phobic behavior. *Journal of Abnormal Psychology*, 1970, *75*, 104–112.

Humphreys, C. *Concentration and meditation*. Baltimore: Penguin, 1935.

Hussain, M.Z. Desensitization and flooding (implosion) in the treatment of phobias. *American Journal of Psychiatry*, 1971, *127*, 1509–1514.

Hutson, M.F. The relationship of anxiety level to learning skills in beginning horseback riding. Unpublished master's thesis, University of North Carolina, Greensboro, 1965.

Illovsky, J., & Fredman, N. Group suggestion in learning disabilities of primary grade children: A feasibility study. *International Journal of Clinical and Experimental Hypnosis*, 1976, *24*, 87–97.

Isen, A.M., Shalker, T.E., Clark, M., & Karp, L. Affect, accessability of material in memory, and behavior: A cognitive loop? *Journal of Personality and Social Psychology*, 1978, *36*, 1–12.

Jackson, J.A., Gass, G.C., & Camp, E.M. The relationship between posthypnotic suggestion and endurance in physically trained subjects. *International Journal of Clinical and Experimental Hypnosis*, 1979, *27*, 278–293.

Jacobson, E. *Progressive relaxation*. Chicago: University of Chicago Press, 1929.

Jakibchuk, Z., & Smeriglio, V.L. The influence of symbolic modeling on the social behavior of pre-school children with low levels of social responsiveness. *Child Development*, 1976, *47*, 838–841.

James, W. *The principles of psychology* (Vol. 1). New York: Holt, 1890.

Jaynes, J. *The origin of consciousness in the breakdown of the bicameral mind*. Boston: Houghton, Mifflin, 1976.

Jencks, B. Utilizing the phases of the breathing rhythm. In F.H. Frankel & H.S. Zamansky (Eds.), *Hypnosis at its bicentennial*. New York: Plenum Press, 1978.

Jersild, A.T., & Holmes, F.B. Methods of overcoming children's fears. *Journal of Psychology*, 1935, *1*, 75–104.

Johnson, A. School phobia: Discussion. *American Journal of Orthopsychiatry*, 1957, *27*, 307–309.

Johnson, A.M., Falstein, E.I., Szurek, S.A., & Svendson, M. School phobia. *American Journal of Orthopsychiatry*, 1941, *11*, 702–707.

Johnson, L.S. Self-hypnosis: Behavioral and phenomenological comparisons with heterohypnosis. *International Journal of Clinical and Experimental Hypnosis*, 1979, *27*, 240–264.

Johnson, L.S. Current research in self-hypnotic phenomenology: The Chicago paradigm. *International Journal of Clinical and Experimental Hypnosis*, 1981, *29*, 247–258.

Johnson, L.S., & Weight, D.G. Self hypnosis versus heterohypnosis: Experimental and behavioral comparisons. *Journal of Abnormal Psychology,* 1976, *85,* 523–526.

Jones, M.C. The elimination of children's fears. *Journal of Experimental Psychology,* 1924, *7,* 382–390. (a)

Jones, M.C. A laboratory study of fear: The case of Peter. *Journal of Genetic Psychology,* 1924, *31,* 308–315. (b)

Kahn, J.H., & Nursten, J.P. School refusal: A comprehensive review of school phobia and other failures of school attendance. *American Journal of Orthopsychiatry,* 1962, *32,* 707–718.

Kallman, W.M., & Feuerstein, M. Psychophysiological procedures. In A. Ciminero, K.S. Calhoun, & H.E. Adams (Eds.), *Handbook of behavioral assessment.* New York: Wiley, 1977.

Kamin, L.J. Predictability, surprise, attention, and conditioning. In B.A. Campbell and R.M. Church (Eds.), *Punishment and Aversive Behavior.* New York: Appleton-Century-Crofts, 1969.

Kanfer, F.H., Karoly, P., & Newman, A. Reduction of children's fear of the dark by competence-related and situational threat-related verbal cues. *Journal of Consulting and Clinical Psychology,* 1975, *43,* 251–258.

Kanfer, F.H., & Phillips, J.S. *Learning foundations of behavior therapy.* New York: Wiley, 1970.

Kazdin, A.E., & Wilcoxin, L.A. Systematic desensitization and non specific treatment effects: A methodological evaluation. *Psychological Bulletin,* 1976, *83,* 729–758.

Kelley, G.A., Kern, G.M., Kirkley, B.G., Patterson, J.M., & Keane, T.M. Reactions to assertive versus unassertive behavior: Differential effects for males and females and implications for assertiveness training. *Behavior Therapy,* 1980, *11,* 670–682.

Kendall, P.C., & Hollon, S.D. Cognitive-behavioral interventions: Overview and current status. In P.C. Kendall & S.D. Hollon (Eds.), *Cognitive-behavioral interventions.* New York: Academic Press, 1979.

Kennedy, W.A. School phobia: Rapid treatment of 50 cases. *Journal of Abnormal Psychology,* 1965, *70,* 285–289.

Kiesler, D.J. Some myths of psychotherapy and the search for a paradigm. *Psychological Bulletin,* 1966, *65,* 110–136.

Kihlstrom, J.F. Context and cognition in posthypnotic amnesia. *International Journal of Clinical and Experimental Hypnosis,* 1978, *26,* 246–267.

King, N.J. The therapeutic utility of abbreviated progressive relaxation: A critical review with implications for clinical practice. In M. Hersen, R.M. Eisler, and P.M. Miller (Eds.), *Progress in Behavior Modification* (Vol. 10). New York: Academic Press, 1980.

Kintsch, W. *Learning, memory, and conceptual processes.* New York: Wiley, 1970.

Klein, D.F. Delineation of two drug responsive anxiety syndromes. *Psychopharmacology* (Berlin), 1964, *5,* 397–408.

Klein, D.F. Importance of psychiatric diagnosis in prediction of clinical drug effects. *Archives of General Psychiatry,* 1967, *16,* 118–126.

Klein, D.F., & Fink, M. Psychiatric reaction patterns to imipramine. *American Journal of Psychiatry,* 1962, *119,* 432–488.

Kondas, O. Reduction of examination anxiety and stage fright by group desensitization and relaxation. *Behavior Research and Therapy,* 1967, *5,* 275–281.

Kornhaber, R.C., & Schroeder, H.E. Importance of model similarity on extinction of avoidance behavior in children. *Journal of Consulting and Clinical Psychology,* 1975, *43,* 601–607.

Kosslyn, S. Information representation in visual images. *Cognitive Psychology,* 1975, *7,* 341–370.

Kramer, E. Hypnotic susceptibility and previous relationship with the hypnotist. *American Journal of Clinical Hypnosis,* 1969, *11,* 175–177.

Kroger, W.S., & Fezler, W.D. *Hypnosis and behavior modification: Imagery conditioning.* Philadelphia: J.B. Lippincott Company, 1976.

Lader, M.H., & Mathews, A.M. A physiological model of phobic anxiety and desensitization. *Behaviour Research and Therapy,* 1968, *6,* 411–421.

Landers, D.M. Motivation and performance: The role of arousal and attentional factors. In W.F. Straub (Ed.), *Sport psychology: An analysis of athlete behavior.* New York: Mouvement Publications, 1978.

Lang, P.J. The mechanics of desensitization and the laboratory study of human fear. In C.M. Franks (Ed.), *Behavior therapy: Appraisal and status.* New York: McGraw-Hill, 1969.

Lang, P.J. Imagery in therapy: An information-processing analysis of fear. *Behavior Therapy,* 1977, *8,* 862–886.

Lang, P.J., Lazovik, A.D., & Reynolds, D.J. Desensitization, suggestibility, and pscudotherapy. *Journal of Abnormal Psychology,* 1965, *70,* 395–402.

Lange, A.J., & Jakubowski, P. *Responsible assertive behavior.* Champaign, Illinois: Research Press, 1976.

LaPouse, R., & Monk, N. Fears and worries in a representative sample of children. *American Journal of Orthopsychiatry,* 1959, *29,* 803–818.

Lavoie, G., & Sabourin, M. Hypnosis and schizophrenia: A review of experimental and clinical studies. In G.D. Burrows & L. Dennerstein (Eds.), *Handbook of hypnosis and psychosomatic medicine.* Amsterdam, Elsevier/North-Holland Biomedical Press, 1980.

Lazarus, A. *Psychological stress and the coping process.* New York: McGraw-Hill, 1965.

Lazarus, A.A. *Behavior therapy and beyond.* New York: McGraw-Hill, 1971.

Lazarus, A.A. "Hypnosis" as a facilitator in behavior therapy. *International Journal of Clinical and Experimental Hypnosis,* 1973, *21,* 25–31.

Lazarus, A.A. *Multimodal behavior therapy.* New York: Springer, 1976.

Lazarus, A. Has behavior therapy out lived its usefulness? *American Psychologist,* 1977, *32,* 550–554.

Lazarus, A.A., & Abromovitz, A. The use of "emotive imagery" in the treatment of children's phobias. *Journal of Mental Science,* 1962, *108,* 191–195.

Ledwidge, B. Cognitive behavior modification: A step in the wrong direction? *Psychological Bulletin,* 1978, *85,* 353–375.

Lefcourt, H.M. The function of the illusions of control and freedom. *American Psychologists,* 1973, *28,* 417–425.

LeShan, L. *How to meditate.* New York: Bantam Books, 1975.

Levis, D.J., & Hare, D.J. A review of the theoretical rationale and empirical support for the extinction approach of implosive (flooding) therapy. In M. Hersen, R.M. Eisler, & P.M. Miller, *Progress in behavior modification* (Vol. 4). New York; Academic Press, 1977.

Liberman, R.P., & Davis, J. Drugs and behavior analysis. In M. Hersen, R.M. Eisler, & P.M. Miller, *Progress in behavior modification* (Vol. 1). New York: Academic Press, 1975.

Libet, B., Alberto, W.W. Wright, E.W., & Feinstein, B. Responses of human somato-sensory cortex to stimuli below threshold for conscious sensation. *Science,* 1967, *158,* 1597–1600.

Liébault, A.A. *Du sommeil et des états analogues considérés surtout au point de rue de l'action moral sur le physique.* Paris: V. Massow, 1866.

Linehan, M.M. Structured cognitive-behavioral treatment of assertion problems. In P.C. Kendall & S.D. Hollon (Eds.), *Cognitive-behavioral interventions.* New York: Academic Press, 1979.

London, P. Subject characteristics in hypnosis research: Part 1. Survey of experience, interest, and opinion. *International Journal of Clinical & Experimental Hypnosis,* 1961, *9,* 151–161.

London, P. *The Children's Hypnotic Susceptibility Scale.* Palo Alto, Calif.: Consulting Psychologists Press, 1963.

London, P. The induction of hypnosis. In J.E. Gordon (Ed.), *Handbook of clinical and experimental hypnosis.* New York: Macmillan, 1967.

London, P., & Fuhrer, M. Hypnosis, motivation, and performance. *Journal of Personality,* 1961, *29,* 321–333.

London, P., Hart, J.T., & Leibovitz, M.P. EEG alpha rhythms and susceptibility to hypnosis. *Nature,* 1968, *219,* 71–72.

London, P., & Madsen, C.H. Effect of role playing on hypnotic susceptibility in children. *Journal of Personality and Social Psychology,* 1968, *10,* 66–68.

Lorenz, K. Innate bases of learning. In K. Pribram (Ed.), *On the biology of learning.* New York: Harcourt Brace Jovanovich, 1969.

Lovibond, S.H.L. Current status of behavior therapy. *Canadian Psychologist,* 1966, *7,* 93–101.

MacFarlane, J.W., Allen, L., & Honzik, M.P. *A Developmental Study of the Behavior Problems of Normal Children Between 21 Months and 14 Years.* Berkeley: University of California Press, 1954.

Malmo, R.B. *On emotions, needs, and our archaic brain.* New York: Holt, Rinehart & Winston, 1975.

Mandler, G. *Mind and emotion.* New York: Wiley, 1975.

Marks, I. *Fears and phobias.* London: Academic Press, 1969.

Marks, I.M. Flooding (implosion) and allied treatments. In W.S. Agras (Ed.), *Behavior modification: Principles and clinical applications.* Boston: Little, Brown, 1972.

Marks, I. Behavioral treatments of phobic and obsessive-compulsive disorders: A critical appraisal. In M. Hersen, R.M. Eisler, & P.M. Miller (Eds.), *Progress in behavior modification* (Vol. 1). New York: Academic Press, 1975.

Marks, I.M., Gelder, M.G., & Edwards, G. Hypnosis and desensitization for phobias: A controlled prospective trial. *British Journal of Psychiatry,* 1968, *114,* 1263–1274.

Marshall, W.L., Gauthier, J., & Gordon, A. The current status of flooding therapy. In M. Hersen, R.M. Eisler, & P.M. Miller (Eds.), *Progress in behavior modification* (Vol. 7). New York: Academic Press, 1979.

Marshall, W.L., Stoian, M., & Andrews, W.R. Skills training and self-administered desensitization in the reduction of public speaking anxiety. *Behaviour Research and Therapy,* 1977, *15,* 115–117.

Martens, R. Anxiety and motor behavior: A review. *Journal of Motor Behavior,* 1971, *3,* 151–179.

Martens, R., & Landers, D.M. Motor performance under stress: A test of the inverted-u hypothesis. *Journal of Personality and Social Psychology,* 1970, *16,* 29–37.

Mathews, A.M., Gelder, M.G., & Johnston, D.W. *Agoraphobia: Nature and treatment.* London: The Guilford Press, 1981.

May, J.R. Psychophysiology of self-regulated phobic thoughts. *Behavior Therapy,* 1977, *8,* 150–159.

May, J.R., & Johnson, H.J. Psychological activity to internally elicited arousal and inhibitory thoughts. *Journal of Abnormal Psychology,* 1973, *82,* 239–245.

McCutcheon, B.A., & Adams, H.E. The physiological basis of implosive therapy. *Behavior Research and Therapy,* 1975, *74,* 587–592.

Meares, A. *A system of medical hypnosis.* Philadelphia: W.B. Saunders, 1960.

Meichenbaum, D. Toward a cognitive theory of self-control. In G. Schwartz & D. Shapiro (Eds.), *Consciousness and self-regulation: Advances in research* (Vol. 1). New York: Wiley, 1976.

Meichenbaum, D., & Cameron, R. Stress inoculation: A skills training approach to anxiety management. Unpublished manuscript. University of Waterloo, 1973.

Meichenbaum, D.H., & Tuck, D. The cognitive behavioral management of anxiety, anger, and pain. In P. Davidson (Ed.), *The behavioral management of anxiety, depression, and pain.* New York: Bruner/Mazel, 1976.

Melamed, B.G., & Siegel, L.J. Reduction of anxiety in children facing hospitalization and surgery by use of filmed modeling. *Journal of Consulting and Clinical Pscyhology,* 1975, *43,* 511–521.

Miller, B.V., & Levis, D.J. The effects of varying short visual exposure times to a phobic test stimulus on subsequent avoidance behavior. *Behavior Research and Therapy*, 1971, *9*, 17–21.

Miller, G.A. The magical number seven, plus or minus two: Some limits on our capacity for processing information. *Psychological Review*, 1956, *63*, 81–97.

Miller, L.C., Barrett, C.L., & Hampe, E. Phobias of childhood in a prescientific era. In A. Davids (Ed.), *Child personality and psychopathology: Current topics*. New York: Wiley, 1974.

Miller, L.C., Barrett, C.L., Hampe, E., & Noble, H. Comparison of reciprocal inhibition, psychotherapy, and waiting list control for phobic children. *Journal of Abnormal Psychology*, 1972, *79*, 269–279.

Millon, T. *Modern psychopathology*. Philadelphia: W.B. Saunders, 1969.

Mischel, W. *Personality and assessment*. New York: Wiley, 1968.

Moore, N. Behavior therapy in bronchial asthma. A controlled study. *Journal of Psychosomatic Research*, 1965, *9*, 257–276.

Morgan, A.H. The heritability of hypnotic susceptibility in twins. *Journal of Abnormal Psychology*, 1973, *82*, 55–61.

Morgan, A.H., & Hilgard, E.R. Age differences in susceptibility to hypnosis. *International Journal of Clinical and Experimental Hypnosis*, 1973, *21*, 78–85.

Morgan, A.H., Johnson, D.L., & Hilgard, E.R. The stability of hypnotic susceptibility: A longitudinal study. *International Journal of Clinical and Experimental Hypnosis*, 1974, *22*, 249–257.

Morgan, A.H., & Hilgard, J.R. The Stanford Hypnotic Clinical Scale. Appendix in E.R. Hilgard & J.R. Hilgard, *Hypnosis in the relief of pain*. Los Altos, Calif.: William Kauffman, 1975.

Morgan, A.H., & Hilgard, J.R. The Stanford Hypnotic Clinical Scale for Children. *American Journal of Clinical Hypnosis*, 1979, *21*, 148–169.

Morgan, A.H. MacDonald, H., & Hilgard, E.R. EEG alpha: Lateral asymmetry related to task, and hypnotizability. *Psychophysiology*, 1974, *11*, 275–282.

Morgan, W.P. Pre-match anxiety in a group of college wrestlers. *International Journal of Sports Psychology*, 1970, *1*, 7–13.

Morganstern, K.D. Implosive therapy and flooding procedures: A critical review. *Psychological Bulletin*, 1973, *79*, 318–334.

Morganstern, K.P. Issues in implosive therapy: Reply to Levis. *Psychological Bulletin*, 1974, *81*, 380–382.

Murphy, L.E. Muscular effort, activation level, and reaction time. *Proceedings of the 74th Annual Convention of the American Psychological Association*, 1966, pp. 1–2.

Myers, T., Murphy, D., & Smith, S. The effect of sensory deprivation and social isolation on self-exposure to propaganda and attitude change. *American Psychologist*, 1973, *18*, 440.

Naruse, G. The hypnotic treatment of stage fright in champion athletes.

International Journal of Clinical and Experimental Hypnosis, 1965, *13*, 63–70.

Neale, J.M., & Oltmans, T.F. *Schizophrenia.* New York: Wiley, 1980.

Neisser, V. *Cognitive psychology.* New York: Appleton-Century-Crofts, 1967.

Nideffer, R.M. The relationship of attention and anxiety to performance. In W.F. Straub (Ed.), *Sport psychology: An analysis of athlete behavior.* New York: Mouvement Publications, 1978.

Nisbett, R., & Wilson, T. Telling more than we can know: Verbal reports on mental processes. *Psychological Review*, 1977, *84*, 231–259.

Ohman, A. Fear relevance, autonomic conditioning, and phobias: A laboratory model. In S. Bates, W.S. Dockers, K. Gotestam, L. Melin, & P.O. Sjoden (Eds.), *Trends in behavior therapy.* New York: Academic Press, 1979.

Ohman, A., Eriksson, A., & Olofsson, C. One-trial learning and superior resistance to extinction of autonomic response conditioned to potentially phobic stimuli. *Journal of Comparative and Physiological Psychology*, 1975, *88*, 619–627.

Ollendick, T.H. Fear reduction techniques with children. In M. Hersen, R.M. Eisler, & P.M. Miller (Eds.), *Progress in behavior modification* (Vol. 8). New York: Academic Press: 1979.

Olness, K. The use of self-hypnosis in the treatment of childhood nocturnal enuresis: A report on forty patients. *Clinical Pediatrics*, 1975, *14*, 273–279.

Orme-Johnson, D. W. Autonomic stability and Transcendental Meditation. *Psychosomatic Medicine*, 1973, *35*, 341–349.

Orne, M.T. The nature of hypnosis: Artifact and essence. *Journal of Abnormal and Social Psychology*, 1959, *58*, 277–299.

Orne, M.T. On the social psychology of the psychological experiment: with particular reference to demand characteristics and their implications. *American Psychologist*, 1962, *17*, 776–783.

Orne, M.T. On the mechanisms of posthypnotic amnesia. *International Journal of Clinical and Experimental Hypnosis*, 1966, *14*, 121–134.

Orne, M.T. On the simulating subject as a quasi-control in hypnosis research: What, why, and how. In E. Fromm & R.E. Shor (Eds.), *Hypnosis: Research developments and perspectives.* Chicago: Aldine-Atherton, 1972.

Orne, M.T. Communication by the total experimental situation: Why it is important, how it is evaluated, and its significance for the ecological validity of findings. In P. Pliner, L. Krames, & T. Alloway (Eds.), *Communication and effect.* New York: Academic Press, 1973.

Orne, M.T. On the construct of hypnosis: How its definition affects research and its clinical application. In G.D. Burrows & L. Dennerstein (Eds.), *Handbook of hypnosis and psychomatic medicine.* Amsterdam: Elsevier/North-Holland Biomedical Press, 1980.

Orne, M.T., & Evans, F.J. Social control in the psychological experiment. *Journal of Personality and Social Psychology*, 1965, *1*, 189–200.

Orne, M.T., Hilgard, E.R., Spiegel, H., Spiegel, D., Crawford, H.J., Evans, F.J., Orne, E.C., & Frischholz, E.J. The relation between the Hypnotic Induction Profile and the Stanford Hypnotic Susceptibility Scales, Forms A and C. *International Journal of Clinical and Experimental Hypnosis,* 1979, *27,* 85–102.

Orne, M.T., & Wender, P. Anticipatory socialization for psychotherapy: Method and rationale. *American Journal of Psychiatry,* 1968, *124,* 88–98.

Ornstein, R.E. *The psychology of consciousness.* New York: Harcourt Brace Jovanovich, 1977.

Overton, D.A. State-dependent learning produced by depressant and atropine-like drugs. *Psychopharmacologia,* 1966, *10,* 6–31.

Page, J.D. *Psychopathology.* Chicago: Aldine Publishing, 1975.

Paivio, A. *Imagery and verbal processes.* New York: Holt, 1971.

Patmore, A. *Playing on their nerves: The sport experiment.* London: Stanley Paul, 1979.

Patterson, G.R., & Guillion, M.E. *Living with children: New methods for parents and teachers.* Champaign, Illinois: Research Press, 1968.

Paul, G.L. *Insight versus desensitization in psychotherapy.* Stanford, Calif.: Stanford University Press, 1966.

Paul, G.L. Outcome of systematic desensitization. II. Controlled investigations of individual treatment variations, and current status. In C.M. Franks (Ed.), *Behavior therapy: Appraisal and status.* New York: McGraw-Hill, 1969.

Pavlov, I.P. *Conditioned reflexes.* Oxford: Oxford University Press, 1927.

Perry, C. Is hypnotizability modifiable? *International Journal of Clinical and Experimental Hypnosis,* 1977, *25,* 125–146.

Perry, C., Gelfand, R., & Marcovitch, P. The relevance of hypnotic susceptibility in the clinical context. *Journal of Consulting and Clinical Psychology,* 1979, 592–603.

Perry, C., & Mullen, G. The effect of hypnotic susceptibility on reducing smoking behavior treated by an hypnotic technique. *Journal of Clinical Psychology,* 1975, *31,* 498–505.

Pinneo, L.R. The effects of induced muscle tension during tracking on level of activation and on performance. *Journal of Experimental Psychology,* 1961, *62,* 523–531.

Platonov, K. *The word as a physiological and therapeutic factor.* Moscow: Foreign Language Publishing House, 1959.

Poser, E.G., & King, M.C. Strategies for the prevention of maladaptive fear response. *Canadian Journal of Behavioral Science,* 1975, *7,* 279–294.

Postman, N. *Crazy talk, stupid talk.* New York: Delta Books, 1976.

Pribram, K., & McGuiness, D. Arousal, activation, and effort in the control of attention. *Psychological Review,* 1975, *82,* 116–149.

Price, R., Glickstein, M., Horton, D., & Bailey, R. *Principles of psychology.* New York: Holt, Rinehart & Winston, 1982.

Rachlin, H. *Introduction to modern behaviorism.* San Francisco: W.H. Freeman, 1970.

Rachman, S., & Hodgson, R. Synchrony and desynchrony in fear and avoidance. *Behavior Research and Therapy,* 1974, *12,* 311–318.

Rachman, S.J., & Hodgson, R.J. *Obsessions and compulsions.* Englewood Cliffs, N.J.: Prentice-Hall, 1980.

Rathus, S.A. A 30-item schedule for assessing assertive behavior. *Behavior Therapy,* 1973, *4,* 398–406.

Rawlings, R.M. The genetics of hypnotisability. Unpublished honours thesis. University of New South Wales, January, 1977.

Redlich, F.C., & Freedman, D.X. *The theory and practice of psychiatry.* New York: Basic Books, 1966.

Reiss, S. Pavlovian conditioning and human fear: An expectancy model. *Behavior Therapy,* 1980, *11,* 350–396.

Riddick, C., & Meyer, R.G. The effect of automated relaxation training with response contingent feedback. *Behavior Therapy,* 1973, *4,* 331–337.

Rimm, D.C., Janda, L.H., Lancaster, D.W., Nahl, M., & Dittman, K. An exploratory investigation of the origin and maintenance of phobias. *Behavior Research and Therapy,* 1977, *15,* 231–238.

Rimm, D.C., & Masters, J.C. *Behavior Therapy.* New York: Academic Press, 1979.

Rodriguez, R., Nietzel, M.T., & Berzins, J.I. Sex role orientation and assertiveness among female graduate students. *Behavior Therapy,* 1980, *11,* 353–367.

Rogers, T., & Craighead, W.E. Physiological responses to self-statements: The effects of statement valence and discrepancy. *Cognitive Therapy and Research,* 1977, *1,* 99–108.

Rohrbaugh, M., Riccio, D.C., & Arthur, A. Paradoxical enhancement of conditioned suppression. *Behaviour Research and Therapy,* 1972, *10,* 125–130.

Rosen, G.M. Subjects' initial therapeutic expectancies and subjects' awareness of therapeutic goals in systematic desensitization: A review. *Behavior Therapy,* 1976, *7,* 14–27.

Rosenthal, T.L., & Reese, S.L. The effects of covert and overt modeling on assertive behavior. *Behavior Research and Therapy,* 1976, *14,* 463–469.

Roth, M. The phobic anxiety depersonalization syndrome. *Proceedings of the Royal Society of Medicine,* 1959, *52,* 587–595.

Ruch, J.C. Self-hypnosis: The result of heterohypnosis or vice versa? *International Journal of Clinical and Experimental Hypnosis,* 1975, *23,* 282–304.

Russell, P.L., & Brandsma, J.M. A theoretical and empirical integration of the rational-emotive and classical conditioning theories. *Journal of Consulting and Clinical Psychology,* 1974, *42,* 389–397.

Russell, R.K. & Sipich, J.F. Cue-controlled relaxation in the treatment of test anxiety. *Journal of Behavior Therapy and Experimental Psychiatry,* 1973, *4,* 47–49.

Sachs, L., & Anderson, W. Modification of hypnotic susceptibility. *International Journal of Clinical and Experimental Hypnosis,* 1967, *15,* 172–180.

Sallis, J.F., Lichstein, K.L., & McGlynn, F.D. Anxiety response patterns: A comparison of clinical and analogue populations. *Journal of Behavior Therapy and Experimental Psychiatry*, 1980, *11*, 179–183.

Salter, A. Three techniques of autohypnosis. *Journal of General Psychology*, 1941, *24*, 423–438.

Salter, A. *Conditioned reflex therapy.* New York: Farrar, Straus and Giroux, 1949.

Sanders, R.S., & Reyher, J. Sensory deprivation and the enhancement of hypnotic susceptibility. *Journal of Abnormal Psychology*, 1969, *74*, 375–381.

Sarbin, T.R. Contributions to role-taking theory: I. Hypnotic behavior. *Psychological Review*, 1950, *57*, 255–270.

Sarbin, T.R., & Coe, W.C. Hypnosis: A social psychological analysis of influence communication. New York: Holt, Rinehart & Winston, 1972.

Sarbin, T.R., & Slagle, R.W. Hypnosis in psychophysiological outcomes. In E. Fromm & R.E. Shor (Eds.), *Hypnosis: Research developments and perspective.* Chicago: Aldine-Atherton, 1972.

Sartory, G., Rachman, S., & Grey, S. An investigation of the relation between reported fear and heart rate. *Behavior Research and Therapy*, 1977, *15*, 435–438.

Schacter, S. The interaction of cognitive and physiological determinants of emotional state. In C.D. Spielberger (Ed.), *Anxiety and behavior.* New York: Academic Press, 1966.

Schacter, S., & Singer, J.E. Cognitive, social, and physiological determinants of emotional state. *Psychological Review*, 1962, *69*, 379–399.

Schafer, D.W. Hypnosis in a burn unit. *International Journal of Clinical and Experimental Hypnosis*, 1975, *23*, 1–14.

Scheier, I.H., & Cattell, R.B. *Handbook and test kit for the IPAT 8-parallel-form anxiety battery.* Champaign, Ill.: Institute for Personality and Ability Testing, 1960.

Schubot, E.D. The influence of hypnotic and muscular relaxation in systematic desensitization of phobic behavior. Unpublished doctoral dissertation, Stanford University, 1966.

Schultz, J.H., & Luthe, W. *Autogenic methods.* New York: Grune & Stratton, 1969.

Schwartz, R., & Gottman, J. Toward a task analysis of assertive behavior. *Journal of Consulting and Clinical Psychology*, 1976, *44*, 910–920.

Scovern, A.W., & Kilmann, P.R. Status of electroconvulsive therapy: Review of outcome literature. *Psychological Bulletin*, 1981, *87*, 260–303.

Seligman, M.E.P. On the generality of the laws of learning. *Psychological Review*, 1970, *77*, 406–418.

Seligman, M.E.P. Phobias and preparedness. *Behavior Therapy*, 1971, *2*, 307–320.

Seligman, M.E.P. *Helplessness.* San Francisco: W.H. Freeman & Co., 1975.

Seligman, M.E.P., & Hager, J.L. *Biological boundaries of learning.* New York: Appleton-Century-Crofts, 1972.

Sells, S.B. On the nature of stress. In J.E. McGrath (Ed.), *Social and psychological factors in stress.* New York: Holt, Rinehart & Winston, 1970.

Shapira, K., Kerr, T.A., & Roth, M. Phobias and affective illnesses. *British Journal of Psychiatry,* 1970, *117,* 25–32.

Sheehan, P.W., & Perry, C.W. Research in hypnosis: An overview of current methods. In G.D. Burrows & L. Dennerstein (Eds.), *Handbook of hypnosis and psychosomatic medicine.* Amsterdam: Elsevier/North-Holland Biomedical Press, 1980.

Shervin, H., & Dickman, S. The psychological unconscious: A necessary assumption for all psychological theory. *American Psychologist,* 1980, *35,* 421–434.

Shipley, R.H., & Boudewyns, P.A. Flooding and implosive therapy: Are they harmful? *Behavior Therapy,* 1980, *11,* 503–508.

Shor, R.E. Hypnosis and the concept of the generalized reality-orientation. In C.T. Tart (Ed.), *Altered states of consciousness.* New York: Wiley, 1969.

Shor, R.E. *The Inventory of Self-Hypnosis (Form A): Breaths Version.* Palo Alto, Calif.: Consulting Psychologists Press, 1970.

Shor, R.E., & Easton, R.D. A preliminary report on research comparing self- and heterohypnosis. *American Journal of Clinical Hypnosis,* 1973, *16,* 37–44.

Shor, R.E., & Orne, E.C. *The Harvard Group Scale of Hypnotic Susceptibility, Form A.* Palo Alto, Calif.: Consulting Psychologists Press, 1962.

Shor, R.E., Orne, M.T., & O'Connell, D.N. Psychological correlates of plateau hypnotizability in a special volunteer sample. *Journal of Personality and Social Psychology,* 1962, *3,* 80–95.

Sidman, M. *The tactics of scientific research.* New York: Basic Books, 1960.

Singer, J.L., & Pope, K.S. Daydreaming and imagery skills as predisposing capacities for self hypnosis. *International Journal of Clinical and Experimental Hypnosis,* 1981, *29,* 271–281.

Skinner, B.F. *Science and human behavior.* New York: Macmillan, 1953.

Skinner, B.F. A case history in scientific method. In S. Koch (Ed.), *Psychology: A study of a science* (Vol. 2). New York: McGraw-Hill, 1959.

Slater, E., & Roth, M. *Clinical psychiatry.* London: Baillière, Tindall, & Cassell, 1969.

Smith, M.J. *Kicking the fear habit.* New York: Bantam Books, 1977.

Smith, M.L., & Glass, G.V. Meta-analysis of psychotherapy outcome studies. *American Psychologist,* 1977, *32,* 752–760.

Spanos, N.P., & Barber, T.X. Behavior modification and hypnosis. In M. Hersen, R.M. Eisler, & P.M. Miller (Eds.), *Progress in behavior modification* (Vol. 3). New York: Academic Press, 1976.

Sperry, R.W. A modified concept of consciousness. *Psychological Review,* 1969, *76,* 532–536.

Spiegel, H. The grade 5 sydrome: The highly hypnotizable person. *International Journal of Clinical and Experimental Hypnosis,* 1974, *22,* 303–319.

Spiegel, H., & Spiegel, D. *Trance and treatment: Clinical uses of hypnosis.* New York: Basic Books, 1978.

Speilberger, C.D. Theory and research on anxiety. In C.D. Spielberger (Ed.), *Anxiety and behavior.* New York: Academic Press, 1966.

Stampfl, T.G., & Levis, D.J. Essentials of implosive therapy: A learning-theory-based psychodynamic behavioral therapy. *Journal of Abnormal Psychology,* 1967, *72,* 496–503.

Steffens, J.J. Covert reinforcement: Two studies and a comment. *Psychological Reports,* 1977, *40,* 291–294.

Stern, D.B., Spiegel, H., & Nee, J.C.M. The Hypnotic Induction Profile: Normative observation, reliability, and validity. *American Journal of Clinical Hypnosis,* 1978, *21,* 109–133.

Strosahl, K.D., & Ascough, J.C. Clinical uses of mental imagery: Experimental foundations, theoretical misconceptions, and research issues. *Psychological Bulletin,* 1981, *89,* 422–438.

Strupp, H. Specific vs. nonspecific factors in psychology and the problem of control. *Archives of General Psychiatry,* 1970, *23,* 393–401.

Suedfeld, P. *Restricted environmental stimulation: Research and clinical applications.* New York: Wiley, 1980.

Suinn, R., & Richardson, F. Anxiety management training. A nonspecific behavior therapy program for anxiety control. *Behavior Therapy,* 1971, *2,* 498–510.

Sulzer-Azaroff, B., & Mayer, G.R. *Applying behavior-analysis procedures with children and youths.* New York: Holt, Rinehart & Winston, 1977.

Sutcliffe, J.P. "Credulous" and "skeptical" views of hypnotic phenomena. A review of certain evidence and methodology. *International Journal of Clinical and Experimental Hypnosis,* 1960, *8,* 73–100.

Sutcliffe, J.P., Perry, C.W., & Sheehan, P.W. Relation of some aspects of imagery and fantasy to hypnotic susceptibility. *Journal of Abnormal Psychology,* 1970, *76,* 279–287.

Tart, C.T. Psychedelic experiences associated with a novel procedure, mutual hypnosis. *American Journal of Clinical Hypnosis,* 1967, *10,* 65–78.

Tart, C.T. *States of consciousness.* New York: E.P. Dutton, 1975.

Tasto, D.L. Systematic desensitization, muscle relaxation and visual imagery in the counterconditioning of a four-year-old child. *Behavior Research and Therapy,* 1969, *7,* 409–411.

Tellegen, A., & Atkinson, G. Openness to absorbing and self-altering experiences ("absorption"), a trait related to hypnotic susceptibility. *Journal of Abnormal Psychology,* 1974, *83,* 268–277.

Terrace, H.S. Stimulus control. In W.K. Honig (Ed.), *Operant behavior: Areas of research and application.* New York: Appleton-Century-Crofts, 1966.

Thorndike, E.L. *The psychology of wants, interests, and attitudes.* New York: Appleton Century, 1935.

Tinbergin, N. *The study of instinct.* Oxford: Clarendon Press, 1951.

Tinkler, S. The use of hypnosis in dental surgery. In J. Hartland, *Medical and dental hypnosis and its clinical applications.* London: Baillière Tindall, 1971.

Tinterow, M.M. (Ed.), *Foundations of hypnosis: From Mesmer to Freud.* Springfield, Ill.: Charles C. Thomas, 1970.

Ullmann, L.P., & Krasner, L. *A psychological approach to abnormal behavior.* Englewood Cliffs, N.J.: Prentice-Hall, 1975.

Unestahl, L.E. Hypnotic preparation of athletes. In G.D. Burrows, D.R. Collison, & L. Dennerstein (Eds.), *Hypnosis 1979.* Amsterdam: Elsevier/ North-Holland Biomedical Press, 1979.

Valentine, C.W. The innate bases of fear. *Journal of Genetic Psychology,* 1930, *37,* 394–419.

Valentine, C.W. *The psychology of early childhood.* London: Methuen, 1946.

Vaughn, F. School phobia (1954), cited by W. Talbot, Panic in school phobia. *American Journal of Orthopsychiatry,* 1957, *27,* 286–295.

Veltens, E. A laboratory task for induction of mood states. *Behavior Research and Therapy,* 1968, *6,* 473–482.

Vogt, O. Zur Kenntnis des Wesens und der psychologischen Bedeutung des Hypnotismus. *Zeitschrift fuer Hypnotismus,* 1894–95, *3,* 277.

Wachtel, P.L. Anxiety, attention, and coping with threat. *Journal of Abnormal Psychology,* 1968, *73,* 137–143.

Wade, T.C., Malloy, T.E., & Proctor, S. Imaginal correlates of self- reported fear and avoidance behavior. *Behavior Research and Therapy,* 1977, *15,* 17–22.

Waldfogel, S. Emotional crises in a child. In A. Burton (Ed.), *Case studies in counseling and psychotherapy.* Englewood Cliffs, N.J.: Prentice-Hall, 1959.

Walker, W.L., & Diment, A.D. Music as a deepening technique. *Australian Journal of Clinical and Experimental Hypnosis,* 1979, *1,* 35–36.

Wallace, B. *Applied hypnosis.* Chicago: Nelson-Hall, 1979.

Watkins, J.G. Antisocial behavior under hypnosis. Possible or impossible? *International Journal of Clinical and Experimental Hypnosis,* 1972. *20,* 95–100.

Watson, J.B. *Behaviorism.* New York: W.W. Norton, 1930.

Watson, J.B., & Marks, I.M. Relevant and irrelevant fear in flooding. A crossover study of phobic patients. *Behavior Therapy,* 1971, *2,* 275–293.

Watson, J.B., & Rayner, R. Conditioned emotional reactions. *Journal of Experimental Psychology,* 1920, *3,* 1–14.

Watts, F.N. Habituation model of systematic desensitization. *Psychological Bulletin,* 1979, *86,* 627–637.

Weekes, C. *Agoraphobia: Simple, effective treatment.* London: Angus & Robertson, 1977.

Weiss, J.M. Effects of coping response on stress. *Journal of Comparative and Physiological Psychology,* 1968, *65,* 251–260.

Weiss, J.M. Effects of coping behavior with and without a feedback signal on stress pathology in rats. *Journal of Comparative and Physiological Psychology,* 1971, *77,* 22–30.

Weitzenhoffer, A.M. *General techniques of hypnotism.* New York: Grune & Stratton, 1957.

Weitzenhoffer, A.M., & Hilgard, E.R. *Stanford Hypnotic Susceptibility Scale, Forms A and B.* Palo Alto, Calif.: Consulting Psychologists Press, 1959.

Weizenhoffer, A.M., & Hilgard, E.R. *Stanford Hypnotic Susceptibility Scale, Form C.* Palo Alto, Calif.: Consulting Psychologists Press, 1962.

Weitzman, B. Behavior therapy and psychotherapy. *Psychological Review,* 1967, *74,* 300–317.

Wenger, M.A., & Bagchi, B.K. Studies of autonomic functions in a practitioner of yoga in India. *Behavioral Science,* 1961, *6,* 312–332.

Westbrook, R.F., Clarke, J.C., & Provost, S. Long-delay learning in the pigeon: Flavor, color, and flavor-mediated color aversions. *Behavioral and Neural Biology,* 1980, *28,* 398–407.

Westphal, C. (1871) cited in Marks, I.M. *Fears and phobias.* London: Academic Press, 1969.

White, R.W. A preface to the theory of hypnotism. *Journal of Abnormal and Social Psychology,* 1941, *36,* 477–505.

White, R.W. Motivation reconsidered: The concept of competence. *Psychological Review,* 1959, *66,* 297–333.

Whitehurst, G.J., & Vasta, R. *Child behavior.* Boston: Houghton-Mifflin, 1977.

Wickramasekera, I. The effects of electromyographic feedback on hypnotic susceptibility: More preliminary data. *Journal of Abnormal Psychology,* 1973, *82,* 74–77.

Willis, R.G.D. *Diary of a cricket season.* London: Pelham Books Ltd., 1979.

Windheuser, H.J. Anxious mothers as models for coping with anxiety. *Behavioral Analysis and Modification,* 1977, *1,* 39–58.

Wolberg, L.R. *Medical hypnosis* (Vols. 1 & 2). New York: Grune & Stratton, 1948.

Wolfenstein, M. *Disaster.* London: Routledge, 1957.

Wolpe, J. *Psychotherapy by reciprocal inhibition.* Stanford: Stanford University Press, 1958.

Wolpe, J. The conditioning and deconditioning of neurotic anxiety. In C.D. Speilberger (Ed.), *Anxiety and behavior.* New York: Academic Press, 1966.

Wolpe, J. *The practice of behavior therapy.* New York: Pergamon Press, 1969.

Wolpe, J. The experimental model and treatment of neurotic depression. *Behavior Research and Therapy,* 1979, *17,* 555–565.

Wolpe, J. The dichotomy between clinical conditioned and cognitively learned anxiety. *Journal of Behavior Therapy and Experimental Psychiatry,* 1981, *12,* 35–42.

Wolpe, J., & Rachman, S. Psychoanalytic "evidence": A critique based on Freud's case of Little Hans. *Journal of Nervous and Mental Disease,* 1960, *131,* 135–148.

Wood, C.G., & Hokanson, J.E. Effects of induced muscular tension on performance and the inverted-u function. *Journal of Personality and Social Psychology,* 1965, *1,* 506–510.

Woodworth, R.W., & Schlosberg, H. *Experimental psychology.* New York: Henry Holt, 1954.

Yates, A.J. *Theory and practice in behavior therapy.* New York: Wiley, 1975.

Yates, A. *Biofeedback and the modification of behavior.* New York: Plenum Press, 1980.

Yerkes, R.M., & Dodson, J.D. The relation of strength of stimulus to rapidity of Lakit-formation. *Journal of Comparative Neurology of Psychology.* 1908, *18,* 459–482.

Young, P.C. Is rapport an essential characteristic of hypnosis? *Journal of Abnormal and Social Psychology,* 1927, *22,* 130–139.

Zettle, R.D., & Hayes, S.C. Conceptual and empirical status of rational-emotive therapy. In M. Hersen, R.M. Eisler, & P.M. Miller (Eds.), *Progress in behavior modification* (Vol. 9). New York: Academic Press, 1980.

Zitrin, C.M. Combined pharmacological and psychological treatment of phobias. In M. Mavissakalian & D.H. Barlow (Eds.), *Phobia: Psychological and pharmacological treatments.* New York: Guilford Press, 1981.

Zubek, J.P. (Ed.). *Sensory deprivation: Fifteen years of research.* New York: Appleton-Century-Crofts, 1969.

Index

Index

Abreactions, 68–69
Agoraphobia, 190, 263–264
  behavior therapies for, 263–264
  clinical picture of, 264–268
  cognitive therapies for, 280–281
  counter-anxiety measures, 283–
    285
  counterproductive suggestions,
    283
  definitional problems, 270–271
  depression and, 269–270
  ECT and, 269
  exposure therapies for, 285–287
  eye closure and, 282–283
  fear of open spaces, 268–269
  flooding, 286
  hierarchy for, 315–318
  hypnotic techniques for, 282–285
  in vivo exercises for, 285–287
  model of, 271–273
  onset of, 266–268
  panic attacks in, 264–266, 274
  panic attack therapies, 278–282
  pharmacological management,
    278–279
  prevalence of, 266–268
  rationale therapy, 275–278
  syndrome vs. phobic, 271–273
  therapies for, 273–275
  visual contact problems, 286

Amnesia, 5–7, 66
Analgesia, hypnotic, 18–21
Anxiety
  arousal and, 290–293
  cognitive, see Cognitive anxiety
  cognitive theory of, 168, 185–190
  conditioning theory of, 168, 170–
    178
  definition of, 169n., 236
  depression and, 260–261
  fear and, 169
  measurement of, 169–170
  multiprocess model of, 190, 193,
    194
  panic, 190–192
  perseverance, 190–192
  phobic vs. nonphobic, 178–179,
    185–186. See also Phobic
    anxiety
  problem of, 169–170
  in sports, see Sports anxiety
  state, 292–293
  theoretical and clinical status of,
    169–170
  trait, 292–293
  volunteer-based studies of, 168
Anxiety reduction (Dimension 1),
    25, 26, 31–32, 53, 79, 114,
    222–224
Arm levitation, 69–72, 76–77

Arousal
    anxiety and, 290–293
    in sports anxiety, 297
Arousal, reduction in (Dimension
        2), 26, 27, 31–32, 53, 79,
        114, 222–224
Assertion therapy, 13
Assertive behavior, cognitive anxiety
        and, 255–261
Assessment, *see* Measurement
Attentional processes, sports anxiety
        and, 294–295, 298
Audiotapes, use of, in induction,
        164–166
Autogenic training, 84
Autonomic responses, 23
Autosuggestion, 156–158, 163. *See
        also* Self-hypnosis
Aversive therapy, 145

Behavioral inertia (Dimension 4),
        26, 28–29, 31–32, 79, 114
Behavior therapy, 289–290
    vs. cognitive therapy, 187, 238
    for panic attacks, 281–282
Biofeedback procedures, 51–53,
        120–121
Breathing
    deepening and, 84–85
    in meditation, 125–126, 128,
        132–133
    rapid, 76–78

Children
    phobic anxiety in, 228–235
    phobic reactions in, 180–181
    role of parents, in treatment of
        phobias and fears, 234–235
    school phobia, 230–231
Children, hypnosis in, 93–94
    adult induction techniques for,
        109–110
    assessment scales, 94–97

deepening techniques, 109–110
dropped-coin induction, 107–109
duration of hypnotic episodes,
        101
eye-fixation induction, 105–107
hypnotizability, 94
imaginal induction, 102–105
induction techniques for, 102–
        110
parental expectations, 98–100
parental role in children's self-
        hypnosis, 112
preparation, 97–98
resistance to self-hypnosis home
        practice, 113
self-hypnosis, 110–113
Children's Hypnotic Susceptibility
        Scale (CHSS), 94–95
Classical conditioning, 56–58
Claustrophobia, hierarchy for, 320–
        321
Cognitive, definition of, 187, 236–
        237, 244
Cognitive activities in meditation,
        126–127, 128
Cognitive anxiety, 185–186
    based on misinformation, 189–
        190
    coexistence with panic and phobic
        anxieties, 194–195
    definition of, 236–237
    distinctions and pseudo battles
        over, 186–187
    vs. phobic anxiety, 178–179,
        185–187, 261–262
    RET for, *see* Rational-emotive
        therapy
    self-statements, 187–188
    set, 188–189
    therapy for, *see* Cognitive therapy
        for anxiety
    unassertiveness and, 255–256
Cognitive avoidances, 227–228
Cognitive-hypnotic techniques for
        assertive problems, 256–261

Cognitive therapy, 30–31
  for anxiety, *see* Cognitive therapy
    for anxiety
  behavior therapy and, 187, 238
  for panic attacks, 280–281
  see also Rational-emotive therapy
Cognitive therapy for anxiety
  aims of, 237–238
  application, 254–255
  modification of self-statements,
    254–255
  nonverbal cognitions and, 244–
    248
  objections to, 252–253
  rationale, 248–249
  stages of, 248–255
  see also Cognitive anxiety
Complex agoraphobia, *see* Agora-
    phobia
Conditioning theory of anxiety,
    170–178, 184, 185, 189
  conditioning and evolution, 174–
    175
  elements and limitations of, 172–
    173
  evaluation, 173–174
  evolution and phobias ("pre-
    paredness"), 175–177
  phobias and modeling, 177–178
Conditioning theory of prephobic
    stimuli, 184
Control, *see* Transfer of control
Covert reinforcement for anxiety
    control, 226
Cue-controlled relaxation, 312

Dangers of hypnosis, 10–11
Deepening procedures, 81–89
  breathing methods, 84–85
  definition of, 81*n*.
  descending steps method, 85–87
  fractionation method, 87–89
  hypnotizability vs. depth of hyp-
    nosis, 81

  music in, 90–91
  relaxation method, 83–84
  variability of depth of hypnosis,
    82
Depression
  agoraphobia and, 269–270
  anxiety and, 260–261
  hypnosis and, 12
Descending steps method of deep-
    ening, 85–87
Desensitization, *see* Systematic
    desensitization
Dimension 1, *see* Anxiety reduction
Dimension 2, *see* Arousal, reduction
    in
Dimension 3, *see* Focused attention
Dimension 4, *see* Behavioral inertia
Dimension 5, *see* Uncritical thinking
Dimension 6, *see* Transfer of
    control
Direct-stare induction technique, 78
Disengagement, 55–56
  in hypnosis vs. meditation, 117–
    118
  see also Induction techniques
Dishabituation, phobias and, 182–
    184
Distancing for anxiety control, 225–
    226
Dropped-coin induction technique,
    107–109

EEG, 4, 97
Effort in hypnosis, 9
Evolution, phobias and, 176–177
Expectations, *see* Therapeutic
    outcome
Exposure therapies
  for agoraphobia, 274, 285–287
  for children with fear and pho-
    bias, 231–233
  duration of exposure, 219–222
  hierarchical construction, 215–
    216

Exposure therapies (*cont.*)
  imagery in, 217–218
  for phobic anxiety, 195–207
  sheer exposure, 223
  for sports anxiety, 299–302
  see also Flooding; Systematic
    desensitization
Eye closure
  agoraphobia and, 282–283
  in meditation, 135–136
Eye-fixation technique of induction,
    72–73
  for children, 105–107

Fear
  in children, 228–235
  definition of, 169*n.*
  phobic, 181
Flooding
  for phobic anxiety, 196–198
  therapeutic and iatrogenic out-
    comes, 198–202
Focused attention (Dimension 3),
    26, 27–28, 31–32, 54, 79,
    114–115
  in meditation, 117–119, 128–130,
    132
  in self-hypnosis, 157–158
Fractionation method of deepening,
    87–89

Generalized reality orientation, 33
General-process conditioning the-
    ory, 173, 175

Habituation, phobias and, 182–184
Hallucination, 24, 85–87
Harvard Group Scale of Hypnotic
    Susceptibility (HGSHS), 43,
    44, 49, 154
Heightened suggestibility, 15–16,
    41

Heterohypnosis
  clinical use of, 150–151
  induction taught for self-hypno-
    sis, 155–156
  vs. self-hypnosis, 144–147, 148–
    151
  see also Hypnosis
Hierarchy construction
  for agoraphobia, 315–318
  for claustrophobia, 320–321
  general guidelines for, 218–219
  in phobic anxiety treatment, 215–
    216
  for public speaking anxiety, 322–
    323
  sample scenes, 313–323
  for social phobia, 318–320
  for test (exam) anxiety, 321–322
Hoax in hypnotic performance, 17
Humor for anxiety control, 226–
    227
Hyperventilation, 76–78. *See also*
    Breathing
Hypnosis
  for agoraphobia, 282–285
  anxiety reduction, 25, 26, 31–32,
    53, 79, 114, 222–224
  arousal, reduction in, 26, 27, 31–
    32, 53, 79, 114, 222–224
  assessment and modification, 38–
    60
  behavioral inertia, 26, 28–29, 31–
    32, 79, 114
  in children, *see* Children, hypno-
    sis in
  cooperative theory of, 21
  credulous view of, 19
  danger of, 10–11
  definition of, 114–115
  dictionary definition of, 15
  early references to, 2–3
  effort expenditure in, 9
  focused attention, 26, 27–28, 31–
    32, 54, 79, 114–115
  hoax and, 17

Hypnosis (*cont.*)
  immobility and, 7–8
  induction procedures, *see* Induction procedures
  integrative approach to, 21–24
  level of performance during, 19–20
  measurement of, *see* Measurement
  meditation and, *see* Meditation
  memory and, 5–7
  motivated behavior and, 300–302
  myths about, *see* Myths and misconceptions
  operations and processes, 25–30
  role-playing interpretations, 20
  skeptical view of, 18–21
  sleep state and, 2–5
  special-state theory of, 21–23
  for sports anxiety, 299–302
  three stages of, 15
  transfer of control, 26, 29–30, 31–32, 55–58, 114
  transcience/permanence of treatment effects, 9–10
  uncritical thinking, 26, 29, 31–32, 52–53, 79, 114
  uses of, *see* Anxiety
  see also Exposure therapies
Hypnotic analgesia, 18–21
Hypnotic Induction Profile (HIP), 50, 81
Hypnotic relaxation via sensory awareness, 78–81
Hypnotic stability, 42–44
Hypnotic techniques, reliability of, 39–40. *See also* Induction procedures
Hypnotic trance, *see* Trance
Hypnotizability, 38–39
  assessment of, 2
  of children, 94
  clinical scales, 49–50
  vs. depth of hypnosis, 81
  distribution of, 41–42

  and focused attention, 115
  measurement of, 47–49
  measurement of, in children, 94–97
  modification of, 40, 50–55
  therapeutic outcome and, 44–47, 81

Iatrogenic outcomes, 198–202
Idiosyncratic reactions to induction, 66–67
Imaginal induction, 73–75, 115
  for children, 102–105, 110–111
  deepening, 85–87
  exposure techniques, 217–218
  for self-hypnosis in children, 110–111
Immobility, myth about, 7–8
Induction procedures, 15
  anxiety reduction, 25, 26, 31–32, 53, 79, 114, 222–224
  arm levitation, 69–72
  arousal, reduction in, 26, 27, 31–32, 53, 79, 114, 222–224
  audiotapes, 164–166
  behavioral inertia, 26, 28–29, 31–32, 79, 114
  breathing method of deepening, 84–85
  deepening procedures, 81–89
  descending step method of deepening, 85–87
  direct-stare technique, 78
  first induction, 64–69
  focused attention, 26, 27–28, 31–32, 54, 79, 114–115
  fractionation method of deepening, 87–89
  gradual transition in, 62
  hypnotic relaxation via sensory awareness, 78–81
  idiosyncratic reactions, 66–67
  imaginal techniques, 73–75, 115. *See also* Imaginal induction

Induction procedures (*cont.*)
   indirect eye-fixation technique,
     72–73
   nonverbal techniques, 89–91
   operating principles, 61–64
   permissive vs. authoritarian ap-
     proaches, 62
   perseverative reactions, 68–69
   rapid, 75–78
   recall and, 66
   relaxation method of deepening,
     83–84
   self-hypnosis, 63, 147–148
   suiting techniques to patient, 62–
     63
   termination, 91–92
   trance, 30–36
   transfer of control, 26, 29–30,
     31–32, 55–58, 114
   uncritical thinking, 26, 29, 31–32,
     52–53, 79, 114
   value of, 24
Inertia, *see* Behavioral inertia
Instincts, phobias and, 179–182
Integrative approach to hypnosis,
   21–24
Inventory of Self-Hypnosis (ISH),
   153
In vivo exercises for agoraphobia,
   285–289

Legal issues in hypnosis, 11
Lucid sleep, 3

Management and procedures, *see*
   Agoraphobia; Cognitive therapy for anxiety; Induction
   procedures; Phobic anxiety
   management and proce-
   dures; Sports anxiety
Mantra, 127, 129–130, 132, 134–
   135, 137
   movement, 136
   see also Meditation

Measurement, 40–41
   children's assessment scales, 94–97
   clinical hypnotizability scales, 49–
     50
   concerns of, 44
   hypnotic stability, 42–44
   hypnotizability, 47–49
   modification of hypnotizability,
     50–55
   therapeutic outcome and, 44–47
Medical issues in hypnosis, 11
Meditation, 79, 84, 224
   abreactions, 138–139
   breathing in, 125–126, 128, 132–
     133
   cognitive activities in, 126–127,
     128
   common element in diverse prac-
     tices, 116–117
   common misconceptions about,
     139
   conceptualization of, 116–119
   control of physiological reactions,
     119–120
   count-out technique, 128, 131,
     134–135
   disengagement in, 117
   effects of, 119–122
   enhanced control of attention,
     121–122
   eye closure in, 135–136
   focused attention, 117–119, 128–
     130, 132
   and hypnosis, comparison of,
     116–119
   increase in hypnotizability and,
     139–140
   mantra, 127, 129–130, 132, 134–
     135, 136, 137
   mini-meditation exercises, 140–
     141
   modifications and special tech-
     niques, 131–137
   muscle relaxation for, 133–134
   need for a rationale for, 131
   outside use of, 139–141

Meditation (*cont.*)
  posture for, 117, 124
  preparation for, 122–123
  problems in, 137–139
  psychological effects of, 120–122
  self-hypnosis and, 157
  sense of failure in, 137
  for sports anxiety, 302–303
  structured approach to, 128–130
  take-home exercise schedule for
    daily, 142
  tension release reactions, 138
  time of, 123–124
  types of, 116
  unstructured approach to, 127
  use of the term, 141, 143
  visual, 136
Memory
  cognition and, 23
  hypnosis and, 5–7
Misconceptions, *see* Myths and
  misconceptions
Misinformation and cognitive anxiety, 189–190
Mobile attention, 28
Modeling
  for anxiety control, 204–205
  for children with fear and pho-
    bias, 233–234
  phobias and, 177–178
Modification of hypnotizability, 40,
  50–55
Motivated behavior and hypnosis,
  300–302
Muscle relaxation, *see* Progressive
  muscular relaxation
Music in induction, 90
Myths and misconceptions, 1–2
  discussing, at first induction, 64–
    65
  hypnosis can uncover and poten-
    tiate psychological disorders,
    12–13
  hypnosis impairs memory, 5–7
  hypnosis is dangerous, 10–11
  hypnosis is a sleep state, 2–5

  hypnosis makes the patient more
    difficult to live with, 13–14
  hypnosis requires effort, 9
  hypnosis requires immobility, 708
  hypnotic treatment effects are
    transient/permanent, 9–10
  about self-hypnosis, 151–153

Neurypnology, 3
Nonphobic anxieties, *see* Cognitive
  anxiety; Panic anxiety
Nonverbal cognitions, 244–248
Nonverbal techniques of induction,
  89–91
No-treatment control group, 202

Operant behavior modification, 145
Operant conditioning, 56
Organismic variables, 15
Orienting reflex, 27

Panic anxiety, 190–192
  coexistence with phobic and cog-
    nitive anxieties, 194–195
  see also Agoraphobia
Panic attacks in agoraphobia, 264–
  266, 274
Panic attack therapies, 278–282
  behavioral techniques, 281–282
  cognitive techniques, 280–281
  pharmacological methods, 278–
  279
Parents, *see* Children
Perception and cognition, 23
Performance efficiency and arousal,
  290–293, 294
Permanence of hypnotic treatment
  effects, 9–10
Perseverance anxiety, 190–192
Perseverative reactions after termination, 68–69
Pharmacological therapy for panic
  attacks, 278–279

Phenothiazines, 279
Phobias, 46–47
  evolution and, 175–177
  habituation and dishabituation,
      182–184
  instincts and, 179–182
  modeling and, 177–178
  see also Phobic anxiety
Phobic agoraphobia, 271–273
Phobic anxiety
  in children, 228–235
  clinical definition of, 176
  coexistence with cognitive and
      panic anxieties, 194–195
  cognitions and, 192
  vs. cognitive anxiety, 178–179,
      185–187, 261–262
  conditioning theories of, 180–181
  definitional problems, 204–205
  elaboration of, 192
  ethological position, 178–182
  evolution and phobias ("pre-
      paredness"), 175–177
  inhibition and, 192
  management and procedures, *see*
      Phobic anxiety management
      and procedures
  vs. nonphobic anxiety, 178–179,
      185–186
  phobic fear and, 181
  uncovering the dimensions of,
      207–211
Phobic anxiety management and
      procedures
  anxiety control methods, 224–
      228
  arousal and anxiety control: re-
      duction and elimination,
      222–224
  cognitive avoidance, 227–229
  cognitive therapy, 195
  covert reinforcement, 226
  distancing, 225–226
  exposure durations, 220–222
  exposure techniques, 195–207,
      212, 214–215

exposure techniques for children,
      231–233
exposure therapy and patient ex-
      pectancies, 202–207
flooding and systematic desensi-
      tization, 196–202
guessing techniques, 211–214
hierarchy construction, 215–216
hierarchy scene construction:
      general guidelines, 218–219
humor, developing sense of,
      226–227
hypnosis, use of, 200–202, 211–
      214, 227–228
imaginal exposure, 207, 212,
      214–215, 217–218
in vivo exposure, 214–215
metaphor for treatment, 205
modeling, 224–225
modeling for children, 233–234
patient expectancies, 202–207
patient models of change, 205–
      207
therapeutic and iatrogenic out-
      comes of flooding and sys-
      tematic desensitization, 198–
      202
treatment considerations, 195–
      196
treatment for children, 231–235
type of exposure: imaginal vs. *in
      vivo*, 214–215
Phobic fear, 181
Phobic stimuli, 176–177, 178, 179,
      185
Placebo control groups, 202–203,
      205
Posthypnotic amnesia, 5–7
Posthypnotic recall, 66
Posthypnotic suggestion, 34
Posture in meditation, 117, 124
Progressive muscular relaxation, 79,
      83–84, 222, 224
  additions and variations, 312
  for anxiety, 120–121
  duration, 310

Progressive muscular relaxation
(*cont.*)
   meditation and, 133–134
   problems, 310–311
   quantitative or qualitative esti-
      mates of muscle tension,
      307–308
   rationale, 305–307
   sample exercise, 311–312
   tension changes: gradual vs.
      abrupt, 308–309
Psychoanalysis vs. cognitive therapy,
   237–238
Psychological disorders, myth that
   hypnosis can uncover and
   potentiate, 12–13
Psychotropic drugs for panic attacks, 279
Public speaking anxiety, hierarchy
   for, 322–323

Rapid-breathing induction, 76–78
Rapid-induction technique, 75–78
Rapport, importance of, 35–36
Rational-emotive therapy (RET),
   145, 188, 238–241, 244
Recall, posthypnotic, 66
Relaxation method of deepening,
   83–84
Relaxation therapies, 84, 145. *See
   also* Progressive muscular
   relaxation
Response, 15
   spontaneous vs. evoked, 16
Response-inhibition model of unas-
   sertiveness, 255–256
Role-playing in hypnosis, 20, 24

School phobia, 230–231
Self-hypnosis, 9, 63
   assessment issues and clinical ap-
      plications, 153–159
   audiotapes and, 164–166
   vs. autohypnosis, 110

   autosuggestion, 156–159, 163
   in children, 110–113
   clinical use of, 150–151
   disengagement, 156
   focused attention in, 115–116,
      157–158
   vs. heterohypnosis, 144–147,
      148–151
   home use of, 4–5, 161–164
   induction procedures, 147–148
   meditation and, 157
   myths and misconceptions about,
      151–153
   nature of, 148–151
   overt behavior and, 159–160
   possibility of, 146–148
   rationale for operation and uses
      of, 156–157
   resistance to, in children, 113
   role of parents in children's,
      112
   sleep and, 164
   for sports anxiety, 302–303
   structured, 153–159
   studies of, 145, 147–148, 149,
      153
   task-relevant self-suggestions, 163
   taught with heterohypnotic in-
      duction, 155–156
   teaching, 156–161
   technical aids to, 164–166
   termination procedures, 152
   transfer of control, 58
   transfer of training, 160–161
   unstructured, 153–159
Self-statements
   changing, about arousal, 242–243
   cognitive anxiety and assertive be-
      havior, 255–256
   modification of, in cognitive ther-
      apy, 242, 254–255
   stress inoculation and cognitive-
      hypnotic techniques for as-
      sertive problems, 256–258
Sensory awareness, hypnotic relaxation via, 78–81

Sensory deprivation and modifica-
    tion, 51, 52–53
Separation phobias, 264, 271–272.
    See also Agoraphobia
Sets, modifications of, 258–260
Skills deficit model of unassertive-
    ness, 255–256
Sleep state, hypnosis and, 2–5
Social phobia, hierarchy for, 318–
    320
Somnambulism, artificial, 3
S-O-R model of behavior therapy,
    30
Spatial hierarchies, 216
Special-state theory, 21–23
Sports anxiety, 289–290
    arousal and anxiety, 290–293
    attentional processes, 294–295
    exposure techniques, 299–302
    hypnotic management, 296–299
    influence of stress, 295–296
    meditation, role of, 302–303
    self-hypnosis, role of, 302–303
S-R model of behavior therapy, 30
Stability, hypnotic, 42–44
Stanford Hypnotic Clinical Scale for
    Adults (SHCS:Adult), 49, 95
Stanford Hypnotic Clinical Scale for
    Children (SHCS:Child), 94–
    97, 102, 106
Stanford Hypnotic Susceptibility
    Scale
    Form A (SHSS:A), 43, 44, 47–49,
        95, 153
    Form B (SHSS:B), 43, 44, 47–49,
        95
    Form C (SHSS:C), 49, 95, 154
State anxiety, 292–293
Stress, sports anxiety and, 295–296
Stress inoculation for assertive
    problems, 256–261
Structuralists, 188–189
SUDS (subjective units of discom-
    fort), 252, 256, 308, 313–315
Suicide, hypnosis and, 12

Symptom removal, hypnosis and,
    12–13
Symptom substitution, 198–199
Syndrome agoraphobia, 271–273
Systematic desensitization, 145, 222
    for phobic anxiety, 196–198
    therapeutic and iatrogenic out-
        comes, 198–202

Tapes, use of, in induction, 164–
    166
Temporal hierarchies, 216
Termination
    idiosyncratic reactions, 66–67
    perseverative reactions, 68–69
    recall after, 66
    techniques for, 91–92
Test (exam) anxiety, hierarchy for,
    321–322
Tests, *see* Measurement
Thematic hierarchies, 216
Therapeutic outcome
    discussing, at first induction,
        65
    expectations and response to
        hypnosis, 2
    flooding and systematic desensi-
        tization, 198–202
    hypnotizability and, 81
    measurement and, 44–47
Trait anxiety, 292–293
Trance, 30–36
    vs. non-trance behavior, 22–23
    special-state theory, 21–23
    use of term, 19
Transfer of control (Dimension 6),
    26, 29–30, 31–32, 55–58,
    114
    classical conditioning and, 56–58
    operant conditioning and, 56
Transcendental Meditation (TM),
    119, 127, 141
Transience of hypnotic treatment
    effects, 9–10

Tricyclic drugs for agoraphobic, 269–270

Unassertiveness and cognitive anxiety, 255
Uncritical thinking (Dimension 5), 26, 29, 31–32, 52–53, 79, 114

Watsonian conditioning, *see* Conditioning theory of anxiety
Wurzburg School, 188–189

Yerkes-Dodson hypothesis, 290–292, 294, 297
Yoga, 84–85. *See also* Meditation